COGNITIVE-BEHAVIORAL THERAPY FOR OCD

DAVID A. CLARK

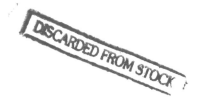
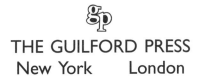

THE GUILFORD PRESS
New York   London

Paperback edition 2007

Printed in the United States of America

This book is printed on acid-free paper.

Last digit is print number: 9 8 7 6

Library of Congress Cataloging-in-Publication Data

Clark, David A., 1954–
  Cognitive-behavioral therapy for OCD / David A. Clark.
    p. cm.
  Includes bibliographical references and index.
  ISBN-10: 1-57230-963-6 ISBN-13: 978-1-57230-963-0 (hardcover: alk. paper)
  ISBN-10: 1-59385-375-0 ISBN-13: 978-1-59385-375-4 (paperback)
  1. Cognitive therapy. 2. Obsessive–compulsive disorder. I. Title.
  RC489.C63C57 2004
  616.85′2270651–dc22

                                                              2003020283

To my parents, Albert and Ardith,
for their support and encouragement

About the Author

David A. Clark, PhD, is a professor in the Department of Psychology, University of New Brunswick, Canada. He received his PhD from the Institute of Psychiatry, University of London, England. Dr. Clark has published numerous articles on cognitive theory and therapy of depression and obsessive–compulsive disorders (OCD), and is a Founding Fellow of the Academy of Cognitive Therapy. He is coauthor, with Aaron T. Beck, of *Scientific Foundations of Cognitive Theory and Therapy of Depression* and coeditor, with Mark Reinecke, of *Cognitive Therapy across the Lifespan: Evidence and Practice*. Drs. Clark and Beck recently developed the Clark–Beck Obsessive–Compulsive Inventory to assess self-reported severity of obsessive and compulsive symptoms. Dr. Clark has received a number of research grants to study the cognitive basis of emotional disorders, the most recent being a Canadian federal grant to investigate intentional control of unwanted intrusive thoughts. He is also a founding member of the Obsessive Compulsive Cognitions Working Group, an international research group devoted to the study of the cognitive aspects of OCD, and the past Associate Editor of *Cognitive Therapy and Research*.

Preface

The cognitive-behavioral perspective is a relatively new development in the theory and treatment of obsessive–compulsive disorders (OCD). The possibility that a greater emphasis on cognitive factors might enhance a behavioral account of OCD can be traced back to Carr (1974), McFall and Wollersheim (1979), Rachman and Hodgson (1980), and Salkovskis (1985). Behavior therapy in the form of exposure and response prevention (ERP), which emerged in the 1960s and 1970s, proved to be a highly effective treatment for many forms of OCD. Behavioral research on obsessions and compulsions offered new insights into the pathogenesis of the disorder. Yet, by the early 1980s, behavioral research into OCD had stagnated. The "cognitive revolution" that led to advances in the treatment of depression and other anxiety disorders, such as panic, had little impact on the research and treatment of OCD. However, by the late 1980s and early 1990s, behavioral researchers like Paul Salkovskis and Jack Rachman were advocating a more integrative theory and treatment of OCD, an approach that amalgamated the behavioral treatment of OCD with Beck's (1976) cognitive theory of emotional disorders. From these two theoretical perspectives on clinical disorders, a new cognitive-behavioral approach to obsessions and compulsions was born.

In many respects, my own professional development has taken a path similar to that seen in cognitive-behavioral therapy (CBT) for obsessional states. My roots are in the behavioral tradition, dating back to the early 1980s when I was a graduate student at the Institute of Psychiatry in London, England. My interest in OCD and unwanted intrusive thoughts was sparked by the stimulating discussions and innovative research of the clinical faculty, most notably Jack Rachman and Padmal de Silva. My doctoral thesis on the psychophysiology of mental control and unwanted intrusive thoughts was an outgrowth of their insights into the pathology of obsessional thought.

In the late 1980s, I was introduced to the cognitive perspective on clinical disorders by Aaron T. Beck. I was privileged to spend a few months at the Center for Cognitive Therapy in Philadelphia, where I received training in Beck's therapy approach. Over the last 15 years I have participated with Tim Beck on a number of collaborative research projects dealing with the cognitive basis of depression and anxiety disorders. One of our most recent projects was the development of a self-report OCD screening measure called the Clark–Beck Obsessive–Compulsive Inventory (Clark & Beck, 2002). Tim Beck's insights into the nature of psychopathology and its treatment have been inspiring and have challenged me to consider new avenues of inquiry and treatment innovation. The cognitive-behavioral perspective taken in this book is a product of my early behavioral training and of the mentoring of Dr. Beck.

My purpose in writing this book is to provide a comprehensive account of contemporary cognitive-behavioral theory, research, and treatment of OCD. Written with a scientist-practitioner orientation, it assumes that psychological treatment of OCD will be effective only if it is theoretically guided and empirically verified. As a result, half of the book is devoted to cognitive-behavioral theory and research of OCD, whereas the rest of the book constitutes a CBT treatment manual for obsessional disorders. I am convinced that clinicians must understand the nature of OCD and the theoretical framework of CBT before they can utilize this treatment approach effectively in the clinical setting. To this end, the book adopts an applied science perspective that continues throughout even the practice-oriented chapters.

Chapter 1 provides an overview of the diagnosis, psychopathology, and phenomenology of OCD. Chapter 2 focuses on the most recent psychological research on the nature and persistence of obsessions, compulsions, and neutralization responses. Chapter 3 presents the behavioral theory and treatment of OCD, with particular attention to their shortcomings that led to a greater emphasis on the cognitive approach among behavioral researchers of OCD. Chapter 4 examines whether a general cognitive deficit might account for the persistence of obsessive–compulsive symptoms, and Chapters 5 through 7 discuss current theories and research that are the basis of contemporary CBT for OCD. Chapter 7 presents an expanded cognitive-behavioral model that might provide a more complete account of obsessional phenomena. This new formulation of obsessions emphasizes the importance of faulty secondary appraisals of mental control, as well as the erroneous primary appraisals of the obsession itself.

Chapters 8 through 13 provide step-by-step, detailed descriptions of cognitive and behavioral strategies for the assessment and treatment of OCD. Chapter 8 offers an evaluation of various assessment instruments for OCD and provides individualized self-monitoring forms and rating scales for an idiographic assessment of obsessions and compulsions. Chapter 9 presents the underlying assumptions and rationale for the cognitive–behavioral treatment of OCD, as well as methods for establishing a healthy therapeutic relationship. Chapters 10, 11, and 12 describe specific cognitive and behavioral intervention tactics that can be used to modify directly the faulty appraisals and beliefs in OCD. Case illustrations, sample therapeutic questions, and clinical resource materials (i.e., handouts) are provided to facilitate the implementation of CBT for obsessional states. Chapter 13 concludes with a review of the empirical status of cognitive-behavioral treatment for obsessions and compulsions and a consideration of the future direction of this new approach to OCD.

As I complete this project, I wish to acknowledge my indebtedness to a number of people. First and foremost, this book is dedicated to my parents, for their important role in launching my academic quest. I thank the Department of Psychology of the University of New Brunswick for being my academic home for the last 15 years. I am grateful to my colleague and former graduate student, Christine Purdon, for sharing her advice and clinical insights, and to my current graduate students, Lorna Scott, Natasha Crewdson, Adrienne Wang, and Shelley Rhyno, whose contributions to my research on intrusive thoughts and obsessions have been invaluable. I also want to acknowledge the financial support I received from a grant awarded by the Social Sciences and Humanities Research Council of Canada. I am most grateful for the assistance, advice, and support of the staff at The Guilford Press—in particular, Jim Nageotte. Jim's editorial guidance and the helpful advice of anonymous reviewers made an important contribution to the organization and direction of the book. Finally, I wish to thank my wife, Nancy, and daughters, Natascha and Christina, for their love, encouragement, and patience as I toiled long hours writing this book.

Contents

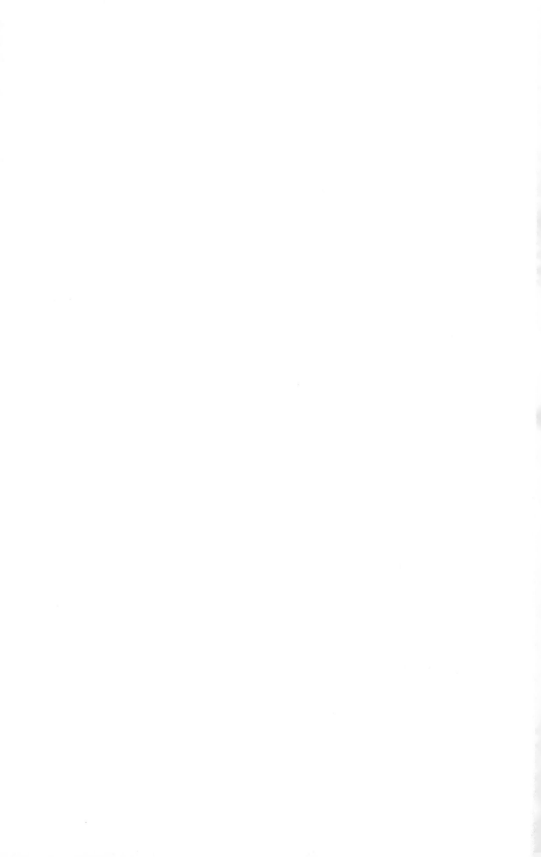

PART I

The Nature of OCD

CHAPTER 1

Obsessive–Compulsive Disorder

A Diagnostic Enigma

Mike, a 35-year-old married engineer, has not worked for many years because of chronic and debilitating obsessions and compulsions. For the last 9 years he has been tormented almost continuously by a variety of unwanted and upsetting intrusive violent thoughts or images such as "I'll stab someone," "I might accidentally contaminate someone's food," "I might cause harm to pets by being careless with cleaning agents," or "I will inadvertently steal items from stores." Overwhelmed with distress, Mike developed a number of counting and repeating compulsions, as well as extensive avoidance behavior, in an effort to neutralize the obsessions. He believed he had to repeat a task until he no longer had an obsession so that he could break the association between the task and the intrusive thought. This would then ensure that the task would not become a trigger for the obsession. As a result of his erroneous belief, Mike would repeat phrases, retrace his steps, wash repeatedly, even hold his breath, in response to the obsession. This behavior would continue until he felt less anxious or the obsession subsided. In addition, Mike developed extensive avoidance of any stimulus or object that might remind him of a particular obsession, such as certain items in his house, a particular subway stop, the number 8, or specific types of information. Mike expressed many beliefs about the threatening nature of his disturbing thoughts, his responsibility to prevent possible harm occurring to himself or others, and his need to gain better control over his tormented mind. Despite his best efforts, Mike was paralyzed by the relentless onslaught of his unforgiving mind.

Anxiety, and the more basic emotion of fear, is a universal human experience that plays a central role in human adaptation and survival. The basic function of fear is to signal a threat or impending danger (Barlow, 2002). The feeling of anxiousness associated with making a speech before

3

a large audience or going for a job interview is understandable, given the potential for embarrassment or rejection. Even some of the phobias that are well known to clinicians, such as acrophobia (fear of heights) or claustrophobia (fear of enclosed places), are understandable. But what if the fear is of one's own thoughts? And what if the thoughts are about actions or circumstances that are highly improbable, if not impossible? In response to this intense anxiety, individuals learn that certain rituals or habitual ways of responding appear to bring temporary relief from their distress, even though the response may not be logically connected to the fear. This unusual, seemingly inexplicable, anxiety disorder is what has been labeled obsessive–compulsive disorder (OCD).

Why would a highly intelligent professional become so consumed with improbable, even nonsensical, thoughts of harm, sex, and violence that his or her ability to function in daily life is in serious jeopardy? How can these mental intrusions cause so much anxiety and lead to the irresistible urge to carry out time-consuming compulsive rituals? How can a reasonable, logical person draw such flimsy and farfetched inferences and associations between entirely unrelated ideas when it comes to his or her primary obsessive–compulsive concerns? All of this occurs, however, even though individuals are fully aware that the events or actions represented in such thoughts are imagined, highly improbable, and entirely uncharacteristic of their personalities and values. In the case of Mike, his fears that he would harm others occurred without a shred of external evidence that he was violent.

The case illustrates the symptom profile associated with OCD, one of the nine major types of anxiety disorders in the text revision of the fourth edition of the *Diagnostic and Statistical Manual of Mental Disorders* (DSM-IV-TR; American Psychiatric Association [APA], 2000). The hallmark of the disorder is the presence of recurrent or persistent obsessions or compulsions that are severe enough to be time-consuming, or to cause marked distress or significant impairment, but are perceived by the patient to be excessive or unreasonable (APA, 2000). Understanding and treating OCD can be one of the greatest challenges facing mental health practitioners, given the idiosyncratic, highly persistent, and entirely irrational nature of these conditions.

When confronted with a severe case of OCD, a clinician might assume that obsessive phenomena have no counterpart in normal human functioning. However, obsessions and compulsions can be found in most individuals to varying degrees. Who hasn't had an unwanted intrusive thought, image, or impulse that pops into the mind for no apparent reason? Examples include the urge to jump in front of an approaching train even though you are not suicidal, the thought of blurting out a rude or embarrassing comment to someone you have just met, or an annoying tune that keeps running through your head. And what about the superstitious, repetitive behaviors we perform to relieve anxiety? For example, consider the baseball player who taps the base a certain number of times before the first pitch or the routines a person may have when sitting down to take an exam.

In reality, obsessions and compulsions can occur as normal as well as abnormal phenomena. Yet when does an obsession or compulsion become pathological? And how can we effectively treat these conditions when they cause significant personal distress and interference in daily functioning? These are the two overarching questions that guide this book. I approach these issues with new research findings on the cognitive basis of OCD. The emerging theory and research have given cognitive-behavioral therapists a new understanding and innovative interventions for the treatment of OCD. First, however, I offer a brief overview of the diagnostic literature on OCD; a consideration of the critical characteristics and issues that surround obsessions and compulsions follows in Chapter 2. This sets the stage for an extended discussion of the new cognitive theory, research, and treatment of OCD in the chapters to follow.

DIAGNOSIS OF OCD

Overview

The essential features of OCD are the repeated occurrence of obsessions and/or compulsions of sufficient severity that they are time-consuming (> 1 hour per day) or cause marked distress or impairment (DSM-IV-TR; APA, 2000). Obsessions are unwanted, unacceptable intrusive and repetitive thoughts, images, or impulses that are associated with subjective resistance, are difficult to control, and generally produce distress even though the person having such thoughts may recognize their senselessness (Rachman, 1985). Their content often focuses on troubling, repugnant, or even nonsensical themes about dirt and contamination, aggression, doubt, unacceptable sexual acts, religion, and orderliness, symmetry, and precision.

Compulsions, on the other hand, are repetitive, stereotyped behaviors or mental acts that are usually performed in response to an obsession in order to prevent or reduce anxiety or distress (APA, 2000). A compulsion is generally accompanied by an especially strong urge to carry out the ritual resulting in a diminished sense of voluntary control over the ritual (Rachman & Hodgson, 1980). Subjective resistance is often present, but the person eventually gives in to the overpowering urge to perform the ritual. Washing, checking, repeating specific behaviors or phrases, ordering (rearranging objects to restore balance or symmetry), hoarding, and mental rituals (i.e., repeating certain superstitious words, phrases, or prayers) are the most common compulsions.

Anxiety and OCD

The most common view is that OCD should be classified as an anxiety disorder, because it has a symptom profile similar to those of disorders like generalized anxiety disorder (GAD), specific phobias, hypochondriasis, and body dysmorphic disorder, which suggests the possibility of a common diathesis (Brown, 1998). More specifically, features consistent with an anxiety disorder classification include (1) a subjective feeling of anxiety or distress, which is elicited by most obsessions, (2) a behavioral or cognitive compulsion in response to the obsession, (3) an internal or external trigger for the obsession or compulsive urge, (4) anxiety or discomfort arising from a provocation, (5) anxiety reduction with completion of the compulsion, (6) reassurance seeking, (7) fear of disaster, (8) occurrence of disruptive events that can interfere or invalidate the compulsion, and (9) avoidance behavior (de Silva, 1986). Consistent with these considerations, DSM-IV-TR (APA, 2000) situates OCD within the anxiety disorder classification.

Some clinical researchers have challenged the prevailing view of OCD as an anxiety disorder. Summerfeldt and Endler (1998) concluded that OCD, with the possible exception of washing compulsions, may not be an anxiety disorder because the selective bias for threat seen in most anxiety states is not always present in obsessional states. Enright (1996) points out that there are important differences between OCD and other anxiety disorders, including possible differences in biochemistry, presence of greater functional impairment in OCD, and the increased complexity and vagueness of the fear-eliciting stimuli in OCD. Others suggest that OCD may share a common etiology with chronic (multiple) tic disorder and Gilles de la Tourette syndrome (see review by O'Connor, 2001). It is also possible that the greater symptom variability and abstract nature of many obsessions have led to the speculation of links with other classes of psychopathology. At the very least, the increased heterogeneity of obsessive–compulsive symptoms suggests that OCD is a less unified and homogeneous diagnostic entity than other anxiety disorders.

The DSM-IV diagnosis of OCD is adopted in this book because it is the prevailing perspective accepted in cognitive-behavioral theory and therapy of the disorder. Moreover, there is strong empirical evidence that OCD can be reliably diagnosed when DSM-IV-TR criteria are utilized by trained interviewers using a structured clinical interview (Brown, Di Nardo, Lehman, & Campbell, 2001). Table 1.1 presents a summary of the DSM-IV-TR diagnostic criteria (APA, 2000).

According to DSM-IV, a person must have either obsession(s) or compulsion(s) in order to have a diagnosis of OCD, and the vast majority of diagnosable individuals experience both types of symptoms (Foa & Kozak, 1995). To qualify as an obsession, the thought, image, or impulse

TABLE 1.1. Summary of DSM-IV-TR Diagnostic Criteria for OCD

Criterion A

Presence of obsessions and/or compulsions:
Obsessions are repetitive and persistent thoughts, images, or impulses that, at some point, are considered intrusive and inappropriate and cause marked distress; they are not worries about real-life problems; they are accompanied by attempts to ignore, suppress, or neutralize (i.e., subjective resistance); and they are acknowledged as a product of the person's mind.

Compulsions are repetitive behaviors or mental acts that the person feels compelled to perform in response to an obsession or certain rigidly applied rules; and the function of the behaviors or mental acts is to prevent or reduce distress or some dreaded event or situation. The rituals either are not connected in a realistic way with what they are intended to neutralize or are clearly perceived as excessive.

Criterion B

Recognition at some point during the disorder that the obsessions or compulsions are excessive or unreasonable.

Criterion C

Obsessions or compulsions cause marked distress, are time-consuming (at least 1 hour per day), or significantly interfere with daily activities or with social or occupational functioning.

Criterion D

Content of the obsessions or compulsions is not restricted to another Axis I disorder if present. (Obsessions and compulsions must be evident outside the context of a co-occurring condition.)

Criterion E

Obsessions or compulsions are not due to direct physiological effects of a substance or a general medical condition.

Specifier

With poor insight: For most of the current episode, the person does not consider his or her obsessions and compulsions excessive or unrealistic.

Note. Based on DSM-IV-TR diagnostic criteria from the American Psychiatric Association (2000, pp. 462–463).

must be (1) persistent, intrusive, inappropriate, and distressing, (2) subject to control efforts, (3) recognized as having an internal origin (i.e., not due to thought insertion), and (4) distinct from worries about daily problems. Overt compulsions, on the other hand, are fairly easy to recognize, although mental (covert) rituals can present a more complicated picture. The purpose of an overt or covert compulsion is to relieve distress associated with the obsession or to prevent some anticipated dreaded outcome.

It is not performed to obtain pleasure or gratification and so can be distinguished from impulse control disorders like sexual addictions or gambling.

As stated in DSM-IV-TR, for a diagnosis of OCD, it is necessary that at some point in the illness the person recognizes that the obsession(s) or compulsion(s) are excessive or unreasonable. However, many individuals with OCD are not certain that their obsessive–compulsive symptoms are senseless, unreasonable, or excessive (see Foa & Kozak, 1995). In these cases clinicians may indicate that patients have "poor insight" into their obsessional fears (see Table 1.1 for "insight specifier"). The third diagnostic criterion (Criterion C) indicates that the disturbance is of sufficient intensity to warrant an Axis I diagnosis. Inasmuch as milder forms of obsessions and compulsions have been reported in the general population, this severity criterion is important for establishing that the threshold for disorder has been met. As with most other DSM-IV-TR disorders, Criteria D and E (see Table 1.1) are included to ensure that the obsessive–compulsive symptoms are not the result of another Axis I or II disorder.

EPIDEMIOLOGY AND DEMOGRAPHY OF OCD

Prevalence

Estimates of the lifetime prevalence of OCD have varied across epidemiological studies, depending on diagnostic criteria and interview method. Early research concluded that OCD was relatively rare, with general population estimates as low as 0.05% (see Karno & Golding, 1991). However, the more rigorous Epidemiologic Catchment Area (ECA) Study determined that the lifetime prevalence of OCD was much higher, with a rate of 2.5% based on DSM-III criteria (Karno, Golding, Sorenson, & Burnam, 1988). Other more recent studies have also confirmed this higher rate for OCD (for review see Antony, Downie, & Swinson, 1998). Nevertheless, it may be that the higher prevalence reported in the ECA study is an overestimation because its lay interview method tended to produce unreliable OCD diagnoses (Antony et al., 1998). Lay interviewers may overdiagnose OCD because they mistake worries for obsessions and have difficulty in assessing the degree of disability or distress (Stein, Forde, Anderson, & Walker, 1997). Two recent epidemiological studies reported a lower 1-year prevalence rate (0.7%) than the 1-year rate (1.6%) found in the ECA study (Kringlen, Torgersen, & Cramer, 2001; Andrews, Henderson, & Hall, 2001). Although these results are by no means conclusive, it is reasonable to place the lifetime prevalence for OCD between 1 and 2% of the general population.

Gender, Age, and Onset

Most studies report a slightly greater incidence of OCD in women. In their review, Rasmussen and Eisen (1992) noted that 53% of their OCD sample were women, a gender difference confirmed in the epidemiological research (Andrews et al., 2001; Karno & Golding, 1991; Kringlen et al., 2001). Men typically have an earlier age of onset than women and therefore begin treatment at a younger age (e.g., Lensi et al., 1996; Rasmussen & Eisen, 1992). However, it is unclear whether gender has any impact on the course of the disorder. There is some evidence of gender differences in symptom expression, with women displaying more washing and cleaning rituals and men reporting more sexual obsessions (Lensi et al., 1996; Rachman & Hodgson, 1980; Steketee, Grayson, & Foa, 1985).

Young adults between 18 and 24 years are at the highest risk for developing OCD (Karno et al., 1988). Sixty-five percent develop the disorder before age 25, with less than 5% of patients reporting an initial onset of OCD after 40 years of age (Rachman & Hodgson, 1980; Rasmussen & Eisen, 1992). Moreover, a substantial number of adults report onset in childhood or adolescence, and children and adolescents with severe OCD will continue to experience symptoms for many years (Rettew, Swedo, Leonard, Lenane, & Rapoport, 1992; Thomsen, 1995). OCD clearly appears to be a disorder of the young, with some evidence that rates may even decline with age (Karno & Golding, 1991).

There does not appear to be a typical mode of onset in OCD. A substantial number of patients experience a gradual onset of the disorder, whereas others report an acute onset, often in response to a particular life experience (Black, 1974; Lensi et al., 1996; Rachman & Hodgson, 1980). Half to two-thirds of patients with OCD report a significant life event prior to the onset of illness, such as the loss of a loved one, severe medical illness, or major financial problems (Lo, 1967; Lensi et al., 1996). In a more systematic study of life events, McKeon, Roa, and Mann (1984) found that patients with OCD experienced significantly more life events in the 12 months before the onset of illness than the nonclinical comparison group. There is also evidence that a significant number of women with OCD report initial onset during pregnancy (Neziroglu, Anemone, & Yaryura-Tobias, 1992). In a recent review, Abramowitz, Schwartz, Moore, and Luenzmann (2003) concluded that a subset of patients with OCD experience an onset or worsening of symptoms during pregnancy or the puerperium, but it is unclear whether this might be related to postpartum depression. Although life circumstances such as pregnancy may increase vulnerability to OCD, it is important to remember that many individuals cannot identify an environmental trigger for their illness (Rasmussen & Tsuang, 1986).

Ethnicity, Marital Status, and Family Involvement

Cultural differences in the rate of OCD may not be as pronounced as might be expected. In the cross-national collaborative study (Weissman et al., 1994), prevalence, age of onset, and comorbidity were quite consistent across seven national sites (United States, Edmonton, Puerto Rico, Munich, Taiwan, Korea, and New Zealand). The lifetime prevalence rate for Taiwan was substantially lower, but this was true for all psychiatric disorders. Likewise, African Americans may have a lower lifetime prevalence of OCD, but this is not unique to this particular disorder (Karno et al., 1988). As discussed in the next chapter, culture does play a bigger role in determining the content of obsessions and compulsions.

Individuals with OCD have a high rate of celibacy, marry at an older age, and have a low fertility rate (Rachman, 1985). Rates of separation or divorce, marital dysfunction, and sexual dissatisfaction are common in OCD, but the rates do not appear greater as compared with those of other anxiety disorders or depression (Black, 1974; Coryell, 1981; Freund & Steketee, 1989; Karno et al., 1988; Rasmussen & Eisen, 1992).

Considerable stress is placed on family members living with an individual with severe OCD. Family members may be directly drawn into the illness either by trying to stop the symptoms or by cooperating with the patient's ritualistic behavior. Family members and relatives frequently make accommodations for the patient's rituals, which in turn increases family stress and dysfunction (Calvocoressi et al., 1995). A higher rate of critical and rejecting comments may have a limited negative impact on the patient's symptom severity, and the level of depression and anxiety in family members influences how they respond to the patient's obsessions and compulsions (Amir, Freshman, & Foa, 2000). Clearly, family members are caught in a difficult dilemma. Regardless of whether they refuse to be drawn into the patient's rituals or whether they accommodate to the rituals, they end up feeling the ill effects of living with OCD.

Education and Employment Status

At one time it was thought that individuals with OCD have higher intelligence and attain a higher level of education than individuals with other psychiatric disorders (e.g., Black, 1974). However, more recent empirical research indicates that educational attainment in OCD is consistent with that of other disorders and is lower as compared with nonclinical comparison groups (Andrews et al., 2001; Karno & Golding, 1991; Kringlen et al., 2001). Any evidence of higher scores on standardized intelligence tests is only slight and nonsignificant when compared with matched nonclinical controls (Rasmussen & Eisen, 1992).

OCD has a significant negative impact on a person's ability to function socially and occupationally, especially in more severe cases. However, when common indices of employment are used, it is unclear whether OCD is associated with worse employment outcomes as compared with other psychiatric disorders. Generally, employment status and level of income did not differ when OCD was compared with other anxiety disorders (Antony et al., 1998; Karno et al., 1988), although contrary findings have been reported with higher rates of unemployment and lower income in OCD relative to other anxiety conditions (Steketee, Grayson, & Foa, 1987). Research will continue to investigate whether there is evidence of a detrimental effect on occupational attainment that is specific to OCD. In the meantime, the clinician must be aware that many patients with severe OCD are often unable to carry out their usual work or social activities shortly after onset of the illness (Pollitt, 1957).

COURSE AND OUTCOME IN OCD

Investigation of the natural course of OCD is difficult because most individuals with the disorder eventually seek treatment. Moreover, the treatment regimens for OCD have improved substantially over the years, thereby affecting the natural course and outcome of the disorder. Even though individuals with OCD may delay treatment onset by 2 to 7 years (Lensi et al., 1996; Rasmussen & Tsuang, 1986), OCD is associated with a high rate of mental health service utilization (Regier et al., 1993). Yet it is important to note that, like those with other mental health problems, most individuals with OCD do not seek treatment (Pollard, Henderson, Frank, & Margolis, 1989).

Despite the challenges facing researchers, a few observations can be made about the natural course of OCD. A long-term follow-up (mean = 47 years) study by Skoog and Skoog (1999) demonstrates that OCD tends to take a chronic course, with a waxing and waning of symptoms over a lifetime. After nearly five decades, half of their sample of patients with OCD (*n* = 122) continued to experience clinically significant symptoms and another one-third had subclinical features (although 83% showed improvement in the 40-year period). Complete recovery occurred in only 20% of the sample. These results are entirely consistent with other research showing that OCD episodes tend to be lengthy and that spontaneous remission of symptoms is low (Demal, Lenz, Mayrhofer, Zapotoczky, & Zitterl, 1993; Foa & Kozak, 1996; Karno & Golding, 1991).

There have been attempts to characterize the typical course of OCD symptoms. The majority of patients with OCD show a fairly chronic, continuous course with the disorder, with a small minority (10%) actually ex-

periencing a deterioration over time. A large minority of patients experience an intermittent course with obsessive–compulsive symptoms waxing
and waning, possibly in response to stressful life experiences (Demal et
al., 1993; Lensi et al., 1996; Rasmussen & Tsuang, 1986). Rachman and
Hodgson (1980) distinguished between patients who exhibited a part-
time or a full-time OCD lifestyle. For "full-timers" the disorder can be ma-
lignant, affecting all aspects of a person's life, whereas "part-timers" have
relatively benign obsessive–compulsive symptoms that allow them to lead
productive and satisfying lives. Analysis revealed that full-time patients
with OCD were more likely compulsive washers than checkers and that
they had poorer treatment outcomes than those who had a more limited
form of the disorder.

Although it is difficult to reach a definitive conclusion about the natural course of OCD, it may be said that the majority of individuals with
the disorder experience a fairly early but insidious onset in adolescence or
early adulthood, with a mixture of obsessive and compulsive symptoms
that build during periods of stress and possibly subside during intervals of
relative stability. This pattern of waxing and waning symptoms can continue over a number of years until their severity progresses to the point
where the person finally seeks treatment.

COMORBIDITY IN OCD

Clinical disorders rarely occur in isolation. Individuals who meet the diagnostic criteria for one disorder have a much higher probability of meeting
the criteria for two or more disorders (L. A. Clark, Watson, & Reynolds,
1995; Maser & Cloninger, 1990). In fact, patients with a single diagnosis
are less common in treatment settings than patients with two or more diagnoses. The term *diagnostic comorbidity* refers "to the co-occurrence of
two or more current or lifetime mental disorders in the same individual"
(Brown, Campbell, Lehman, Grisham, & Mancill 2001, p. 585). Interest in
current comorbidity is important because the presence of a secondary coexisting disorder is usually associated with greater symptom severity,
poorer response to treatment, and poorer prognosis (Bronisch & Hecht,
1990; Brown & Barlow, 1992; Clark, Beck, & Stewart, 1990). Research on
lifetime comorbidity in which two disorders covary at different points of
time in the same individual (i.e., one disorder may precede or follow another) is significant because it suggests that the disorders may share a
common underlying etiology.

Like other anxiety disorders, OCD has a very high rate of diagnostic
comorbidity. Although there is some discrepancy across studies, the most
consistent finding is that half to three-quarters of individuals with OCD
are seen to have at least one additional current disorder (Antony et al.,

1998; Brown, Campbell, Lehman, Grisham, & Mancill, 2001; Karno & Golding, 1991; see Yaryura-Tobias et al., 2000, for lower comorbidity rates). When lifetime comorbidity is considered, fewer than 15% of cases have a sole diagnosis of OCD (Brown, Campbell, et al., 2001; Crino & Andrews, 1996). These findings indicate that more often than not the clinician will have to contend with other disorders when treating OCD.

Comorbidity of OCD with other disorders appears to be asymmetrical. Whereas additional diagnoses of depression or other anxiety disorders have a high rate of occurrence in OCD, obsessional disorder, as a co-occurring condition with major depression or other anxiety disorders, is less common, even when lifetime rates are considered (Antony et al., 1998; Brown, Campbell, et al., 2001; Crino & Andrews, 1996). Moreover, the temporal order of lifetime comorbidity may differ between disorders. Brown, Campbell, et al. (2001) found that comorbid anxiety disorders tended to temporally precede index cases of OCD, whereas comorbid depression tended to occur after the onset of an obsessional disorder. With onset of an obsessional episode, an individual remains at elevated risk for developing anxiety, mood disorders, eating disturbance, and tic disorders as long as the episode persists (Yaryura-Tobias et al., 2000).

Researchers have been particularly interested in the lifetime co-occurrence of OCD with psychosis because of its etiological implications. Early psychiatric writing proposed a relationship between obsessional thinking and the thought disturbance seen in schizophrenia (for discussion, see Lewis, 1936; Stengel, 1945). However, only a minority of patients with OCD (15–20%) show any symptoms of psychosis, and these are usually in the form of poor insight or lack of resistance to the obsession (Insel & Akiskal, 1986). A small number of individuals with OCD have obsessional ideation that meets the criteria for delusion, but the number of individuals with OCD who progress to schizophrenia is no greater than the number of those with other anxiety disorders (Rachman & Hodgson, 1980; Stein & Hollander, 1993).

Depression

For decades clinical researchers have recognized a close relationship between OCD and depression (e.g., Lewis, 1936; Rosenberg, 1968; Stengel, 1945). The co-occurrence of current major depressive episode or dysthymia in persons with OCD is very high, ranging from 30 to 50% (Bellodi, Sciuto, Diaferia, Ronchi, & Smeraldi, 1992; Brown, Moras, Zinbarg, & Barlow, 1993; Lensi et al., 1996; Karno & Golding, 1991). These rates are even higher (65 to 80%) for lifetime prevalence of depressive disorder (Brown, Campbell, et al., 2001; Crino & Andrews, 1996; Rasmussen & Eisen, 1992). In addition, the presence of depression increases obsessional symptoms, thereby contributing to an exacerbation of the disorder. However, the more usual pattern is that the persistent and debilitating effects of the OCD lead to the development of a secondary depressive disorder (Demal et al., 1993; Rasmussen & Eisen, 1992; Welner, Reich, Robins, Fishman, & van Doren, 1976). The progression from obsessive–compulsive symptoms to depression occurs three times more often than the reverse pattern. On the other hand, obsessional symptoms, and even obsessional disorder, can be found in diagnosable depressive disorders, although much less frequently than the incidence of depressive disorders in patients with OCD (Lewis, 1936; Kendell & Discipio, 1970; Gittleson, 1966).

The impact of depressive symptoms and disorder on treatment response in OCD is complicated. Depression may have a greater negative impact on obsessive than compulsive symptoms (Ricciardi & McNally, 1995); thus, improvement in mood state can have a beneficial impact on obsessive–compulsive symptoms (Rachman, 1985). In terms of treatment effects, it appears that individuals with OCD and comorbid major depression can show significant gains in treatment, but the posttreatment symptom level is still significantly greater than in patients without concurrent depression (e.g., Abramowitz & Foa, 2000). Finally, severe levels of depressive symptoms are associated with a poor response to treatment, whereas mild to moderate depression may not substantially interfere with treatment gains (Abramowitz, Franklin, Street, Kozak, & Foa, 2000; see review by Steketee & Shapiro, 1995).

Anxiety Disorders

It might be expected that OCD would have a high rate of concurrent and lifetime comorbidity with other anxiety disorders, given that they share the same diagnostic classification. This is exactly what was found. Many individuals with a principal diagnosis of OCD experience additional anxiety symptoms and disorders. Social phobia consistently emerged as having a high rate of comorbidity with OCD (35–41%), with specific phobias (17–21%) having the next highest rate of co-occurrence. Results are more mixed concerning panic disorder, with some studies showing moderately high comorbidity rates (29%) and other studies reporting relatively low rates of co-occurrence (12%). It is still unclear whether GAD is rare (7%) or, at the very least, occurs somewhat less frequently (12–22%) in patients with OCD (Antony et al., 1998; Brown et al., 1993; Brown, Campbell, et al., 2001; Crino & Andrews, 1996).

Obsessive and compulsive symptoms often co-occur with other anxiety symptoms, so that the more anxiety exhibited by an individual, the greater the negative impact on functioning (Welkowitz, Struening, Pittman, Guardino, & Welkowitz, 2000). Although other anxiety disorders are frequently found in persons with OCD, obsessions and compulsions are rarely evident in other anxiety disorders (another example of the asymmetrical comorbidity pattern in OCD). Brown et al. (1993), for example, found that OCD rarely occurred (2%) in patients with a principal diagnosis of GAD. This asymmetry was also evident at the symptom level, with 41% of the patients in the OCD sample reporting worry but only 15% of the GAD patients having obsessions. Overall, evidence of symptom overlap and diagnostic co-occurrence of anxiety disorders with OCD indicates that these disorders are sufficiently related to suggest that they may share a common underlying diathesis or higher-order trait like negative affect or neuroticism (Brown, 1998).

OCD Spectrum Disorders

There is increasing recognition of a broad range of psychological and neuropsychiatric disorders that are related to OCD but that span various DSM-IV diagnostic classifications. Together these disorders have been referred to as the obsessive–compulsive spectrum disorders (OCSDs). Largely on the basis of clinical observations, this group of disorders is thought to share phenomenological features, course of illness, family history, comorbidity, and treatment response with OCD (Goldsmith, Shapira, Phillips, & McElroy, 1998; Neziroglu, Stevens, Yaryura-Tobias, & Hoffman, 1999). OCSDs include somatoform disorders (i.e., body dysmorphic disorder, hypochondriasis), eating disorders (anorexia and bulimia), impulse control disorders (i.e., trichotillomania, kleptomania, patholgical gambling), paraphilias and nonparaphilic sexual addictions (also called sexual compulsions), and movement disorders such as tics and Tourette's syndrome (Goldsmith et al., 1998; Hollander, 1993; Hollander & Wong, 2000). According to Hollander and Wong (2000), OCSDs share many characteristics with OCD in (1) symptom profile, which involves intrusive obsessive thoughts and repetitive behaviors, (2) associated features such as demography, family history, comorbidity, and clinical course, (3) neurobiology, (4) response to certain behavioral and pharmacological treatments specific to obsessional problems, and (5) genetic and environmental etiology.

It is beyond the scope of this discussion to deal with the conceptual and empirical evidence for a shared etiology, neurobiology, family history, and treatment response in OCSDs (for reviews, see Black, 1998; Goldsmith et al., 1998; Hollander, 1993; Hollander & Wong, 2000). However, evidence of increased comorbidity between OCD and OCSDs is relevant to the current discussion of disorders that may be associated with an obsessive–compulsive condition.

Elevated comorbidity rates have been reported for OCSDs in samples of patients with a principal diagnosis of OCD. Within samples of patients with OCD 15–37% have an associated body dysmorphic disorder (preoccupation with an imagined or slight defect in physical appearance; Gold-smith et al., 1998). The somatic obsessions that are common in OCD are similar to hypochondriasis (Fallon, Rasmussen, & Liebowitz, 1993; Rasmussen & Eisen, 1992; Rasmussen & Tsuang, 1986), and higher rates of aberrant eating behavior and anorexia or bulimia have been found in samples of patients with OCD relative to controls (O'Rourke et al., 1994). Pathological gamblers experience more obsessions, compulsions, and avoidance behaviors (Frost, Meagher, & Riskind, 2001). Higher rates of lifetime diagnosis of OCD may be found in trichotillomania (chronic hair pulling; Swedo, 1993), even though trichotillomania and OCD are clearly more distinct than similar (see review by Elliott & Fuqua, 2000).

Relatively high rates of tics or tic disorders, including Tourette's syndrome, have been found in individuals, especially children and adolescents, with OCD (Goldsmith et al., 1998; March & Mulle, 1998). Thirty to 40% of adults with Tourette's syndrome experience obsessive and compulsive symptoms (Leckman, 1993). Although this might be taken as evidence of a link between OCD and OCSDs, it must be remembered that the comorbidity rate for spectrum disorders is generally not as high as the co-occurrence of depression or other anxiety disorders. It may also be that individuals with OCSDs have higher rates of co-occurring obsessions and compulsions than the reverse. At this point, then, it is unclear how often obsessive–compulsive spectrum disorders will be found in samples of patients with OCD. The clinician should be aware that spectrum disorder symptoms and disorders may be present in patients with OCD. Black (1998) provides a helpful list of screening questions that can be used to rule out the presence of OCSDs.

Obsessive–Compulsive Personality Disorder

A final comorbidity issue that deserves particular mention is the relationship between OCD and obsessive–compulsive personality disorder (OCPD). DSM-IV-TR describes OCPD in terms of "a preoccupation with orderliness, perfectionism, and mental and interpersonal control, at the expense of flexibility, openness, and efficiency" (APA, 2000, p. 725). The concept of OCPD is rooted in Freud's notion of the anal personality, characterized by a tendency to be parsimonious, obstinate, and orderly (Freud, 1959/1908). Originally, the obsessional personality or anal character was considered the premorbid personality for OCD, and some early studies suggested a strong link between the presence of OCD symptoms and obsessional personality traits (Ingram, 1961a; Kline, 1968; Sandler & Hazari, 1960).

A number of later empirical studies found that obsessional personality characteristics were quite distinct from obsessive–compulsive symptoms and that the majority of patients with OCD do not have a premorbid obsessional personality (for reviews, see Pollak, 1979; Rachman & Hodgson, 1980). Despite an Axis II comorbidity rate of 50–65%, the most common personality disorders in OCD are the dependent and avoidant patterns, with OCPD being less prevalent than one might expect (see the review by Summerfeldt, Huta, & Swinson, 1998). However, other studies continue to find elevated levels of OCPD in clinical samples of patients with OCD (e.g., Samuels et al., 2000). It may be that OCPD traits are more closely associated with a particular subset of obsessive–compulsive symptoms, such as doubting and checking, rather than other symptoms, such as washing (Gibbs & Oltmanns, 1995; Tallis, Rosen, & Shafran, 1996). Moreover, certain features of OCPD may be more relevant to OCD than other characteristics of the personality category. For example, perfectionism, a characteristic of OCPD, is significantly elevated in OCD relative to nonclinical controls (Frost & Steketee, 1997).

In sum, it is clear that OCPD is not a preexisting condition with etiological significance for OCD. The situation is most succinctly summed up by Rasmussen and Eisen (1992), who concluded that (1) OCPD occurs in many people who never develop an Axis I disorder, (2) OCPD frequently occurs in psychiatric conditions other than OCD, (3) the majority of patients with OCD do not have compulsive personalities, but (4) there is no overwhelming empirical support for the discontinuity of OCPD and OCD. I further suggest that certain aspects of OCPD, like perfectionism, may be more relevant to OCD than is the entire obsessive–compulsive personality constellation. In addition, certain symptoms of OCD, like checking and doubting, may be more closely related to the compulsive personality than other symptoms, like washing. Future research that takes a more fine-grained approach to this issue is clearly needed.

SUBTYPES OF OCD

As compared with other anxiety disorders, the symptom presentation in OCD is much more diverse and idiosyncratic to the personal concerns and life experiences of individuals. An argument could be made against treating OCD as a unitary diagnostic category with a common etiology, clinical presentation, and response to treatment. However, there may be a limited number of different types of obsessive and compulsive symptoms that are quite consistent across time and cultures (Rasmussen & Eisen, 1998). If individuals can be categorized into homogeneous symptom types, it may be possible to look for a common etiology and develop specialized treatment protocols for particular OCD subtypes. An alternative to the use of symptom subtypes is the dimensional approach, in which individuals vary along a prescribed set of symptom dimensions.

Symptom Subtypes

Rasmussen and Eisen (1992, 1998) report on one of the most extensive studies of symptom subtyping based on more than 1,000 patients with OCD seen at Butler Hospital, Brown University. The seven OCD subtypes described by Rasmussen and Eisen are summarized in Table 1.2.

The two most common symptom types, compulsive washing and checking, account for the majority of OCD cases. Recurrent and abhorrent thoughts of committing violent acts toward others or engaging in personally disgusting sexual acts are the third most common type of obsession seen in OCD. These obsessions usually elicit patients' compulsive urge to seek reassurance from others or to repeatedly confess their troubling thoughts to friends and family. Somatic obsessions, involving a persistent fear of developing a life-threatening illness (e.g., cancer, heart attack, AIDS), are most often associated with checking and reassurance seeking. Obsessions concerned with symmetry and precision refer to a need to have objects or events in a certain order or position. This can result in the repetition of certain actions in an exact fashion or a compulsion to straighten things so they appear exactly symmetrical. Often a "just right feeling" is the motive for a person's compulsive reordering and repeating rituals, rather than a reduction in tension or anxiety. In compulsive hoarding, the person feels compelled to repeatedly check his or her possessions to ensure that nothing is missing. Finally, the OCD subtype least often encountered in the clinical setting is religious obsession. Individuals of this subtype obsess over the meaning of morality, sins, and whether they have been diligent in keeping religious law. Sometimes referred to as *scrupulosity,* this type of obsessional rumination may be on the decline as a result of increased liberalization of church laws and morality (Rasmussen & Eisen, 1998).

TABLE 1.2. OCD Symptom Subtypes Described by Rasmussen and Eisen (1998)

Prevalence	Obsession	Compulsion
Most common	Fear of contamination (50%)	Washing/cleaning (50%)
	Pathologic doubt (42%)	Checking (61%)
	Sex (24%) or aggression (31%)	Need to ask/confess (34%)
	Somatic (33%)	
	Need for symmetry/precision (32%)	Symmetry/precision (28%)
		Hoarding (18%)
Least common	Religious/blasphemy (10%)	

Note. Because many individuals with OCD have multiple obsessions and compulsions, percentages do not add to 100.

There is considerable clinical and experimental evidence that compulsive washing and checking are distinct subtypes of OCD. Rachman and Hodgson (1980) compared the clinical presentation of compulsive cleaning and checking in a number of studies. Cleaning compulsions have a stronger phobic component involving escape responses (i.e., an attempt to restore a safe state of cleanliness), whereas checking is more often associated with doubting and indecision accompanied by active-avoidance behavior (i.e., checking prevents some future negative outcome). Checking rituals take longer to complete, have a slow onset, evoke more internal resistance, and are more likely accompanied by feelings of anger or tension than cleaning compulsions. In addition, the compulsive checker has more difficulty obtaining the required certainty or assurance that the possible negative future event has been averted or prevented from occurring. Steketee et al. (1985) also reported significant differences in symptoms and the fear structure of individuals with cleaning versus checking compulsions. Clearly, then, there is strong support for considering compulsive washing and checking distinct subtypes of OCD.

It has been well known that a small number of individuals have obsessional ruminations without overt compulsions (Akhtar, Wig, Varma, Pershad, & Verma, 1975; Ingram, 1961b; Rachman, 1985; Rasmussen & Tsuang, 1986; Welner et al., 1976). More recently it has been suggested that a much higher proportion of individuals with OCD (approximately 20%) might fall into the category of obsessional ruminators (see Freeston & Ladouceur, 1997a), although Foa, Steketee, and Ozarow (1985) speculated that most individuals in these pure obsessional subtypes do exhibit mental compulsions. This was borne out in the DSM-IV field trial for OCD, in which only 2.1% of the sample had obsessions without compulsions (Foa & Kozak, 1995). Because overt and covert (mental) compulsions/neutralization perform the same role and function in OCD, it is still not clear whether obsessional rumination should be considered distinct from other subtypes of OCD. The requirement of a specialized treatment protocol tailored to obsessional ruminators would support the view that it is a specific symptom subtype of OCD. However, the necessary clinical comparison studies have not been done to show that pure obsessional rumination has a distinct phenomenology from other OCD subtypes.

Hoarding behavior occurs in 20–31% of OCD patients (Frost, Krause, & Steketee, 1996; Rasmussen & Eisen, 1992), although it is also fairly common in nonclinical samples of individuals. As noted in Table 1.2, hoarding as the primary clinical presentation is not common and hoarding behavior is evident in other psychiatric disorders such as anorexia nervosa, psychotic disorders, depression, and organic disorders (Frost, Steketee, & Greene, 1999). Frost and Hartl (1996) proposed that clinical compulsive hoarding be defined as:

(1) the acquisition of, and failure to discard a large number of possessions that appear to be useless or of limited value; (2) living spaces sufficiently cluttered so as to preclude activities for which those spaces were
designed, and (3) significant distress or impairment in functioning
caused by the hoarding. (p. 341)

A critical feature of clinical compulsive hoarding is that it leads to
clutter. It is this outcome that determines whether hoarding behavior is
considered pathological. A second primary assumption is that the hoarding involves saving useless objects, to which the individual has an excessive emotional attachment (Frost & Hartl, 1996). A number of associated
features have been identified with compulsive hoarders, including compulsive acquisition or buying, inability to discard possessions, lack of organization, and avoidance of decision making (e. g., avoidance of making decisions to discard objects; Frost & Steketee, 1999).

There is considerable debate on whether hoarding should be considered a subtype of OCD or an entirely different disorder. Evidence that
hoarding may be a variant of OCD includes (1) the high correlation between hoarding and obsessive–compulsive symptom measures, (2) higher
rates of hoarding behavior in samples of individuals with OCD, (3) elevated scores of hoarders on obsessive–compulsive symptom measures,
and (4) an association between hoarding and impaired impulse control
(Frost & Gross, 1993; Frost et al., 1996; Frost et al., 1998). There may be
some functional similarity between OCD and some forms of hoarding
(Shafran & Tallis, 1996). Nevertheless, there are other significant factors
that suggest hoarding is not a variant of OCD. The ego-syntonic nature of
hoarding and checking of one's possessions, the fact that hoarding is
rarely the dominant clinical presentation in OCD, and the relative lack of
response to treatments effective for other OCD subtypes suggests that
hoarding may be distinct from OCD (Black et al., 1998; Frost et al., 1996;
Rasmussen & Eisen, 1998). Moreover, a separate hoarding dimension was
found on some OCD measures, such as the Yale–Brown Obsessive–Compulsive Scale (YBOCS), which suggests that hoarding may be distinct from
other obsessive and compulsive symptoms (Calamari, Wiegartz, & Janeck,
1999; Leckman et al., 1997; Summerfeldt, Richter, Antony, & Swinson,
1999). At this point, it is not at all clear whether hoarding should be included as a subtype of OCD. The program of research on compulsive
hoarding undertaken by Frost, Steketee, and colleagues will lead to further clarification of the diagnostic status of this condition.

Despite the widespread acceptance of symptom subtyping in OCD,
this approach has a number of serious limitations. It assumes that patients
in general have one primary obsessive or compulsive symptom, when in
reality many patients have multiple obsessions and compulsions (e.g.,
Akhtar et al., 1975) that may cut across different subtypes. Moreover,

most individuals with OCD show substantial changes in their obsessive-compulsive symptoms over time (Skoog & Skoog, 1999). The cross-sectional nature of most subtype research ignores the dynamic changing nature of obsessive–compulsive symptoms. It also tells us little about the underlying processes and etiology of symptom development. For these reasons, a dimensional analysis may offer a more accurate analysis of symptom presentation in OCD.

Symptom Dimensions

The dimensional perspective does not assume that individuals can be categorized into specific symptom subtypes. Instead, distinct symptom dimensions are identified on which individuals may differ to varying degrees (i.e., present high, medium, or low on each dimension). These dimensions are usually investigated by factor analyzing obsessive-compulsive symptom measures.

An example of this approach is an early study by Hodgson and Rachman (1977), in which they factor analyzed the 30-item Maudsley Obsessional Compulsive Inventory (MOCI). Four symptom dimensions were derived: checking, cleaning, obsessive slowness, and excessive doubting. Three of the dimensions appear quite robust, whereas the last, obsessional slowness, has not consistently emerged (Taylor, 1998). This may be due to the poor item composition of the MOCI Slowness subscale or the rarity of primary obsessional slowness (Rachman, 1974). Factor analyses of other self-report obsessive–compulsive symptom measures, such as the Padua Inventory, have revealed multiple symptom dimensions that correspond to washing, checking, obsessional rumination, and precision (e.g., van Oppen, Hoekstra, & Emmelkamp, 1995). Chapter 8, on cognitive-behavioral assessment, discusses in greater detail the factor analytic research performed on various interview and self-report obsessive–compulsive symptom measures.

Four studies, each involving large samples of patients with OCD, have recently reported on various types of structural analyses of the obsessions and compulsions symptom checklist of the YBOCS (Goodman et al., 1989a, 1989b). Generally, four symptom dimensions were discovered: (1) aggressive, sexual, religious, somatic obsessions and checking compulsions, (2) symmetry, exactness obsessions and counting, ordering compulsions, (3) dirt, contamination obsessions and cleaning compulsions, and (4) hoarding (Baer, 1994; Leckman et al., 1997; Summerfeldt et al., 1999). However, some inconsistencies have emerged across studies. For example, based on a cluster analysis of the YBOCS symptom checklist, Calamari et al. (1999) were able to only partially replicate the previous four-symptom structure. In other cases the YBOCS four symptom dimensions emerged only in a second-order factor analysis based on a priori symptom categories. When the original symptom items were factor analyzed, the symptom dimensions were not replicated (Summerfeldt et al., 1999).

Research on the symptom dimensions of OCD is only in its infancy. Recent studies using more sophisticated statistical methods on well-standardized measures of obsessive–compulsive symptoms are too few to allow firm conclusions. There does seem to be fairly consistent evidence for distinct washing and checking dimensions. Beyond these two dimensions (or subtypes?), differences emerge across studies. It may be that the lower frequency of other types of obsessive–compulsive symptoms makes their reliable identification in empirical studies more difficult.

Certainly, we often see individuals in whom the primary clinical presentation is obsessional rumination, without overt compulsions, symmetry or precision obsessions, hoarding, or abhorrent religious or sexual obsessions. What is at issue is whether these symptom presentations constitute distinct subtypes or dimensions of obsessive–compulsive phenomena. As discussed previously, the dimensional approach to symptom classification may rest on a firmer conceptual basis than the subtype perspective. However, problems have emerged with the dimensional approach. It has been difficult to replicate the same obsessive–compulsive dimensions across studies even when the same assessment measure is used. Moreover, we have not progressed to proposing individual symptom profiles based on a dimensional symptom analysis. If a consensus can emerge on the salient symptom dimensions of OCD, could individuals with particular symptom profiles be matched to a specific treatment regimen? Might certain etiological, pathogenic, or prognostic implications be associated with particular symptom profiles? Although much remains unknown about the critical symptom dimensions of OCD, more progress is likely to result from adopting a dimensional perspective on symptom presentation than from continuing the search for stable OCD subtypes.

SUMMARY AND CONCLUSION

There are many characteristics of OCD that make it a diagnostic enigma. It takes a chronic, often debilitating, course, affecting 1–2% of the general population. The disorder strikes individuals during their youth and then persists, often for a lifetime, with an intermittent worsening of symptoms that can have severe and fairly generalized negative effects on daily living and personal attainment. OCD also has such a diverse, idiosyncratic clinical presentation that it is not possible to consider the disorder a single homogeneous diagnostic entity. Various subtypes of the disorder have been identified that may differ in the psychological processes and fear structure that maintain obsessional symptoms. Although consensus on OCD subtypes has eluded researchers, it is evident that some variations in treatment protocol will be needed for compulsive cleaning and checking, obsessional rumination without overt compulsions, and hoarding. In the end, the explication of salient symptom dimensions may prove more profitable than the continued search for stable OCD subtypes.

The high comorbidity rate within OCD for depression and other anxiety disorders, especially social phobia and possibly panic disorder, makes assessment and treatment of the disorder more difficult. Characteristics associated with other related disorders are common in OCD such as worry, dissatisfaction with physical appearance, health concerns, eating disturbance, tics, and perfectionism. This highly variegated mixture of cognitive, behavioral, and affective symptoms, which falls under the rubric of OCD, presents special challenges for clinical researchers and practitioners concerned with understanding and treating this psychological condition. More specific issues in the identification and conceptualization of obsessions and compulsions are discussed in the next chapter.

CHAPTER 2

Phenomenology of Obsessions and Compulsions

Obsessions can be difficult to distinguish from other types of negative cognition such as worry, negative automatic thoughts, or anxious rumination. The following examples illustrate this point: (1) A person with an HIV infection develops a preoccupation with whether he is spreading infection to others; (2) a wife is fearful that her husband will be killed in a plane crash while on business trips; (3) a businessman is afraid of vomiting and so is preoccupied with whether he is getting sick. In each case these individuals suffered from OCD but described a variety of persistent, unwanted, and distressing thoughts that could be experienced as obsessions, worries, or depressive rumination, depending on the context and the functional characteristics of the thought. The problem of distinguishing obsessions from other types of negative cognition is complicated by the presence of concurrent symptoms and disorders (see Chapter 1).

Unlike obsessions, overt or behavioral compulsions are relatively easy to identify. However, recent studies indicate that individuals with OCD engage in a broad range of behavioral and mental responses that are functionally related to the obsession in the same way as compulsive rituals. It is not enough to focus on the presence of overt compulsions; rather, the full range of responses aimed at controlling the obsession and reducing subjective distress must be considered. There is a paradoxical element to compulsive phenomena. Individuals experience an irresistible urge to engage in activities (i.e., compulsions) that lead to substantial interference and impairment in daily living, and yet they usually consider these actions irrational, even senseless. This is evident in the 52-year-old government official who had repeated thoughts of being responsible for fatal accidents happening to others and so felt compelled to check newspapers and other sources to determine whether he had inadvertently harmed someone. In another example, a 41-year-old homemaker had an irresistible urge to check her freezer to ensure that no one was locked inside, even though she realized this was a silly idea.

This chapter deals with key issues related to the nature of obsessions and compulsions. The critical defining features of obsessional phenomena are presented, as well as the differences between pathological and nonpathological obsessions. The problem of overvalued ideation and delusional thought content is contrasted with obsessional ruminations. In addition, the similarities and differences between obsessions, worry, and negative automatic thoughts are discussed. The section on compulsions examines the nature and function of various types of responses to obsessions, including compulsive rituals, avoidance behavior, covert neutralization, cognitive avoidance, and reassurance seeking. The salient features of neutralization and other cognitive control strategies must be understood before a proper cognitive-behavioral assessment of OCD can be implemented.

OBSESSIONS

Defining Obsessions

Obsessional Content

The clinical presentation in OCD may involve a single primary obsession occurring as a repetitive, distressing thought, image, or impulse, or it may involve multiple obsessions and compulsions. Although there is some disagreement across studies, approximately half to three-quarters of individuals with OCD have multiple obsessions (Akhtar et al., 1975; Rasmussen & Eisen, 1998). Individuals most often report obsessional thoughts; obsessive images (7%) and impulses (17%) are reported much less frequently (Akhtar et al., 1975). It may be that obsessional phenomena in the imagery modality are sufficiently different from the thought or mentation form that a different etiology is implicated and modifications in treatment will be required (de Silva, 1986). Because so little research has investigated obsessional imagery, clinicians must continue to assume that the form of the obsession, whether thought, image, or impulse, is of little consequence in understanding or treating the disorder.

Table 2.1 presents clinical examples of the most prominent obsessional content encountered in clinical practice. The content of obsessional thoughts, images, or impulses is highly individualistic and is shaped by personal experiences, sociocultural influences and critical life incidents. Various sociocultural and demographic variables may influence the focus of an individual's obsessive rumination. There is some evidence of gender differences in obsessional content. Men may more often report sexual, symmetry, and exactness obsessions, whereas women may report more in-

TABLE 2.1. Clinical Examples of Different Types of Obsessions

Type of obsession	Clinical example
Dirt/ contamination	"I may have become contaminated by human dirt because I touched these books."
	"The clothes I am wearing touched the floor, so I'm contaminated."
	"I am seating in a public place that is contaminated by other people's germs, so I may get ill."
Harm/injury to self/others	"Have I accidentally killed someone?"
	"It would be easy to take this knife and stab the person next to me."
	A person has thoughts, impulse to rape a female stranger.
	"My two best friends are going to be murdered."
	"Was I sexually molested by babysitters when I was 4 years old?"
	"Maybe I locked someone in the freezer by mistake."
	"Harm will come to my family if I don't complete tasks like counting or repeating certain conversations or actions."
	"I have accidentally run over someone with the car."
Pathologic doubt	"Did I touch these items in the store and damage them?"
	"Did I make a mistake or not do this task completely?"
	"Maybe I didn't complete the application honestly and accurately before I sealed it in the envelop."
	"Did I turn the dials on the stove burners completely off?"
Symmetry/ exactness	"If I am using the right side of my body too much, I must compensate and use the left side more often."
	"The number 14 is upsetting."
	"I must avoid the words 'power,' 'world,' and 'harvest' because they remind me of the past and this will upset me."
	"I don't understand completely what I just read."
Unacceptable sex	"Did I deliberately touch a child for sexual purposes?"
	"Am I sexually attracted to children?"
	A young heterosexual woman is anxious that she might be sexually aroused by women.
	A married man has intrusive thoughts of oral or anal sex with other men.
Religious	A woman has frequent intrusive words of cursing God or sexual slang while reading the Bible.
	The phrase "god damn" occurs in front of every other thought.
	"Did I displease God?" or "I must have displeased God today."
	"I have not made the right decision that is honoring to God and so the Spirit of God has left me and I am condemned to hell."

(continued)

TABLE 2.1. *(continued)*

Type of obsession	Clinical example
Somatic/health concerns	Repeated images of vomiting.
	Intrusive thoughts of probably getting sick.
Hoarding	"Maybe I will need this sometime in the future."
	"I must make the best possible decision."

trusive thoughts or obsessions having to do with dirt, aggression, and sexual victimization (Byers, Purdon & Clark, 1998; Lensi et al., 1996). Cultural differences also affect the content of obsessions. For example, dirt and contamination obsessions were more prevalent in an Indian OCD sample, whereas sex and religion obsessions were relatively rare (Akhtar et al., 1975). Religious obsessions may be more common in cultures with strict religiously based moral codes (Rasmussen & Eisen, 1992). Although religious devotion is no more prevalent in OCD than in other anxiety disorders, there is evidence of a positive relationship between religiosity, guilt, and obsessive–compulsive symptoms and cognitions (Abramowitz, Huppert, Cohen, Tolin, & Cahill, 2002; Sica, Novara, & Sanavio, 2002; Steketee, Quay, & White, 1991). This suggests that religious experience can have an influence on the content and experience of obsessional symptoms.

Presence of depression and other personal experiences may also influence the content of obsessional ideation. Preoccupation with aggression may be evident in obsessional patients with a primary depressive disorder (Rachman & Hodgson, 1980). The onset of an obsessional episode may be preceded by certain traumatic or critical incidents that are thematically related to the content of the obsession (de Silva & Marks, 1999; Rhéaume, Freeston, Léger, & Ladouceur, 1998). For example, de Silva and Marks (1999) describe the case of a woman who developed a compulsion to pray in order to avoid further harm to herself or her mother after she had been robbed at knife point. Clearly, the traumatic robbery event had a significant impact on the type of obsessional content that later emerged. This suggests that personal experiences can play an important role in shaping the specific obsessional content of some individuals with OCD.

Core Features of Obsessions

Over the years obsessions have been defined in a variety of ways that reflect the theoretical perspective of the researcher. Obsessional phenomena were first recognized as distorted religious experiences until the advent of medical theories in the 19th century. Esquirol was probably the first to describe a case of OCD in 1838, although the term *obsession* is attributed to Morel in 1866 (Black, 1974). In 1878 the German neurologist Karl Westphal offered one of the first comprehensive definitions of obsessions, which emphasized the emergence into consciousness of ideas that are against the will, difficult to control or suppress, but are recognized by the person as abnormal and uncharacteristic of him- or herself (Black, 1974; Rosenberg, 1968).

Contemporary definitions of obsessions emphasize to varying degrees the five core features of obsessional phenomena summarized in Table 2.2. One of the most obvious characteristics of obsessions is their *intrusive quality*. Although obsessions are most often triggered by external stimuli (e.g., touching a public telephone may elicit thoughts of contamination), they intrude into conscious awareness against a person's will. Their occurrence interrupts ongoing activity by capturing attentional resources. Obsessional content is also *unacceptable* to the person, in large part because of the negative affect associated with its occurrence. There is a close association between the degree of discomfort caused by the intrusive thought and its perceived unacceptability (Parkinson & Rachman, 1981a). Unacceptability or distress can vary from mild annoyance to severe anxiety or distress.

TABLE 2.2. The Defining Features of Obsessions

Defining features	Explanation
Intrusive quality	The thought, image, or impulse repeatedly enters consciousness in an unintended manner; that is, it occurs against one's will. A subjective feeling of compulsion is associated with the thought.
Unacceptability	The negative affect associated with the intrusion may vary from an annoyance to unpleasantness or distress to strong fear or anxiety.
Subjective resistance	There is a strong urge to resist, suppress, dismiss, or prevent the obsession from entering consciousness either through avoidance, cognitive control strategies, or overt compulsive rituals.
Uncontrollability	There is a subjective sense of diminished control over the obsession. At the best of times, one's ability to suppress the obsession will be incomplete and temporary.
Ego-dystonicity	The intrusion varies from nonsensical, meaningless mental phenomena that have minimal implication for the self, to ideas, images, or impulses that are entirely inconsistent, possibly even threatening, to core values of the self.

Subjective resistance is one of the hallmarks of obsessions. The individual feels compelled to deal with the obsession, to terminate its dominance of conscious awareness through a variety of control strategies, which include reassurance seeking, avoidance, rationalization, distraction, compulsive rituals, and neutralization. Although the degree of resistance against the obsession varies, there is a motivated effort to ignore, suppress, or neutralize the distressing intrusive thought. The desire to rid the mind of the obsession is related to the person's belief that highly undesirable, even threatening, consequences will befall him or her, or others, if the obsession is not successfully terminated. Despite this motivated resistance, the individual fails to exercise the desired level of control over the obsession. This results in a heightened sense of *uncontrollability* of the thought.

The final characteristic, *ego dystonicity,* refers to the degree that the content of the obsession is contrary to or inconsistent with a person's sense of self as reflected in his or her core values, ideals, and moral attributes. Intrusive thoughts are viewed as occurring outside the context of valued aspects of the self; they are not the type of thought, image, or impulse that a person would expect of him- or herself, and so the obsession represents a threat to the person's self-view (Purdon, 2001; Purdon & Clark, 1999). It is this uncharacteristic or ego-alien quality of the thought that imbues it with special personal significance and importance. The repeated occurrence of these ego-dystonic intrusions may cause individuals to question their true character, thus increasing their desire to suppress the intrusions in order to prove to themselves that they do not possess the undesirable characteristic (Purdon, 2001). The ego-dystonic nature of obsessions is most clearly evident in the harm, injury, and sex obsessions that the patient may consider abhorrent, even repugnant. Intrusive thoughts of child molestation, rape, stabbing individuals, running over pedestrians, and the like are completely at odds with the highly conscientious, passive and moralistic nature of individuals. Such thoughts may cause them to wonder whether they might have latent sexual and aggressive desires that will overtake their egos and cause them to engage in abhorrent acts of harm and injury against self or others. However, other types of obsessions also have this ego-dystonic quality because they may be at variance with the self in more subtle ways. For example, persons who are meticulous, conscientious, and perfectionistic may suffer from obsessive doubt over whether a task is done completely because they believe that mistakes reflect an unacceptable level of personal irresponsibility and carelessness.

The five core features of obsessions (Table 2.2) are dimensions on which specific obsessional content will vary in degree or intensity. Thus, obsessions differ in the composition or relative contribution of each characteristic, although we would expect most obsessions to show all five properties to varying degrees. These constructs are useful in distinguishing obsessions from other types of negative cognition, as well as in distinguishing normal from abnormal obsessions.

Normal and Abnormal Obsessions

Most clinicians assume that OCD is a distinct, categorical psychiatric disorder that affects a small percentage of the population. This categorical perspective is entirely consistent with current psychiatric nosology and diagnostic systems like DSM-IV-TR (APA, 2000). In 1978, Stanley Rachman and Padmal de Silva published a controversial study that challenged the conceptualization of obsessions and compulsions as categorically distinct phenomena with no connection to the nonclinical population. In two studies they compared nonclinical subjects and those with OCD in regard to their experience of unwanted, obsessive-like intrusive thoughts, images, and impulses. The results were rather striking. They found that 84% of their nonclinical participants reported unwanted cognitive intrusions that were qualitatively similar in form and content to the clinical obsessions of patients with OCD. However, the obsessions of patients were rated as more frequent, intense, and uncontrollable, and more likely associated with neutralizing responses, than the unwanted intrusions of nonclinical participants. These findings were more recently replicated in a study by Calamari and Janeck (1997).

Over the years numerous studies have verified that most individuals (80–90%) in the general population experience intrusive, obsessive-like thoughts, images, or impulses (e.g., Clark & de Silva, 1985; Freeston, Ladouceur, Thibodeau, & Gagnon, 1991; Parkinson & Rachman, 1981a; Purdon & Clark, 1993; Salkovskis & Harrison, 1984). The cognitive phenomena investigated in these studies have been labeled *unwanted intrusive thoughts*. They are defined as thoughts, images, or impulses that (1) interrupt ongoing activity, (2) are recognized as having an internal origin, and (3) are difficult to control (Rachman, 1981). Unwanted intrusive thoughts are often triggered by a person's current concerns and situations, including stressful experiences (e.g., Horowitz, 1975; Parkinson & Rachman, 1981b). Moreover, cognitive phenomena of this type have also been found in other clinical states like depression (Brewin, Hunter, Carroll, & Tata, 1996).

Evidence of "normal obsessions" in the general population is important for two reasons. First, it offers some insights into the possible ontogenesis of pathological obsessions. As discussed in later chapters, contemporary cognitive-behavioral theories of OCD postulate that clinical obsessions are derived from the occurrence of normal unwanted intrusive thoughts. If this phenomenon was not present in the nonclinical population, most cognitive-behavioral accounts of OCD would be untenable.

A second important implication of this research is that OCD might be more accurately conceptualized from a dimensional rather than categorical perspective. This suggests that patients with OCD and nonclinical subjects differ in degree rather than kind, with normal unwanted intrusive thoughts lying at one end of the continuum and severe clinical obsessions at the other end. Additional support for this view comes from community-based studies reporting rates of 2–20% of subthreshold OCD (Gibbs, 1996), as well as elevated levels of obsessive and compulsive symptoms in the general population (Nestadt, Samuels, Romanoski, Folstein, & McHugh, 1994; Stein et al., 1997; Welkowitz, et al., 2000). The main difference between clinical and subthreshold OCD is that patients evaluate (appraise) their symptoms more negatively (e.g., as more unacceptable, unpleasant, etc.) and perceive less control over their unwanted intrusive thoughts (Gibbs, 1996).

Unwanted distressing intrusive thoughts are upsetting phenomena for most people, whether or not they suffer an obsessional disorder (e.g., Forrester, Wilson, & Salkovskis, 2002). The critical difference between normal and abnormal obsessions lies in how the unwanted intrusive thought is appraised, evaluated, and responded to, rather than in the content or occurrence of specific types of cognition. Table 2.3 presents various dimensions that can be used to determine the clinical status of unwanted intrusive thoughts, images, or impulses.

TABLE 2.3. Criteria for Distinguishing between Normal and Abnormal Obsessions

Normal obsessions	Abnormal obsessions
Less frequent	More frequent
Less unacceptable/distressing	More unacceptable/distressing
Little associated guilt	Significant feelings of guilt
Less resistance to the intrusion	Strong resistance to the intrusion
Some perceived control	Diminished perceived control over the obsession
Considered meaningless, irrelevant to the self	Considered highly meaningful, threatening important core values of the self (ego-dystonic)
Brief intrusions that fail to dominate conscious awareness	Time-consuming intrusions that dominate conscious awareness
Less concern with thought control	Heightened concern with thought control
Less emphasis on neutralizing distress	Strong focus on neutralizing distress associated with the obsession
Less interference in daily living	Significant interference in daily living

Many of these dimensions of abnormality are fairly obvious and were identified in studies that directly compared patients with OCD and non-clinical subjects (Calamari & Janeck, 1997; Rachman & de Silva, 1978). Clinical obsessions are more frequent, distressing, and unacceptable and are associated with less perceived control than the unwanted intrusions of nonclinical individuals. They are more strongly resisted, more ego-dystonic, and more likely to provoke urges to neutralize than nonclinical obsessions. In addition, individuals with clinical obsessions tend to show greater resistance to the obsessions, are more likely to use maladaptive thought control strategies, and perceive their control efforts as less successful than those in non-OCD groups (Amir, Cashman, & Foa, 1997; Ladouceur et al., 2000).

In nonclinical samples, highly frequent unwanted intrusive thoughts are more likely appraised in a personally significant negative manner and are associated with less subjective control as compared with lower-frequency intrusions (Clark, Purdon, & Byers, 2000; Freeston, Ladouceur, Thibodeau, & Gagnon, 1991, 1992). Moreover, a tendency to interpret the mental intrusion as having some special significance for the self, or as an indication of the likelihood of some negative consequence, is associated with increased uncontrollability and distress (Purdon & Clark, 1994a, 1994b; Purdon, 2001; Wroe, Salkovskis, & Richards, 2000).

The remaining dimensions in Table 2.3 refer to aspects of obsessions that are included in the DSM-IV-TR diagnosis of OCD. Clinical obsessions are more time-consuming and cause greater interference in daily living. Trait guilt, which may be triggered by specific intrusive thoughts, is elevated in patients with OCD (Shafran, Watkins, & Charman, 1996) and may be associated with the frequency, distress, and uncontrollability of these unwanted cognitions (Niler & Beck, 1989; for contrary results see Reynolds & Salkovskis, 1991). Whatever the final status of these variables, it is suggested that clinicians refer to the dimensions presented in Table 2.3 as a guide for determining the clinical status of unwanted, distressing intrusive thoughts.

Overvalued Ideation, Delusions, and Obsessions

Overvalued Ideation

Many early writers assumed that an individual's insight into the excessive or unreasonable nature of his or her obsession was a defining feature of the phenomenon (e.g., Jaspers, 1963; Schneider, 1925, as cited in Black, 1974). However, more recent research indicates that insight is not a necessary criterion for obsessions. In the DSM-IV field trial for OCD, only 13% of patients with OCD were certain that their feared consequences would not occur (i.e., had insight into the unreasonableness of their obsessions), whereas 26% were mostly certain that the consequences would occur and 4% were completely certain that the feared consequences would occur (Foa & Kozak, 1995). The last group of individuals would most certainly meet the DSM-IV-TR (APA, 2000) criterion of *poor insight* into their obsessional state.

Although degree of insight varies between persons, most individuals with OCD generally recognize the unrealistic or excessive nature of their obsessions. In fact, it is this very aspect of the experience that is often most baffling. Frequently, a person with OCD will exclaim, "I know this is so silly, but I get really upset at the thought that this paper might be contaminated with germs." But what can we make of the person with OCD who really believes in the possibility of the negative consequence represented in the obsession? What if the person in the preceding example really believes that the paper is contaminated with germs and that he or she might be "infected with cancer" by touching the paper? In this case the obsessive fear of germs and the subsequent cleaning ritual are not considered unreasonable or excessive by the patient.

It is well known that insight into the unreasonable or senseless nature of a person's obsessions is situation bound, with insight highest in nonthreatening but lower in threatening situations (Kozak & Foa, 1994; Steketee & Shapiro, 1995). As long as the person is not around children, for example, the intrusive thought of being a child molester seems truly absurd. When he or she is in the presence of children, the obsessive thought can be quite convincing, given its persistence and accompanying distress. Fluctuations in insight are to be expected. Of greater interest is the small subgroup of patients who show a fairly constant and unwavering conviction as to the reasonableness and probability of the threat represented by the obsession (i.e., the 4% in the DSM-IV field trial who were convinced of their obsessional fears). For these individuals, the obsession may have developed into an overvalued idea (OVI) or possibly even worse, a delusion.

Wernicke first introduced the term OVI in 1900 to refer to a solitary belief that a person felt justified in holding and that strongly determined the person's behavior (see Kozak & Foa, 1994). Jaspers (1963) later elaborated the concept by noting that overvalued ideas involve strong personal identification and fairly intense affect. However, it was Foa's (1979) research on behavioral treatment failure in OCD that ignited interest in OVI and its relevance to OCD. She found that 4 of the 10 patients with OCD who did not respond successfully to behavior therapy believed that their obsessive thoughts or fears were realistic and that their compulsive behavior actually prevented the occurrence of the perceived negative consequences associated with the obsession.

Research on insight (i.e., fixity of belief) and its more extreme form, OVI, has been impeded by lack of definitional clarity. The relationship of

OVI to concepts like insight, judgment, belief, and delusions has not been well articulated (see discussion by Neziroglu & Stevens, 2002). The most widely accepted view is that OVIs are "strongly held unreasonable beliefs that are not as firmly held as delusional ideas" (Kozak & Foa, 1994, p. 344). According to this view, the main difference between obsessions, OVIs, and delusions is how firmly the erroneous idea is held (i.e., the strength or fixity of belief). More recently, Veale (2002) offered a broader cognitive-behavioral perspective on OVI that emphasizes not only strength of belief but also excessive identification or importance of the value (idea) for the self and the degree of rigidity or inflexibility of the idealized value.

Research on the role of OVI in OCD has also been hampered by the lack of valid and reliable measures. However, two new clinician-administered rating scales were recently developed with improved reliability and validity; the Brown Assessment of Beliefs Scale (Eisen et al., 1998), and the Overvalued Ideas Scale (Neziroglu, McKay, Yaryura-Tobias, Stevens, & Todaro, 1999). The Overvalued Ideas Scale, in particular, has good internal consistency, test–retest stability, and convergent and discriminant validity (Neziroglu, McKay, et al., 1999). Later studies that have used these measures provide a more accurate assessment of the impact of OVI in response to treatment.

Do individuals who believe that their obsessional concerns might be reasonable, and therefore show little resistance to their compulsions, have a poorer response to treatment? Some studies have found that high OVI was associated with poorer (or at least lower) treatment response (Foa, 1979; Foa, Abramowitz, Franklin, & Kozak, 1999; Basoglu, Lax, Kasvikis, & Marks, 1988; Neziroglu, Stevens, McKay, & Yaryura-Tobia, 2001), whereas others did not find that it predicted poor outcome (Lelliott, Noshirvani, Basoglu, Marks, & Monteiro, 1988). In the Neziroglu et al. (2001) study, scores on the Overvalued Ideation Scale were correlated with residual gains in compulsions but not obsessions. Furthermore, there is evidence that OCD patients with OVI can be successfully treated with cognitive and/or behavioral interventions (Lelliott et al., 1988; Salkovskis & Warwick, 1985) or medication (O'Dwyer & Marks, 2000).

Further research is needed to determine the extent that lack of insight or OVI is a poor prognostic indicator for OCD. There is evidence that poor insight is associated with greater symptom severity and a higher incidence of comorbid narcissistic and borderline personality disorders (Türksoy, Tükel, Özdemir, & Karali, 2002). Furthermore, there is fairly strong empirical evidence that individuals with OVI may show a poorer treatment response, although it is also clear that an eventual response to treatment is possible if interventions are tailored to deal with the individual's strong belief in his or her obsessional concerns. Moreover, insight into the senselessness of the obsessive–compulsive symptoms is broadly distributed and varies along a continuum. For most individuals, strength of belief may be unstable, varying across time and situations. Fixity of belief may be more evident in certain types of obsessions, such as religious or harming obsessions (Tolin, Abramowitz, Kozak, & Foa, 2001), and it may have more impact on the treatment of compulsions than obsessions (Neziroglu et al., 2001). Clearly, we have much to learn about the impact of insight and OVI on the course of and treatment response in OCD.

Delusions

Delusions are "erroneous beliefs that usually involve a misinterpretation of perceptions or experiences" (APA, 2000, p. 299). Although their content may vary, DSM-IV-TR emphasizes that the main distinction between a strongly held belief (i.e., OVI) and a delusion is the degree of conviction evident with a delusion despite clear contradictory evidence (APA, 2000).

Over the years a number of writers have proposed a link between OCD and schizophrenia-spectrum disorders (Enright, 1996; Insel & Akiskal, 1986; Stengel, 1945). However, only a small percentage of patients with OCD (12–18%) have psychotic-like symptoms, and for many of these individuals the psychotic symptoms consist of lack of insight and strong conviction of the validity of their obsessional fears (see review by Kozak & Foa, 1994; also Welner et al., 1976). A smaller group has delusions, hallucinations, and/or thought disorder (5–6%) that are more indicative of a psychotic illness. Insel and Akiskal (1986) concluded that 20% of patients with OCD develop psychotic symptoms, although the psychosis in OCD is either a paranoid state or a mood disorder. A true schizophrenic deterioration in OCD is extremely rare.

There is no evidence of an etiological or diagnostic connection between OCD and psychotic disorders (Black, 1974; Salkovskis, 1996c). Nor is there any firm evidence that OVI or delusions develop out of obsessions (Kozak & Foa, 1994; Rachman & Hodgson, 1980). However, Insel and Akiskal (1986) noted that in severe OCD, obsessions can shift into delusions when resistance to the obsession is abandoned and insight into its senselessness is lost.

The clinician may, on occasion, encounter persons with OCD who hold firmly to the veracity of their obsessional fears (e.g., OVI) and, even more rarely, a person whose obsessions take on a delusional quality. For this atypical OCD, response to treatment may be particularly poor (Insel & Akiskal, 1986; Kozak & Foa, 1994). A delusion may be suspected if (1) belief in the obsession is held with such firm conviction that it is entirely unresponsive to clear contradictory evidence, (2) the obsession has a bizarre, implausible quality that is disconnected from ordinary life experience, and (3) the individual does not appear distressed or upset by repeated behavioral response to the obsession (i.e., delusion).

Worry, Negative Automatic Thoughts, and the Specificity of Obsessions

Given the high co-occurrence of anxious and depressive symptoms and disorders in OCD, it is not surprising that other troubling negative cognitions are often present in obsessional states. With GAD possibly present in up to 20% of OCD cases (Abramowitz & Foa, 1998) and significant levels of worry reported in more than 40% of obsessional states (Brown et al., 1993), worry is a common clinical problem in OCD. With its focus on the occurrence of obsessions and their imagined consequences (Wells, 1997), worry content in OCD is often quite different from that in nonobsessional states. Nevertheless worry and obsessions can be difficult to distinguish. Measures of obsessive–compulsive symptoms, worry, and depressive cognition are highly correlated in both clinical and nonclinical samples, and there is considerable similarity in the phenomenological profile of the three types of cognition (Clark, 2002). How can these cognitive phenomena be differentiated so that a precise treatment plan can be formulated?

Worry is a predominantly verbal-linguistic activity (i.e., involving thoughts more than images) that is focused primarily on the actual or potential nonachievement of goals in important life spheres (Borkovec, 1994; M. W. Eysenck, 1992; A. Mathews, 1990; Wells & G. Matthews, 1994). Worry deals with real or imagined threat in regard to a wide variety of personal and social concerns that generally fall within the category of social-evaluative (self-concept) threats or physical threat (M. W. Eysenck, 1992). As a result, subjective anxiety is often high during worry states.

Obsessions and worry have many similarities, as evidenced by the significant correlations between measures of the two types of cognitions (e.g., Freeston et al., 1994; Tallis & de Silva, 1992). At the diagnostic level, OCD and GAD may share the same underlying cognitive processes (Brown, Dowdall, Côté, & Barlow, 1994; Turner, Beidel, & Stanley, 1992). Together, these factors indicate that determining whether a particular pattern of negative thought is worry or obsessional can present special challenges to the clinician.

Table 2.4 presents a tentative list of characteristics that may be used to distinguish obsessions from worry, and from another type of clinical cognition discussed later in this section, negative automatic thoughts. The differentiating features of worry and obsessions are based on empirical studies that directly compared clinical and nonclinical samples of individuals in regard to their self-reported experiences of worries and obsessive thoughts, as well as a literature review published by Turner et al. (1992). The general finding from this research is that worry and obsessions are distinguishable. In terms of their similarities, worry and obsessions are equally intrusive, uncontrollable, distressing, attention grabbing,

TABLE 2.4. Characteristics for Distinguishing Obsessions from Worry and Negative Automatic Thoughts

Obsessions	Worry	Negative automatic thoughts[a]
Ego-dystonic (content tends to be uncharacteristic of the self)	Ego-syntonic content focused on self-relevant concerns)	Ego-syntonic (content is self-referent in nature)
Varied format (includes thoughts, images, and impulses)	Verbal format is most prominent	Mainly verbal format but more images than in worry
Focus on consequences of the thought itself	Focus on consequences of actual situations represented in the worry content	Focus on the consequences to the self
Strong evidence of thought–action fusion	Little evidence of thought–action fusion	Little evidence of thought–action fusion
Greater perceived responsibility	Less perceived responsibility	Less perceived responsibility
Negative affect linked to content of the intrusion	Strong negative affect related to the real-life problem of the worry	Negative affect triggered by the occurrence of the thought
Strongly resisted (effort to control)	Moderately resisted (effort to control)	Little resistance (effort to control)
Highly intrusive and unwanted	Moderately intrusive and unwanted	Tends to run parallel to conscious, intentional thought
Moderate perceived uncontrollability	High perceived uncontrollability	Evaluations of controllability less relevant
Highly accessible to awareness	Highly accessible to awareness	Somewhat inaccessible to awareness
High likelihood of associated neutralization	Moderate likelihood of associated neutralization	Minimal use of associated neutralization
Considered highly unacceptable	Considered moderately unacceptable	Considered quite acceptable
Highly implausible (e.g., senselessness)	Quite plausible although exaggerated	Highly plausible, accepted as self-evident
Less amenable to rational disputation	Somewhat amenable to rational disputation	More responsive to rational disputation

[a]Based on comparison in Salkovskis (1985).

strongly resisted, disapproving, and unacceptable. However, the two types of negative cognitions are also quite different.

Obsessions deal with ego-dystonic themes (i.e, sex, aggression, contamination, etc.) and so their occurrence is interpreted as indicating something meaningful about the person (e.g., "I must have latent aggressive tendencies because I have these intrusive thoughts of harming people"). Obsessions are also more intrusive than worry, more unacceptable, more involuntary, engender a greater sense of responsibility, occur in a variety of mental forms (thoughts, images, or impulses), and more likely elicit a thought–action fusion bias (i.e., that the very act of thinking the obsession increases the likelihood of a negative outcome). Worry, on the other hand, has a predominantly verbal format. It is more realistic, with a focus on normal problems of everyday living (i.e., ego-dystonic), deals with the consequences of negative events, is more voluntary, and is perceived as outside personal control (Clark & Claybourn, 1997; Coles, Mennin, & Heimberg, 2001; Langlois, Freeston, & Ladouceur, 2000a, 2000b; Wells & Morrison, 1994). Although it might be expected that obsessions are probably resisted more strongly and are more likely to lead to neutralization or a compulsion, nevertheless, resistance and compulsive responses have also been reported with worry (Schut, Castonguay, & Borkovec, 2001; Wells & Morrison, 1994).

Beck (1963, 1976) first proposed that negative automatic thoughts about an individual's self, personal world, and future were key symptom features of clinical depression. Over the years considerable empirical support has accumulated to suggest that negative thoughts of personal loss or deprivation are specific to depression and, to a lesser extent, that thoughts of personal threat or danger may be more prominent in anxiety (for reviews see Clark & Beck, 1999; Haaga, Dyck, & Ernst, 1991).

It is now known that negative automatic thoughts (NATs) also occur in obsessional states. The NATs in OCD primarily focus on the occurrence and consequence of obsessional thinking. That is, obsessional individuals generate NATs in the form of interpretations or appraisals about the importance of the obsession (see Chapter 5 on cognitive appraisal theories). The distinction between obsessions and NATs was first proposed by Salkovskis (1985). He argued that obsessions are highly intrusive, easily accessible, irrational, ego-dystonic, and may take the form of thoughts, images, or impulses. Negative automatic thoughts, on the other hand, are less intrusive, more difficult to access, rational, ego-syntonic, and take a predominantly verbal and, to a lesser extent, imaginal form. Unfortunately, the necessary studies directly comparing depressive NATs and obsessions have not been done, so there is no way of empirically verifying Salkovskis's (1985) distinctions. However, Table 2.4 offers some tentative differences that may be apparent, based on what is known about the nature of obsessions and depressive cognition.

COMPULSIONS

Forms of Overt Neutralization

Compulsions

Compulsions are repetitive behaviors (e.g., washing, checking, ordering) or mental acts (e.g., praying, counting, repeating phrases) that are performed to reduce anxiety or prevent some dreaded outcome (DSM-IV-TR; APA, 2000). In most cases individuals feel an urge to perform the compulsion (e.g., an urge or pressure to check once more that the light switch is really turned off). DSM-IV-TR emphasizes that compulsions are not associated with pleasure or gratification, which distinguishes them from other forms of repetitive behavior such as addictions or impulse-control disorders (e.g., kleptomania, pathological gambling, trichotillomania, compulsive masturbation). The classic example of a compulsion is personified by the individual who feels an intense urge to repeatedly wash his or her hands in response to touching a doorknob. Such contact elicits the obsessive thought of contamination, accompanied by repeated washing of the hands until the person experiences a significant decline in subjective anxiety. Once anxiety has declined to an acceptable level, the individual ceases to engage in the compulsive washing ritual.

The salient characteristics of compulsions include (1) a repetitive, stereotypic, and intentional action, (2) a subjective pressure or urge to perform, (3) a diminished sense of voluntary control, and (4) the goal of preventing or reducing distress or a dreaded consequence (Rachman & Shafran, 1998). The compulsion is, at best, only partly acceptable to the person and more often is considered an excessive or exaggerated response. In neutral situations the individual may even admit that the compulsion is senseless or irrational. This may provoke subjective resistance so that the individual delays, extends, or postpones acting on the compulsion, but eventually the urge to carry out the compulsion becomes so strong that the individual gives in to the pressure to execute the compulsion (Rachman & Shafran, 1998). Many individuals with OCD eventually give up their struggle against the compulsion, showing only slight or no resistance (Foa & Kozak, 1995; Stern & Cobb, 1978).

Obsessions and compulsions are functionally related. Generally, obsessions elicit anxiety, whereas the accompanying compulsion is performed to reduce anxiety. The vast majority of patients with OCD (75–91%) have both obsessions and compulsions (Akhtar et al., 1975; Foa & Kozak, 1995). Whether obsessions and compulsions are clearly separate phenomena is questioned by studies showing that they fall on the same factors (e.g., Calamari et al., 1999; Leckman et al., 1997; Summerfeldt et al., 1999). However, factor analytic results of a new obsessive–compulsive symptom measure that my colleagues and I developed revealed that obsessions and compulsions items formed clearly distinct dimensions (Clark, Antony, Beck, Swinson, & Steer, 2003). These latter findings, then, support the clinical practice of treating obsessions and compulsions as functionally related, but distinct, clinical phenomena.

Compulsions are not restricted to clinical OCD samples. Many nonclinical individuals report that they sometimes or often perform ritualistic behaviors involving (1) checking, (2) cleaning, washing, and ordering, (3) "magical" protective behaviors, or (4) avoidance of particular objects (Muris, Merckelbach, & Clavan, 1997; see also Burns, Formea, Keortge, & Sternberger, 1995). Naturally, the compulsions of patients with OCD occur with greater frequency and intensity, elicit more resistance and discomfort, and are more often executed in response to a distressing thought or negative mood state. Compulsions such as checking and reassurance seeking are seen in other clinical disorders such as GAD and hypochondriasis (Fallon et al., 1993; Schut, et al., 2001). Like the findings on obsessions, these results support a dimensional perspective on OCD.

Sometimes the term *compulsive* has been applied to other repetitive behaviors like anxious habits (e.g., nail-biting, trichotillimania), addictive behaviors (e.g., pathological gambling, overeating, alcoholism), or other impulse-control disorders. However, the main difference is that some degree of pleasure seeking is evident in these other behavioral patterns, whereas it is entirely absent in compulsions (Foa & Steketee, 1979; Hollander & Wong, 2000). Another clinical phenomenon that can be confused with compulsions is multiple tic disorder. O'Connor (2001) noted that tics are involuntary, impulsive, and purposeless movements, whereas compulsions are more likely to be intentional or voluntary and to be preceded by intrusive thoughts. Normally, behavioral or overt compulsions can be distinguished from tics with considerable reliability within the clinical setting.

Compulsive Urges

A distinction can be made between a compulsive behavior and the compulsive urge that precedes the ritual. Compulsive urges are "the psychological activity that lies between an obsessional thought and the execution of a compulsive act" (Rachman & Hodgson, 1980, p. 211). The critical defining features of compulsive urges are that (1) they relate to obsessions, (2) they impel toward action, (3) they are internally or externally provoked, (4) they frequently relate to compulsive rituals, (5) they are generally associated with internal resistance, and (6) they can be suppressed so that the compulsive act is not executed. Occurrence of the obsession leads to an intensification of the compulsive urge, whereas execution of the compulsion results in a significant decline in discomfort and the subjective intensity of the urge (Rachman, de Silva, & Roper, 1976). Any assessment of compulsive responses should include an account of the urge to perform the compulsion.

Neutralization

There has been some confusion in the OCD literature over the concept of *neutralization*. Initially, the term referred to any compulsive behavior or cognitive strategy that was an attempt to "put things right" or avert the possibility of blame (Salkovskis, 1985). Later, Salkovskis and Westbrook (1989) proposed a much broader definition, in which anything a person does intentionally or effortfully in response to an obsession is considered neutralization. However, Freeston and Ladouceur (1997b) offered a narrower definition of neutralization that is more useful to clinicians and researchers. They define it as "any voluntary, effortful cognitive or behavioral act that is directed at removing, preventing, or attenuating the thought or the associated discomfort" (Freeston & Ladouceur, 1997b, p. 344).

The distinction between compulsion and neutralization can be difficult to make, especially when the compulsion involves a mental or cognitive ritual. Rachman and Shafran (1998) offered the clearest explanation of the difference between the two concepts. Compulsive rituals are repetitive, fairly stereotypic, intentional, and fixed ways of responding that seek to reduce distress or prevent an anticipated negative outcome linked to the obsession. Neutralization, on the other hand, is a broader, more flexible way of responding that aims to cancel the effects of one's thoughts or actions, to "put right" the obsession. This cancellation effect may or may not be an attempt to prevent the dreaded consequence associated with the obsession. The main objective of neutralization is to undo the effects of one's thoughts or actions. Although neutralization is mainly covert and compulsions are usually overt, both are attempts to reduce anxiety.

The difference between compulsions and neutralization is illustrated in the following example. A young woman had obsessive ruminations that she was getting sick and would vomit. Sometimes, in response to this thought, she repeatedly washed her hands or took long baths to rid her body of contamination. This behavior was clearly compulsive, in that she engaged in a fairly strict sequence of behaviors aimed at reducing her fear of contamination. On other occasions she tried to replace the "getting sick" obsession with a pleasant image. This latter response is an example of neutralization, because the replacement image varied in content and was a deliberate strategy to cancel out the negative, distressing effects of the "getting sick" obsession. In fact, she believed that by forming pleasant thoughts she could prevent the "getting sick" obsession from increasing her chances of actually feeling sick.

Neutralization and compulsions play a similar role in the pathogenesis of obsessions. There is evidence that covert neutralization quickly reduces discomfort caused by an obsession. However, in the longer term (i.e., 30–60 minutes later), it causes more discomfort, a greater urge to neutralize, and an increased likelihood of further neutralization responses (Rachman, Shafran, Mitchell, Trant, & Teachman, 1996; Salkovskis, Westbrook, Davis, Jeavons, & Gledhill, 1997). As Rachman (1998) noted, the very act of neutralizing shields the individual from disconfirming evidence that neutralization did not prevent a feared event from occurring or that it was not responsible for reductions in subjective discomfort.

Reassurance Seeking

Individuals with OCD often resort to repeatedly seeking reassurance from others that the feared consequences associated with an obsession will not occur, or that they have completed their compulsive behavior or neutralization thoroughly and completely. For example, a man with obsessional ruminations had repeated intrusive thoughts and images of his wife having intercourse with a boy she dated during high school. He repeatedly sought reassurance from her on whether she realized she had committed an immoral act (according to his perspective), for which she was regretful. For many years he felt compelled to repeatedly question (i.e., interrogate) her, to the point where she became visibly upset, even though he knew the whole issue was senseless. The husband and wife agreed that his irresistible need to question (to pester) was a pathological compulsion that required treatment. In this case, the person sought reassurance from his wife that the feared consequence, represented in the obsession, did not happen (e.g., "Did you enjoy sex with the high school date?"). It is also possible that in some cases a person who is struggling with terminating a compulsion will seek reassurance that the compulsion can be stopped without negative consequences. Someone with checking compulsions might ask a family member whether the stove is really turned off, whether the door is locked, or whether he or she really did sign the form before putting it in the envelop.

Reassurance seeking is a common response used by individuals both with and without OCD to deal with unwanted intrusive thoughts or obsessions (Freeston & Ladouceur, 1997b; Ladouceur et al., 2000). It appears to have a significant link to the perceived uncontrollability of an obsessive intrusive thought (Purdon & Clark, 1994b) Clinical experience suggests that individuals who continually seek reassurance from others find their obsessions and associated anxiety particularly intense. It is as if the very act of seeking assurance from others confirms the actual dangerousness of the obsession. Functionally, reassurance seeking may be a strategy for spreading responsibility for the feared outcome to others, thereby diluting the sense of personal responsibility for preventing harm to self or others (Salkovskis, 1985). Or, like compulsions, reassurance seeking may be an attempt to reduce anxiety, even though the person seeking the information is often fully aware of the answer (Rachman & Shafran, 1998).

Avoidance

Avoidance is often the first choice of action that obsessional individuals use to manage their obsessive–compulsive symptoms. Although avoidance behavior is common to most forms of OCD, it is particularly evident in certain subtypes, such as compulsive cleaning, in which there is a strong phobic element (Rachman & Hodgson, 1980). Individuals with cleaning compulsions have an intense fear of dirt or disease contamination. They often take extreme care to avoid any situation that might bring them in contact with possible contamination (e.g., public areas, close physical contact with others, hospitals or clinics). Only when avoidance fails do they attempt to "escape" from their anxiety by compulsive cleaning. Avoidance is thought to contribute to the salience of obsessions by preventing exposure to obsessional fears. Moreover, avoidance does not give the individual an opportunity to experience disconfirming evidence against the threatening nature of the obsession. Table 2.5 presents a summary of the different types of overt response strategies used in OCD, along with a definition and clinical example of each strategy.

Function of Neutralization

Given the deleterious impact of compulsions, neutralization, reassurance seeking and avoidance on the persistence of obsessional symptoms, why do individuals continue to engage in these maladaptive forms of behavior? One of the main reasons for the persistence of compulsions and other forms of neutralization is that they reduce anxiety. There is now considerable experimental evidence that compulsions and neutralization reduce anxiety. Individuals with OCD who are exposed to stimuli that provoke their obsessions experience a steep rise in anxiety. Execution of the compulsion leads to a quicker decline in anxiety than delaying the compulsion (Rachman & Hodgson, 1980; Rachman & Shafran, 1998). Other reasons for the persistence of compulsions and neutralization is that they reduce the probability of an unfavorable or harmful event (Carr, 1974) or decrease perceived responsibility for preventing harm to oneself or others (Salkovskis, 1985, 1989a, 1999).

Another motive for engaging in compulsive behavior has been referred to as the *just right* perception. Sometimes individuals with OCD perform a compulsive ritual until they perceive that a "just right" state has been achieved (Leckman et al., 2000). However, this criterion is ill suited

TABLE 2.5. Definition and Clinical Examples of Compulsions and Other Forms of Overt/Covert Neutralization

Response strategy	Definition	Clinical example
Compulsive rituals	Repetitive, stereotyped, intentional responses associated with a subjective pressure to act that is often perceived to be excessive and may provoke, albeit temporary, resistance.	In response to a fear of contamination, individuals repeatedly wash their hands to the point where they are sore and bleeding.
Compulsive urges	The subjective state between an obsession and a compulsion in which, provoked by a internal or external stimulus, one feels impelled toward action.	A person with a checking compulsion questions whether the front door is locked. Even though she recalls locking the door, the urge to check is so strong that she returns to try the doorknob one more time.
Neutralization	Intentional, effortful, and voluntary overt or covert acts directed at canceling out the occurrence of an obsession or its associated discomfort, or to prevent a dreaded outcome symbolized in the obsession.	A young woman has an intrusive thought of harm occurring to her boyfriend. At this, she immediately repeats whatever she was doing and thinks about a positive thought in order to cancel out the negative effects of the harm obsession.
Reassurance seeking	Persistent requests for information that might reduce the anticipated threat associated with the intrusion, even when one is fully aware of the answer.	A severely obsessional patient waits until explicitly told it is time to leave the office, because he is unsure as to whether the session has truly ended.
Avoidance	Any attempted effort or activity intended to avert a perceived internal or external provoking stimulus of the obsession.	A patient avoids particular foods, music, objects in his apartment, the number 14, etc., because they trigger a very upsetting harm and sex obsession.

for judging when neutralizing is complete, because the person is using a vague, indeterminable criterion for completion while at the same time experiencing a high state of anxiety (Richards, 1995). "Just right" perceptions may play a prominent role in symmetry and precision OCD, with its desire to have objects or events in a certain order or precision (Rasmussen & Eisen, 1992; Summerfeldt et al., 1999). Thus, a subjective state of relief or "just right" occurs once things are lined up or placed in their exact position. "Just right" perceptions may also be more apparent in primary obsessive slowness and tic-related OCD (Leckman et al., 2000). Leckman and colleagues commented that the "just right" perception primarily involves a need for things to "look" just right as opposed to "feeling" or "sounding" just right. Thus, compulsions or other forms of neutralization are engaged until a perceived state of "just right" is achieved.

Forms of Covert Neutralization and Mental Control

Cognitive-behavioral researchers emphasize that any response to an obsession can have an impact on the persistence of obsessional symptoms. Thus, investigators have broadened their inquiry to include any mental control strategies used to control obsessions and their associated anxiety, as well as the well-documented overt compulsive rituals. A finding that has emerged from this research is that individuals with OCD rely on a variety of thought control strategies to deal with their obsessions (e.g., behavioral distraction, thought stopping, trying to convince oneself that the thought is not important, thought replacement, talking about it, doing nothing, rationalization) much more often than expected. Freeston and Ladouceur (1997b) found that only a third of the cognitive strategies and one-quarter of the behavioral strategies used by patients with OCD to control obsessions could be considered cognitive rituals (i.e., compulsions) or neutralization.

Another unexpected finding is that the mental control strategies used by patients with OCD are more similar to the strategies used by nonclinical individuals than might be expected. Nonclinical persons and individuals with OCD do not differ in the frequency with which they use rationalization (i.e., trying to convince themselves of the unimportance of their thoughts), reassurance seeking, and possibly distraction, in response to unwanted intrusive thoughts or obsessions. However, individuals with OCD do report a significantly greater use of overt compulsions, mental checking, thought stopping, self-questioning, worry, self-punishment and reappraisal than nonclinical control groups (Abramowitz, Whiteside, Kalsy, & Tolin, 2003; Amir, Cashman, et al., 1997; Ladouceur et al., 2000). "Do nothing" in response to an obsessive intrusive thought was reported significantly more often by the nonclinical groups than the groups with OCD (e.g., Ladouceur et al., 2000; Rachman & de Silva, 1978). In addition, there is indirect evidence that certain mental strategies, such as self-punishment and worry, are particularly ineffective in managing OCD symptoms. However, following successful treatment, individuals with OCD may show a significant increase in use of distraction and a significant decrease in the use of punishment (Abramowitz, Whiteside, et al., 2003).

One of the most important differences between clinical and nonclinical individuals is their perception or evaluation of thought control success. Even though individuals with OCD may try longer and harder to control their obsessions, in the end they rate themselves as significantly less effective in their mental control efforts than do nonclinical individuals (Ladouceur et al., 2000). In addition, some studies have found that certain mental control strategies (e.g., neutralization, reassurance seeking, and thought stopping) may be associated with less perceived control and greater distress (Freeston, Ladouceur, Thibodeau, & Gagnon, 1991, 1992; Freeston & Ladouceur, 1993; Purdon & Clark, 1994b). Other studies suggest that the type of mental control has little association with perceived effectiveness (Clark et al., 2000; Purdon & Clark, 1994a), and Freeston, Ladouceur, Provencher, and Blais (1995) even concluded that there was no evidence that one particular thought control strategy was more effective than another. The particular thought control strategy a person utilizes in response to an unwanted intrusive thought or obsession may depend on contextual factors, the type of obsessional content, and whether the intrusive thought is a worry or an obsession (Freeston et al., 1995; Langlois et al., 2000b; Lee & Kwon, 2003). Table 2.6 summarizes the current status of covert neutralization and mental control of unwanted intrusive thoughts and obsessions.

SUMMARY AND CONCLUSION

The assessment of obsessional thoughts, images, or impulses can be difficult because of the nature of obsessional phenomena. Although the content of obsessions tends to be limited to certain themes, obsessional material is, nevertheless, highly idiosyncratic to the concerns and life experiences of individual patients. Almost any thought, image, or impulse can be an obsession if responded to in a pathologic fashion. The five core features of obsessions in Table 2.2 may be helpful in gauging whether cognitive phenomena are obsessional. However, an accurate assessment of obsessions also depends on the ability to differentiate clinical obsessions from normal unwanted intrusive thoughts, overvalued ideas, delusions, worry, and negative automatic thoughts. The characteristics listed in Tables 2.3 and 2.4 should assist in differentiating obsessions from other cognitive–clinical phenomena.

Past research and treatment tended to focus almost exclusively on the role of overt compulsive rituals in the persistence of OCD. Although the importance of compulsions is not denied, it is quite clear that a much broader array of overt and covert responses must be considered in the pathogenesis and treatment of obsessional states. Overt and covert neutralization, reassurance seeking, and a variety of relatively ineffective mental control strategies must be included in the repertoire of maladaptive responses related to obsessional phenomena. Many of these cognitive

TABLE 2.6. Features of Covert Neutralization and the Intentional Control of Obsessions

Characteristic	Explanation
Prevalence of mental control	In OCD, mental control strategies are used more often in response to obsessions than overt or covert compulsive rituals.
Variety of control strategies	Individuals with OCD use a variety of thought control strategies that do not differ from those used by nonclinical individuals.
Dysfunctional control strategies	Individuals with OCD are more likely to use dysfunctional control strategies like compulsive rituals, thought stopping, punishment and worry than nonclinical individuals.
Do nothing	Obsessional individuals are less likely to do nothing in response to their unwanted intrusions, a response strategy shown to be more effective with unwanted intrusive thoughts.
Ineffective control	In OCD, most thought control strategies are less effective or efficient at controlling the frequency and intensity of unwanted intrusions than with nonclinical individuals.
Relation to distress	Escape/avoidance control strategies are associated with increased general distress, whereas attentive thinking about the intrusion is specifically related to increased anxiousness.
Negative appraisals of intrusions	Certain dysfunctional response strategies such as escape/avoidance may be related to increased appraisals of disapproval, ego-dystonicity, uncontrollability, and responsibility for the intrusion.
Context and content of thought	The context and content of the thought influence the type of thought control strategy selected.
Negative mood	Presence of dysphoria or anxious and depressive symptoms decrease the effectiveness of thought control.

response strategies are found in other clinical disorders and in the normal population. Although each of these strategies seems to be quite ineffective, particularly when applied to frequent and highly distressing obsessions, individuals continue in such efforts because of a temporary decline in distress, a misperceived thwarting of some dreaded outcome, or a reduced sense of responsibility. As discussed in later chapters, cognitive-behavioral therapists must deal with a range of mental control responses, not just compulsive rituals, when treating patients with obsessional states.

PART II

Cognitive-Behavioral Theory and Research

CHAPTER 3

Behavioral Perspectives on OCD

The first credible psychological theory and treatment for OCD emerged in the 1960s and early 1970s from the behavioral perspective on clinical disorders and experimental research on learning. Because OCD was considered an anxiety disorder, behavioral theories of fear acquisition, persistence, and modification were assumed to be entirely applicable to the theory and treatment of obsessions and compulsions.

Early behavioral theories and interventions for OCD focused primarily on overt compulsive behaviors, especially washing and checking rituals. The central concept was the *anxiety reduction hypothesis*. Compulsive rituals persisted because of their anxiety-reducing capability; that is, via a form of avoidance learning. The completion of a compulsive act like handwashing reduced high levels of subjective anxiety caused by the occurrence of obsessions (Carr, 1974; Teasdale, 1974). Because a reduction in anxiety or distress is reinforcing, this ensures that the compulsive ritual will be repeated in the future. However, it also paradoxically preserves the fear-eliciting properties of the obsession, thereby setting up an escalating cycle of ever more frequent and intense obsessions and compulsions (e.g., H. J. Eysenck & Rachman, 1965; Rachman & Hodgson, 1980). Obsessions, like other phobic stimuli, were considered conditioned noxious stimuli that acquire their ability to elicit anxiety or discomfort by an association with a prior traumatic or upsetting experience (Steketee, 1993).

The behavioral theory of OCD was based on O. H. Mowrer's (1939, 1953, 1960) two-stage theory of fear and avoidance. In the first stage obsessional fears develop through classical conditioning in which a neutral object (e.g., knife) acquires the ability to elicit discomfort because of its association with an aversive experience (e.g., a person's sudden thought of stabbing her baby). In the second stage, performance of any behavior that relieves the obsessive fear is negatively reinforced because of its anxiety-reducing effects (Steketee, 1993). Thus, avoidance of knives might be the first line of defense against the obsession, but avoidance is often ineffective or not entirely possible (e.g., knives are needed for preparing food). So, for example, the person's asking for reassurance that she has not harmed the child could be negatively reinforced (e.g., feeling relief after receiving reassurance that the child is unharmed), thereby ensuring that the person will again ask for reassurance when thoughts about harming the child recur in the future.

Prior to the mid-1960s there was no effective psychological or pharmacological intervention for OCD. Applications of early behavioral techniques to OCD, such as systematic desensitization, modeling, operant reinforcement, aversion relief, and relaxation therapy, produced modest and rather mixed benefits (Emmelkamp, 1982; Foa, Franklin, & Kozak, 1998; Kozak & Foa, 1997). However, in 1966 Victor Meyer described a behavioral treatment for OCD called exposure and response prevention (ERP), which substantially altered how behavioral psychologists treated obsessions and compulsions (Meyer, 1966; Meyer, Levy, & Schnurer, 1974). The two-factor theory of fear and avoidance provided the theoretical basis for ERP. In the intervening 30 years, a number of clinical trials indicated that 60–85% of patients who complete ERP show significant symptom improvement (for reviews and meta-analyses see Abramowitz, 1998; Emmelkamp, 1982; Foa & Steketee, 1979; Rachman & Hodgson, 1980; Stanley & Turner, 1995; and van Balkom et al., 1994). Today ERP is an integral component of any effective psychological treatment for OCD, including the new cognitive-behavioral therapy described later in this book.

This chapter presents a brief overview of the behavioral theory of OCD. Empirical support for the model is considered, and shortcomings in the behavioral account that led to the new cognitive-behavioral theories of OCD are discussed. In addition, ERP is described and various behavioral approaches to the treatment of obsessions are reviewed. The chapter concludes with a review of the empirical status and outcome literature for ERP. In addition, limitations of the behavioral treatment of obsessions and compulsions that led to the adoption of a more cognitive approach to OCD are discussed.

BEHAVIORAL THEORY

Obsessions

Rachman (1971) argued that, like other phobic stimuli, obsessions are *conditioned noxious stimuli* that cause pain and/or distress for patients and often result in the production of avoidance behaviors (or compulsions) to relieve that distress. However, obsessions are not identical to phobic responses, in that obsessions are more endogenous and are more often associated with depression. Obsessions persist because individuals fail to habituate to the intrusive thought and show increased sensitization or responsiveness to the cognition. A number of factors may increase a person's responsiveness or sensitivity to an unwanted intrusive thought (i.e., obsession), including presence of dysphoria, pre-existing personality vulnerability (e.g., introversion, excessive conscientiousness, moral rigidity), periods of stress, heightened arousal, and perceived loss of control (Rachman, 1971, 1976a, 1978; Rachman & Hodgson, 1980). In addition, the occurrence of both active (i.e., compulsive ritual) and passive (i.e., avoidance of situations that trigger the obsession) avoidance contribute to a failure of habituation and increased sensitivity to the obsession. Rachman and Hodgson (1980) also proposed that vulnerability to obsessions can be attributed to five factors: (1) presence of dysphoric mood, (2) exposure to stress, (3) intolerance or unacceptability of thoughts, (4) heightened sensitivity to threatening stimuli, and (5) a personality constellation characterized by dysthymia, high emotionality or neuroticism, and introversion.

Compulsions

Compulsive rituals like cleaning, checking, and reassurance seeking persist because of avoidance learning or what Mowrer (1953) called "solution learning." Avoidance learning occurs when a learned activity circumvents or prevents exposure to a noxious or fear stimulus (Teasdale, 1974). The avoidant activity is strengthened through a process of operant conditioning. In the case of OCD, the compulsion takes the form of active avoidance because it reduces anxiety associated with the obsession (Emmelkamp, 1982). However, anxiety reduction is often very short term in patients with severe OCD (i.e., relief may last only a matter of minutes in many cases), and so the whole cycle of anxiety elicitation and relief will be repeated.

Anxiety reduction is a sufficient but not necessary condition for the persistence of compulsions, because a minority of individuals will show no change or even an increase in anxiety following completion of their compulsive rituals. In such cases it may be that the compulsion alleviates other negative emotions like guilt or dysphoria, or that it reduces the probability of longer-term unpleasantness (or attains long-term safety) at the expense of an increment in short-term anxiety (Carr, 1974; Rachman & Hodgson, 1980). For example, a person with compulsive checking may continue to check whether the stove is turned off even though each repetition of the act leads to greater frustration and anxiety. However, the patient is willing to endure immediate distress in order to prevent a more serious long-term consequence—an unattended burner causing a house fire.

Empirical Support

A number of testable hypotheses are derived from the behavioral model of OCD, and these have been subjected to numerous experimental investigations by Rachman, Marks, Foa, Emmelkamp, and others. Because classial conditioning is the process through which obsessions acquire their anxious property, external traumas or stressors should be present in the etiology of obsessions. There is considerable empirical evidence that obsessions can be provoked by external stimuli (e.g., Steketee et al., 1985; Roper, Rachman, & Hodgson, 1973). However, 20–30% of obsessions and unwanted intrusions occur without external triggers and there is often little relationship between the content of obsessions and environmental events (Rachman & Hodgson, 1980). Although stressful life events and the environment do appear to have an influence on OCD, they rarely exert their impact immediately at the onset of obsessive–compulsive symptoms, as implied by the classical conditioning stage of the behavioral model (Steketee, 1993). Overall empirical support for the hypothesis that obsessions are acquired through association with a traumatic or highly aversive experience is not compelling.

There is considerable experimental evidence that obsessions are accompanied by subjective and physiological anxiety or distress. Provocation of an obsession, such as a person's fear of contamination or doubts that he or she has performed a task correctly, will result in a significant increase in subjective distress and heightened physiological arousal prior to that person's engaging in a compulsive ritual (e.g., Boulougouris, Rabavilas, & Stefanis, 1977; Boulougouris & Bassiakos, 1973; Hodgson & Rachman, 1972; Roper et al., 1973; Roper & Rachman, 1976; Rabavilas & Boulougouris, 1974). Furthermore, presence of adverse mood (i.e., dysphoria, anxiety) reduces the individual's ability to prevent or dismiss (remove) unwanted intrusive thoughts from consciousness. An individual who is depressed, for example, is less able to use distraction and thought replacement to deal successfully with unwanted cognitions (e.g., Conway, Howell, & Giannopoulos, 1991; Reynolds & Salkovskis, 1992; Sutherland, Newman, & Rachman, 1982).

The behavioral model predicts that obsession-prone individuals will be more responsive or sensitive to certain unwanted intrusive thoughts or obsessions. Individuals with OCD do rate their unwanted intrusive thoughts or obsessions as more intense, discomforting, distressing, and unacceptable than nonclinical individuals (controls) rate their unwanted thoughts (Calamari & Janeck, 1997; Rachman & de Silva, 1978). However, both patients with OCD and nonclinical individuals (controls) show a decrease in the intensity or responsiveness to an obsession with repeated presentations of an obsession, rather than an increase as predicted by the behavioral model (Janeck & Calamari, 1999; Parkinson & Rachman, 1980; Rachman & de Silva, 1978).

A final hypothesis critical to the behavioral account of OCD is the prediction that compulsions and other neutralizing responses will cause a temporary reduction in distress and an increase in perceived control over obsessions. There is considerable experimental evidence that production of overt compulsions like washing or checking results in an immediate and significant decline in subjective discomfort (for reviews of this experimental literature see Rachman & Hodgson, 1980; Rachman & Shafran, 1998). Moreover, these findings also apply to covert neutralization. In a recent study (Marks et al., 2000), patients with OCD reported a significant decline in subjective discomfort when they generated an image that canceled the effects of the obsession (e.g., someone with exactness obsessions imagines returning home and rearranging the misplaced objects). However, anxiety reduction is not always evident with compulsions or other forms of neutralization. There is a small minority of compulsions (possibly as much as 20%) that result in an elevation in subjective anxiety. Moreover, the temporary anxiety-reducing effects of neutralization may not be specific to obsessions, but instead may be apparent when individuals neutralize other types of thoughts such as anxious images (Marks et al., 2000). These latter findings are more difficult to accommodate within the behavioral account.

In summary, there is considerable empirical support for certain aspects of the behavioral account. Table 3.1 provides a summary of the main empirical support for the behavioral model. Most obsessions do elicit anxiety or discomfort, individuals prone to OCD are more responsive to certain unwanted thoughts or obsessions, and most often compulsions and other forms of neutralization lead to a temporary reduction in discomfort. However, there are important aspects of the behavioral model that are difficult to reconcile with empirical findings. There is little support for the view that obsessions are acquired by association with a traumatic or aversive experience. The presence of nonsensical obsessions (e.g., intrusion of certain phrases or musical tunes) that are not anxiety provoking and the persistence of compulsions that elevate anxiety are difficult to accommodate within the behavioral model.

Another problem for a conditioning theory is that many individuals with OCD report multiple obsessions and the content of obsessions can change over time. It is hard to imagine that obsessional thinking shifts because a person is exposed to numerous pairings of neutral thoughts and different aversive events. In addition, there is a nonrandom distribution of obsessional content that is difficult to reconcile from a classical conditioning perspective (i.e., obsessional fears tend to focus on a limited range of concerns that do not correspond to a conditioning explanation).

TABLE 3.1. Empirical Status of the Behavioral Model of OCD

Positive findings

- Most obsessional thoughts, images, or impulses provoke anxiety or discomfort.
- Individuals prone to OCD are more responsive to certain unwanted intrusive thoughts or obsessions.
- Compulsions and other forms of neutralization most often cause a temporary reduction in anxiety or discomfort.

Negative findings

- There is little evidence that obsessions are acquired via association with a traumatic experience.
- A minority of obsessions (i.e., nonsensical tunes, phrases, exactness/symmetry) do not elicit anxiety or discomfort.
- Sometimes compulsions elevate anxiety or discomfort.
- Many people with OCD have multiple obsessions.
- There is a nonrandom distribution to obsessional content.
- The content and form of obsessions often change over time.
- Compulsions may occur in response to other negative emotions or to reduce the likelihood of some imagined aversive consequence.

Finally, problems raised with the two-factor conditioning theory of phobias are applicable to the behavioral theory of OCD (see Rachman, 1976b, 1977). For all of these reasons, the two-factor conditioning model of obsessions and compulsions is no longer tenable (Carr, 1974; Emmelkamp, 1982; Rachman & Hodgson, 1980; Salkovskis, 1989b).

BEHAVIOR THERAPY FOR OCD

Exposure and Response Prevention (ERP)

Victor Meyer (1966) published the first case report on the use of exposure and response prevention (ERP) to treat OCD. He reasoned that if individuals with OCD are persuaded to remain in a fear situation and prevented from carrying out the compulsive ritual, then they will learn that the feared consequences of not performing the ritual do not occur. This will result in a modification of the obsessive–compulsive-related goal expectation, which in turn should lead to a cessation of the compulsive behavior. Meyer (1966) reported some success in using ERP to treat a patient with compulsive washing and another with blasphemous sexual obsessions, which were neutralized by repeating and redoing rituals. Both patients were treated by this author on an inpatient basis with 20–25 hours of direct exposure and response prevention. Later, in a study involving 15 patients with OCD treated with ERP, 10 were either "much improved" or totally asymptomatic, with treatment gains maintained in two-thirds of the patients over a varying follow-up period (Meyer et al., 1974).

Exposure

The treatment begins by providing patients with a rationale for the two main components of the intervention, exposure and response prevention. A fear hierarchy is first constructed that lists a variety of situations or objects the patient finds distressing and/or avoids because they elicit anxiety and obsessional symptoms. Table 3.2 illustrates a possible fear hierarchy for a patient with compulsive washing rituals. After rating the level of discomfort and compulsive urge associated with each situation, the therapist encourages patients to select their highest-rated fear situation or the most discomforting situation they are willing to tackle (de Silva & Rachman, 1992).

Three elements of exposure must be present for treatment to be effective. First, a high level of anxiety must be elicited and maintained during each exposure session. For example, in one of the between-session homework assignments, the patient with compulsive washing referred to in Table 3.2 was asked to sit in various chairs where other people had previously sat. Given her obsessional thoughts about dirt and contamination, this type of exposure elicited considerable anxiety. Sitting in the manager's chair at work, for example, resulted in a subjective anxiety rating of 90/100. After several minutes in the chair, her anxiety level dropped to 30. For exposure sessions to be effective, it is important that patients are repeatedly exposed to high-anxiety situations and that they remain in

TABLE 3.2. Illustrative Fear Hierarchy of a Patient with Compulsive Washing Rituals

Items in fear hierarchy	Level of anxiety[a]
Sitting in a friend's apartment	10
Wearing the same clothes for two consecutive days	15
Vacuuming the apartment and coming in contact with dirt	25
Noticing dust on furniture at work	30
Handling books that other people probably handled	30
Touching doorknobs in public buildings	50
Seating on a park bench	55
Having one's pyjamas come in contact with the apartment floor	65
Wearing clothes that fell on the floor	65
Washing clothes in a public laundromat	75
Using a public pay phone	90
Shaking hands with a unfamiliar person	90
Using a public toilet	100

[a]0 = no anxiety to 100 = maximum anxiety/panic.

those situations until they experience a significant decline in their level of discomfort (de Silva & Rachman, 1992; Steketee, 1999).

Second, the therapist should provide considerable support and encouragement as patients attempt their distressing situations. Individuals with OCD are often reluctant to expose themselves to situations that cause so much distress. In providing support, the therapist must ensure that the encouragement does not become a neutralizing response that patients can use to reduce their anxiety. Rather, the therapist should remind the patient that the anxiety will dissipate on its own. The therapist must refrain from reassuring the patient that the dire consequences of exposure to the fear stimulus will not occur. This is the core fear that must be targeted by the exposure session. Finally, the therapist should model the most appropriate response by performing each exposure task before the patient engages in the task (Rachman, Hodgson, & Marks, 1971; Rachman, Marks, & Hodgson, 1973; Roper, Rachman, & Marks, 1975). By modeling the appropriate behavioral response, the patient is shown that despite some discomfort, contact with the provoking stimulus can be made without engaging in a compulsive or neutralizing response (e.g., washing hands).

Response Prevention

The response prevention component of ERP involves the suppression of any compulsive ritual or other response that alleviates or neutralizes the discomfort caused by the obsession. Exposure sessions can last approximately 30 minutes, followed by instructions to refrain from carrying out a neutralizing response. Response prevention can last up to 2 hours, with the therapist present during this entire interval. The therapist should not physically restrain the patient from carrying out a compulsion, but should instead use distraction, conversation, and encouragement to assist the patient in refraining from compulsive rituals (de Silva & Rachman, 1992). In addition, every effort must be made to refrain from providing reassurance to the patient. For example, if asked, "Are you sure nothing bad will happen if I don't check?" the therapist should encourage the patient to wait and see what happens. The therapist must also be on the lookout for brief substitute rituals or mental neutralizing that the patient may use to alleviate anxiety during exposure. It is also important to validate the patient's anxiousness during the exposure and response prevention phases of treatment. The therapist should communicate understanding of the distress the patient is experiencing and acknowledge the courage the person needs to face his or her greatest fears.

It is recommended that a graded exposure strategy be employed and that therapists begin with a moderately difficult fear situation. Daily sessions lasting about 90 minutes are recommended for moderate to severe

OCD (Kozak & Foa, 1997; Steketee, 1993, 1999). Weekly sessions may suffice for milder OCD. However, most research treatment studies utilize a daily treatment schedule of 15 sessions over 3 weeks. This type of intensive treatment is not feasible in many clinical settings. Abramowitz, Foa, and Franklin (2003) reported that twice-weekly sessions of ERP can be as effective as intensive daily treatment, especially in the long term. It is unknown whether weekly ERP sessions, which is the likely modus operandi of many practitioners, is sufficient to produce clinically significant treatment effects.

In vivo exposure to actual fear situations is preferred over imaginal exposure, although the latter can be used initially to prepare the patient for *in vivo* exposure (de Silva & Rachman, 1992). Imaginal exposure can also be useful for obsessions based on fearful catastrophes such as disasters or accidents happening to loved ones (de Silva & Rachman, 1992; Foa & Kozak, 1997). Self-controlled exposure is as effective as therapist-assisted exposure (Emmelkamp & Kraanen, 1977; Emmelkamp, van Linden, van den Heuvell, Ruphan, & Sanderman, 1989), and family members or spouses can be used as co-therapists in outpatient ERP (Emmelkamp & De Lange, 1983; see also Emmelkamp, 1982). These studies indicate that the current practice of offering outpatient, self-controlled ERP can be an effective treatment for OCD.

Behavioral Treatment of Obsessions

Approximately 20% of individuals with diagnosable OCD have distressing obsessional ruminations without overt compulsions (Freeston & Ladouceur, 1997a). Unfortunately, ERP appears to have little relevance in directly treating obsessional ruminations (Rachman, 1976a). To address this situation, behavior therapists have proposed other interventions or modifications of ERP for treatment of obsessional ruminations: thought stopping, paradoxical intention, thought satiation or habituation training, and audiotaped habituation training. Each of these treatment approaches is discussed in the following sections.

Thought Stopping

Probably the most widely used intervention by clinicians to deal with obsessional ruminations is *thought stopping*, even though the efficacy of the procedure remains doubtful (Beech & Vaughan, 1978; Emmelkamp, 1982; Rachman, 1983; Reed, 1985). Thought stopping was introduced by Wolpe (1958) as a technique for reducing the frequency of disturbing thoughts that are out of proportion to reality. The patient is asked to verbalize a typical maladaptive thought sequence, and the therapist suddenly shouts, "Stop!" This sequence is repeated several times, with the patient eventually learning to subvocally say, "Stop," whenever the thought intrudes into consciousness. After repeated trials of thought stopping, the thoughts return less readily and become progressively easier to stop. If verbalizing "stop" does not reduce the thought intrusions, Wolpe (1958) suggested, a buzzer may be used to interrupt or block the thought sequence. Others have used more aversive consequences to block obsessional thoughts, such as banging the desk, electric shocks, or snapping the wrist with a rubber band (Reed, 1985).

A number of case reports and a few controlled studies have investigated the effectiveness of thought stopping (e.g., Bass, 1973; Leger, 1978; Likierman & Rachman, 1982; Stern, 1970; Stern, Lipsedge, & Marks, 1973; Tryon & Palladino, 1979; Yamagami, 1971). The results were at best mixed, with a number of studies finding thought stopping relatively ineffective in producing sustained reductions in obsessional rumination. Furthermore, interventions entirely opposite to thought stopping, such as deliberate and repeated exposure to obsessional thinking, proved just as effective as thought stopping (Emmelkamp & Kwee, 1977; Hackmann & McLean, 1975). Salkovskis and Westbrook (1989) calculated treatment effects across studies and concluded that only 46% of patients (13/28) showed improvement in the frequency of their obsessions and only 12% (2/17) were improved on ratings of the distress of obsessions. Rachman (1976a) noted that thought stopping is an ad hoc technique that lacks a theoretical rationale. Even though thought stopping is still used in clinical practice, there is insufficient empirical support to justify its continued use as a direct treatment of obsessional ruminations.

Paradoxical Intention

In *paradoxical intention* patients are given *in vivo* exposure to situations or objects that evoke the obsession with instructions to elaborate the obsessional material. They are told to deliberately dwell on their obsessive ideation and to elaborate and exaggerate it in an effort to be convinced of its validity. Solyom, Garza-Perez, Ledwidge, and Solyom (1972) based their rationale for using paradoxical intention on the observation that contrary or paradoxical thinking is evident in many forms of obsessional thinking. The following is an example of exposure based on paradoxical intention;

> The patient with recurring frightening thoughts of going insane was instructed to tell himself: "It is true, I am going insane, slowly, but surely. I am developing many crazy thoughts and habits. I will be admitted to a mental hospital, put into a straight-jacket and will remain there neglected by everybody until I die. I won't even remember my name. I will forget that I was married, had children and will become a zombie. I will

neglect my appearance and eat like an animal." (Solyom et al., 1972, p. 293)

Except for Solyom et al.'s (1972) report on 10 patients with OCD treated with paradoxical intention, very little research has been published on its effectiveness for obsessional ruminations. However, variations on paradoxical intention have been incorporated into the exposure protocols used in current cognitive-behavioral treatments of obsessional rumination (Freeston & Ladouceur, 1997a; Salkovskis & Westbrook, 1989).

Habituation (Satiation) Training

Rachman (1976a) described another cognitive intervention technique for obsessions based on prolonged exposure. In *satiation training,* patients are instructed to form and then hold onto their obsessions for at least 15 minutes or more per trial. They are encouraged to regard their obsessions as alien and useless and to refrain from all attempts, whether internal or external, to neutralize the obsessional ideation. With successive trials they experience more difficulty in forming and retaining the obsessional ideation. Unlike paradoxical intention, satiation training does not require that individuals exaggerate the consequences of their obsessional thinking. Satiation treatment is most appropriate for obsessional ruminations that are accompanied with strong urges to "put matters right" (Rachman, 1976a).

Likierman and Rachman (1982) later introduced a slight variation on satiation training, which they termed *habituation training.* With habituation training the patient is told to hold onto the obsessional thought or image for a specified period of time (i.e., 5 minutes), whereas in satiation training, the thought or image is retained until it loses most of its associated distress. The few studies that have examined the effectiveness of satiation or habituation training have reported some within-session declines in obsessional thinking, but there is less consistent evidence for between-session improvement (Emmelkamp & Kwee, 1977; Emmelkamp & Giesselbach, 1981; Gurnani & Vaughan, 1981; Likierman & Rachman, 1982; Vogel, Peterson, & Broverman, 1982).

Audiotaped Habituation Training

One reason for the ineffectiveness of habituation training may be that patients are not effectively exposing themselves to the obsession. Because obsessions are private mental events, the therapist cannot be certain that the patient is maintaining full attention to the obsessional thought or image throughout the exposure session. The use of cognitive avoidance strategies like distraction, thought replacement, or rationalization may undermine the effects of exposure to the obsession. To reduce cognitive avoidance, Salkovskis (1983) proposed an audiotaped version of imaginal exposure to obsessions.

In the initial single case study, Salkovskis (1983) used *audiotaped habituation training* to treat a man with compulsive washing and checking. A 10-minute two-track audiotape was made, with channel 1 containing the obsessional rumination recorded in the man's own voice at high frequency (so that covert neutralization after each occurrence was not possible) and channel 2 containing the names of people who had been unpleasant or violent toward him in the past. The patient listened to the tape 20–90 minutes each night at home. Significant reductions were reported in the patient's harming obsessions, and treatment gains were maintained at 6-month follow-up. Since publication of this case, a number of case studies have reported significant treatment effects with audiotaped habituation training (Headland & McDonald, 1987; Martin & Tarrier, 1992; Salkovskis & Westbrook, 1989).

Behavioral Treatment of Obsessions: Current Status

None of the behavioral interventions for obsessional ruminations is sufficiently effective to recommend unqualified adoption by clinicians. Thought-blocking approaches, such as thought stopping, are relatively ineffective (Emmelkamp, 1982; Reed, 1985). Exposure-based treatments, like standard or audiotaped habituation training, have not been sufficiently investigated to allow conclusions about their effectiveness.

It is possible that thought-removal techniques like thought stopping may be appropriate for some circumstances, and thought exposure may be more suitable for other circumstances. It is possible that thought stopping may be useful when the goal is to increase thought control or the ability to remove thoughts when neutralization and resistance to habituation are relatively absent. However, for highly distressing obsessions that are associated with neutralizing responses and avoidance, prolonged exposure to the obsession via habituation training will be more effective (Rachman & Hodgson, 1980). Thought stopping may also be suitable as a type of "covert response prevention" for blocking mental compulsions (e.g., repeating nonsense phrases, rehearsing previous thoughts or verbalizations) (de Silva & Rachman, 1992; Salkovskis & Westbrook, 1989; see case example by Albert & Hayward, 2002). In this situation, the individual is directed to block or remove any thought that might be used to neutralize a prior obsession. Table 3.3 provides some illustrative examples for deciding when thought stopping or exposure-based habituation training may be useful in the treatment of obsessions.

TABLE 3.3. Clinical Illustrations for Differential Use of Thought Stopping and Habituation Training

Clinical example of obsession	Characteristics of obsession	Recommended intervention
Thoughts of accidents and death occurring to family and friends (e.g., parent will die in plane crash)	Moderately distressing intrusion associated with repeating compulsions and avoidance	Habituation training; response prevention
Thoughts of violence and aggression toward others (e.g., "I will molest a child")	High level of distress; often not associated with overt compulsion; usually accompanied by avoidance	Habituation training; response prevention
Must stare at books and magazines that are not symmetrically arranged	No associated anxiety; rearranging compulsion	Response prevention and possibly thought stopping
Preoccupied with thoughts of the movie *Titanic*	No associated anxiety; no overt compulsions; some pleasure	Thought stopping
"I must have the right thought, count, or stare at lines or letters to prevent negative consequences to myself or others."	Intense anxiety and associated repeating, redoing, and counting rituals	Habituation training; response prevention
"God is testing me. Have I pleased Him?"	Response to other thoughts and actions; mental compulsion	Thought stopping
Repeating special phrases or prayers	Mental compulsion or neutralizing response	Thought stopping

Empirical Status of Behavior Therapy (ERP)

Immediate and Long-Term Effectiveness

The efficacy and effectiveness of behavioral treatment (ERP) for OCD is well established. The American Psychological Association Division 12 Task Force on Promotion and Dissemination of Psychological Procedures categorized ERP as a well-established, empirically validated treatment for OCD (Chambless et al., 1998; see also DeRubeis & Crits-Christoph, 1998). The Expert Consensus Guidelines (March, Frances, Carpenter, & Kahn, 1997), based on a survey of 69 experts on OCD, recommended cognitive-behavioral therapy (CBT), which includes a heavy component of exposure and response prevention, the first-line treatment of choice for mild cases of obsessions and compulsions. In more severe cases, CBT should be combined with pharmacotherapy. The expert panel recommended that CBT should begin with weekly individual sessions and between-session homework of self-directed or therapist-assisted *in vivo* exposure and response prevention. Thirteen to 20 sessions was considered the appropriate number of CBT sessions for the typical patient. When a quicker treatment response is needed, or in more severe cases, intensive CBT can be offered, involving daily treatment sessions over 3 weeks (approximately 50 hours of treatment in total).

A number of comprehensive critical reviews have been published on the treatment mechanisms and efficacy of ERP (Abramowitz, 1997, 1998; Foa et al., 1998; Foa & Kozak, 1996; Foa et al., 1985; Foa, Steketee, Grayson, & Doppelt, 1983; Rachman & Hodgson, 1980; Stanley & Turner, 1995; Steketee & Shapiro, 1995; van Balkom et al., 1994). In clinical outcome studies, rates of improvement at posttreatment ranged from 40 to 97%, with a weighted average percentage improvement of 83% (Foa & Kozak, 1996). The number of treatment sessions ranged from 3 to 80 ($M = 15$), and treatments that included both exposure and response prevention were superior to either strategy alone. In an earlier review, Foa et al. (1985) found that 51% of patients with OCD treated with ERP were symptom free or much improved at posttreatment (at least 70% treatment gain), 39% were moderately improved (treatment gains of 31–69%), and 10% failed to respond to ERP.

The long-term effectiveness of ERP has been demonstrated in a number of outcome studies. Foa and Kozak (1996) calculated the average rate of improvement for 376 patients with OCD from 16 studies with a mean follow-up period of 29 months (range 6–72). The percentage of treatment responders who maintained their gains at follow-up was 76%, with a range of 50–100% across studies. Twelve of the studies reported long-term maintenance within the 70–85% of treatment responders. Furthermore, a deliberate focus on relapse prevention significantly improved maintenance of treatment gains (Hiss, Foa, & Kozak, 1994; McKay, 1997).

ERP is at least as effective as, and in most cases superior to, pharmacotherapy at posttreatment (Foa & Kozak, 1996; see also Abramowitz, 1997). When follow-up is considered, patients treated with behavioral therapy maintain their gains much better than patients discontinued from their medication. There is less differential treatment effect when patients treated with ERP are compared with patients who continue on their medication over the follow-up period. In their review, Stanley and Turner (1995) concluded that ERP is associated with an 80–90% improvement rate at posttreatment, as compared with 50–60% for pharmacotherapy, particularly treatment with clomipramine. In addition, dropout and refusal rates are higher for medication than ERP. In their meta-analytic study, van Balkom et al. (1994) found that on self-ratings of obsessional symptoms, behavior therapy produced a significantly greater effect size (d = 1.46) than serotonergic medication (d = 0.95), but there was no significant difference in the effect sizes for the two types of treatment on the independent assessor ratings of symptom severity. Preliminary findings from the National Institute of Mental Health (NIMH)–sponsored collaborative comparison of clomipramine and behavior therapy for OCD indicate that ERP is superior to medication at posttreatment and 3-month follow-up (Kozak, Liebowitz, & Foa, 2000). Yet there is no evidence that the combination of medication and ERP is superior to ERP alone. Nevertheless, individuals who are already taking a serotonin reuptake inhibitor can still show significant benefits from initiating a course of ERP (Franklin, Abramowitz, Bux, Zoellner, & Feeny, 2002). Together these findings indicate that ERP may produce greater immediate and long-term improvement in obsessive–compulsive symptoms than medication alone.

Some qualifications must be noted about the effectiveness of ERP. Approximately 25% of individuals refuse ERP, and another 3–12% will not complete therapy (Foa, Steketee, et al., 1983). If a conservative estimate of 30% is used for refusers and dropouts, then the posttreatment efficacy of ERP is reduced to 63% of patients seeking treatment for their OCD. That is, 36% of patients at posttreatment will have at least a 70% reduction in symptoms, 27% a moderate level of improvement (31% to 69% reduction), and 7% will fail to respond to therapy (Stanley & Turner, 1995). Furthermore, the majority of patients in the ERP outcome studies have cleaning or checking rituals. Much less is known about the efficacy of ERP for other types of OCD such as obsessional doubting, primary obsessional slowness, hoarding, and order and symmetry rituals. ERP is most suitable for patients who have overt compulsions, but it is relatively ineffective for obsessional ruminators without overt compulsions, unless the treatment protocol is substantially altered (Freeston & Ladouceur, 1999; Freeston, Ladouceur, et al., 1997).

Who Benefits from ERP?

A range of variables have been investigated to determine predictors of treatment success with ERP, as well as indicators of poor response. Few sociodemographic characteristics appear predictive, although younger age at symptom and treatment onset may be associated with better treatment gains (Foa, Grayson, et al., 1983; Foa et al., 1985) and lower income may be associated with poorer response to ERP (see review by Steketee & Shapiro, 1995).

Pretreatment severity or duration of obsessive–compulsive symptoms is not predictive of treatment outcome (Foa, Grayson, et al., 1983; Foa et al., 1985; Steketee & Shapiro, 1995). However, the presence of certain symptoms may be related to poor response to ERP. For example, significant hoarding symptoms may be an important predictor of treatment failure (Black et al., 1998; Frost et al., 1999). ERP is better suited for the treatment of obsessive–compulsive disorders with a prominent behavioral component (i.e., overt compulsions) and is less effective in treating the cognitive component of the disorder (Foa et al., 1985; Rachman & Hodgson, 1980; Reed, 1985). Thus, patients with pure obsessions with no overt compulsions, or those with cognitive compulsions or neutralizing responses, will show a poorer response to standard ERP (Rachman, 1983; Salkovskis & Westbrook, 1989). As discussed in the previous chapter, individuals with OVI or lack of insight into the excessive nature of their obsessions and compulsions may show a weaker response to ERP.

There has been considerable research on the impact of depression on response to ERP. The findings are somewhat inconsistent across studies. Generally, mild to moderate levels of depressive symptoms do not appear to interfere with response to ERP. However, as the severity of depression increases, there is a greater likelihood that the mood disturbance will reduce treatment effectiveness (Foa, Franklin, & Kozak, 1998; Stanley & Turner, 1995; Steketee & Shapiro, 1995). For severely depressed patients, ERP should be delayed until they have made at least a partial response to pharmacotherapy (Franklin et al., 2002). On the other hand, high pretreatment anxiety does not preclude a good response to ERP (Foa, Grayson, et al., 1983).

An inability or unwillingness to suspend the performance of rituals, or to tolerate distress during exposure, will undermine the effectiveness of ERP (Rachman & Hodgson, 1980). In addition, low motivation and lack of compliance with treatment procedures will thwart its effectiveness (Foa, Franklin, & Kozak, 1998). Presence of an Axis II personality disorder may be associated with poorer response to ERP. In particular, a schizotypal or borderline personality disorder may predict poorer response to both pharmacotherapy and ERP (Foa, Franklin, & Kozak, 1998). However, prospective studies are needed in which reliable and valid measures of personality disorder are used before any firm conclusions can be reached on the impact of comorbid personality disorder on treatment of OCD.

SUMMARY AND CONCLUSION

The heuristic value of the behavioral perspective on OCD is undeniable. Prior to the development of the behavioral model and its use in treatment of OCD, the contribution of psychology to research on obsessional disorders was negligible. Based on the two-factor theory of fear, the behavioral model offered the first empirically based conceptualization of obsessions and compulsions. The experimental work, derived from the behavioral theory, led to advances in our understanding of the psychological mechanisms involved in the persistence of obsessions and compulsions. We now know that (1) most obsessions are anxiety-provoking stimuli that have many similarities to other phobic stimuli, (2) individuals with OCD are more responsive to their obsessive intrusive thoughts, (3) most compulsive rituals and other forms of neutralization lead to short-term reduction in discomfort, and (4) heightened anxiety and the urge to neutralize will decay spontaneously when overt and covert compulsions are prevented (de Silva, Menzies, & Shafran, 2003; Roper et al., 1973; Rachman et al., 1976).

The most important legacy of the behavioral model is its treatment modality, exposure and response prevention. ERP is considered an empirically supported treatment for OCD, and its effectiveness in treating compulsive washing and checking, in particular, is undisputed. It is the treatment of choice for mild to moderate OCD and should be used in combination with medication in severe cases. Its long-term effectiveness has been empirically verified and its effectiveness demonstrated in terms of symptom improvement and clinically significant recovery.

Despite the advances that can be attributed to the behavioral perspective on OCD, serious limitations are evident in this approach. Table 3.1 summarizes the shortcomings that emerged with behavioral theory and research on OCD. Table 3.4 presents a number of limitations that became apparent with ERP. Together, the problems that emerged in behavioral theory and treatment of OCD led a number of prominent OCD re-

---

TABLE 3.4. Shortcomings of ERP

- A significant minority of patients (20–30%) refuse ERP.
- Approximately 25% of ERP completers fail to improve.
- Behavioral treatment of obsessions is less than adequate.
- Certain subtypes of OCD, such as those with hoarding compulsions, primary obsessional slowness, and symmetry and ordering compulsions, may show less effective response.
- Residual symptoms persist in treated patients.
- Comorbid conditions, like depression, may reduce treatment effectiveness.
- Other negative emotions associated with OCD, like guilt, may be unresponsive to ERP.
- Residual social and occupational impairment is evident at posttreatment.
- Treatment factors, like low motivation, homework noncompliance, and pessimistic attitude toward treatment, can reduce effectiveness.
- Cognitive dysfunctions and biases are prominent in OCD.
- Strict behavioral explanations for the effectiveness of ERP remain unconvincing.

---

searchers to reconsider their approach to the disorder. In the last few years these researchers have shifted their focus to the cognitive basis of OCD. Might cognitive–clinical theory and treatment be integrated with the behavioral perspective to further an understanding of the psychological mechanisms in OCD and enhance our treatment of this disorder? The cognitive-behavioral theory and therapy of OCD discussed in the remaining chapters maintains a strong foundation in the behavioral approach. Its emergence was an attempt to address the limitations of a purely behavioral perspective by integrating cognitive concepts with behavioral approaches to the research and treatment of OCD. And so a dramatic shift has occurred in contemporary psychological theory, research, and treatment toward a strong focus on the cognitive substratum of OCD.

CHAPTER 4

Neuropsychology and Information Processing in OCD

The aberration in thought evident in the symptom presentation of OCD suggests that some type of deficit or deficiency may be present in certain information-processing functions. The cognitive basis of OCD is well illustrated by the 35-year-old woman with checking compulsions who was distressed when leaving the house for fear that she had left a small appliance plugged into the receptacle. What compelled her to return again and again was the erroneous *belief* that even the *slightest possibility* of a disaster (i.e., house fire) must be eliminated because she would be held *responsible* for the occurrence of the negative event. She *believed* that repeated checking lessened the likelihood of the dreaded outcome, and so she had to be *certain* that the appliance was not plugged in. However, she soon experienced distress after completing the compulsion because of *doubt* and *lack of confidence* in her recollection as to whether the appliance was actually plugged in or not.

Long before the advent of CBT, Reed (1968) observed that both psychodynamic and behavioral theorists of OCD focused exclusively on the content, or meaning, of obsessional thought. Much less attention was paid to abnormalities in the formal characteristics of obsessional thinking. For Reed the critical problem in OCD was not *what* people think, but rather *how* they think or reason.

Two different branches of psychology investigate whether individuals with OCD think differently from nonobsessional individuals. Neuropsychology focuses on brain–behavior interactions, in particular "how the brain controls higher cognitive functions such as language, visuospatial ability, memory, and reasoning" (Savage, 1998, p. 254). Neuropsychological studies rely on tests of general cognitive function involving attention, memory, organization, inhibition, and the like. The tests utilize *content independent* material, that is, stimuli unrelated to the current threat concerns in the disorder (McNally, 2001a). Neuropsychological studies of memory in OCD, for example, focus on encoding, storage, and retrieval of standard information, such as objects, words, or phrases, that are entirely unrelated to obsessive–compulsive symptom-related issues (e.g., contamination, doubting, mistakes, etc.). This research, then, examines whether particular impairments in general cognitive functioning may mediate the relationship between brain dysfunction and the symptom features of OCD.

The other research perspective investigates information-processing abnormalities in OCD, using methodologies derived from experimental cognitive psychology (MacLeod, 1993; McNally, 2001a). In this approach information-processing experiments rely on *content-dependent* stimuli to identify specific information-processing biases in OCD. This experimental perspective has been used extensively to investigate information-processing biases in other anxiety disorders (D. M. Clark, 1999; Williams, Watts, MacLeod, & Mathews, 1997) and in depression (Clark & Beck, 1999). Research from this perspective tends to focus on information-processing abnormalities or biases that may account for key features of a disorder, thereby providing insight into its etiology and persistence. Moreover, information-processing experiments can test key hypotheses of cognitive-clinical models in a manner that circumvents the problems encountered with phenomenological self-report research (MacLeod, 1993; McNally, 2000).

This chapter first considers the neuropsychological evidence for general cognitive impairment in OCD. Evidence for a specific neuropsychological profile for compulsive checking is discussed, and a critique of research on general cognitive deficits is offered. This is followed by a critical review of the experimental cognitive research on information-processing bias in OCD and whether these findings shed light on the diagnostic classification of the disorder.

NEUROPSYCHOLOGY OF OCD

Freud and Janet recognized from their clinical observations that fundamental cognitive processing deficits must be present in OCD (Tallis, 1995, 1997). Since then, investigators have focused on impairments in memory functioning, the organization and integration of experience, selective attention, cognitive inhibition, category formation, and frontal lobe function to determine whether OCD is characterized by dysfunction in general cognitive processing. The following section provides an overview of the empirical status of neuropsychological investigations in OCD. More extensive discussions of this research can be found in a number of reviews (Greisberg & McKay, 2003; Savage, 1998; Tallis, 1995, 1997).

General Intellectual Functioning

As noted in Chapter 1, there is some indication that individuals with OCD may exhibit a slight advantage (superiority) in general intelligence. Early studies using standardized intelligence tests tended to support this view (for review see Black, 1974; Rachman & Hodgson, 1980), although more recent research has produced mixed findings (e.g., Coryell, 1981; Steketee et al., 1987). The most cogent conclusion to draw from this literature is that any IQ differences on the Wechsler scales or other standardized intelligence tests tend to be small and insignificant (Rasmussen & Eisen, 1992; Tallis, 1997). Where intelligence test performance is lower, one must rule out the possibility that poor test results are due to the presence of obsessional symptoms like slowness, meticulousness, doubt, and indecision. Obviously, individuals with obsessions would score particularly low on timed subtests.

Difficulties in Executive Function

There is evidence that OCD may be characterized by impairments in executive functioning. *Executive function* describes higher-level control processes that modulate more basic sensory, motor, cognitive, memory, and affective functions. These higher-level functions enable individuals to process all features of a situation so that goals and plans can be prioritized, and behavioral strategies implemented, monitored, and modified in response to the changing demands of the environment (Savage, 1998). In other words, executive functions involve the strategic organization of complex responses or a flexible adaptation to novel stimuli (Purcell, Maruff, Kyrios, & Pantcils, 1998). A number of cognitive tasks fall in this category, including the ability to shift mental sets, inhibit responses, and engage in trial-and-error learning. The most common tests of executive functioning are the Wisconsin Card Sorting Test (WCST) and the Trail Making Test (TMT).

In a number of studies, patients with OCD evidenced greater difficulty shifting to a new rule on the WCST or switching between categories in Category B of the TMT (see reviews by Greisberg & McKay, 2003; Savage, 1998). These findings are consistent with neuroimaging studies in which OCD was characterized by increased metabolism in the frontal–striatal network (i.e., a hyperfrontality profile) (see Cottraux & Gérard, 1998; Savage, 1998).

Savage (1998) presented a neuropsychological model of OCD that illustrates how a cognitive deficit may play a mediating role between an underlying brain dysfunction and clinical symptoms. He proposed that the primary brain dysfunction in OCD is located in the frontal–striatal system. This brain dysfunction leads to a primary impairment in executive function and a secondary disturbance in nonverbal memory. These cognitive dysfunctions, in turn, have an impact on clinical symptoms. For example, difficulty in planning, implementing strategic actions, or switching to a more productive alternative response (i.e., indications of impairment in executive functioning) can lead to automatic, repetitive checking. Changes in clinical symptoms then feed back into the brain dysfunction, so that a vicious cycle of brain dysfunction, cognitive impairment, and clinical symptoms is created. Savage's proposal provides a good illustration of how a neuropsychological deficit may play a central role in the etiology and persistence of OCD. It addresses a criticism often leveled against neuropsychological research in OCD: that demonstrations of general cognitive deficits fail to explain how these dysfunctions relate to the clinical presentation of the disorder (Salkovskis, 1996a).

It would be premature to conclude from these studies that neuropsychological testing confirms the presence of difficulties in executive functioning in OCD. Inconsistent findings are reported across studies. Poor performance on tests such as the WCST or the TMT may be due to the presence of depression rather than obsessional symptoms (Moritz et al., 2001). Moreover, executive function deficits in obsessional disorders may be very specific rather than generalized. For example, Purcell et al. (1998) found that patients in their OCD sample had significant impairment when executive functioning relied on internal representations to guide their response selections, but not when external information was available to guide response organization and selection. Tallis (1995) concluded from his review of research across nine different tests of frontal lobe function that the evidence for cognitive dysfunction was not compelling. The most consistent evidence is for impairment in shifting mental set and poor control over interference effects, whereas deficits in other executive abilities like verbal fluency, abstract reasoning, and problem solving have not reliably emerged across studies (see Greisberg & McKay, 2003).

Memory Impairment

Clinical observation suggests that individuals with OCD, especially those with checking compulsions, exhibit deviations from normal memory functioning. On one hand, it may appear that obsessional individuals are "hypermnesic"; that is, that they have superior recall of details that healthy persons would not remember because such details would be considered insignificant or superfluous (Reed, 1985). On the other hand, the prominence of pathological doubt, indecision, uncertainty, and compulsive checking suggests the possibility of a general memory deficit in OCD (Tallis, 1995). A fairly well-developed experimental literature exists on memory functioning in OCD (see reviews by Amir & Kozak, 2002; Greisberg & McKay, 2003; McNally, 2000; Reed, 1985; Tallis, 1995, 1997).

Some of the earlier research investigated general memory performance, whereas later studies focused on more specific memory deficits. Other research suggests that the deviations in memory functioning may be confined to obsessive–compulsive-relevant concerns or to subjective evaluations of confidence in memory.

Nonverbal Memory Deficits

Individuals with OCD appear to have non-verbal memory deficits (Savage, 1998; Tallis, 1995). Tallis, Pratt, and Jamani (1999) found that patients with OCD had poorer performance on nonverbal immediate and delayed recall and recognition memory, as compared with nonclinical individuals (controls). Sher, Frost, Kushner, Crews, and Alexander (1989) also reported that the only memory test that differentiated a checking from a nonchecking group in a mixed clinical sample was one that involved the recall and reproduction of geometric designs. However, not all studies have reported significant differences. For example, Tolin, Abramowitz, Brigidi, et al. (2001) found that individuals with OCD did not have poorer recall of safe or neutral objects than nonobsessional anxious or nonclinical individuals (controls). In addition, the poorer memory performance in compulsive checking appears specific to nonverbal material. Patients with OCD tend not to differ from nonclinical individuals (controls) on verbal recall or recognition (e.g., MacDonald, Antony, MacLeod, & Richter, 1997; Sher et al., 1989).

It is quite clear that nonverbal memory deficit is not pervasive in OCD. Purcell et al. (1998) found that their sample of patients with OCD performed significantly worse on spatial recognition, but not on delayed recognition or recall of pattern targets, than panic disorder, depressed, and nonclinical groups. Individuals with OCD also scored significantly worse than nonclinical control individuals on immediate recall, but not on delayed recall, of the Rey–Osterrieth figure (Savage et al., 1999). Moreover, it is unclear whether poor nonverbal memory is evident in all subtypes of OCD or whether it is particularly characteristic of compulsive checking (e.g., Sher et al., 1989; Tallis et al., 1999). Tallis et al. (1999), however, found that nonverbal memory deficits were unrelated to scores on the Checking subscale of the Padua Inventory. Nevertheless, Savage et al. (1999) proposed that the immediate nonverbal memory problem in OCD was due to impaired organizational strategies. Individuals with OCD had difficulty encoding information while copying the Rey–Osterrieth figure. This resulted in a lower immediate recall score. Savage and colleagues commented that OCD is not associated with a primary memory deficit (see also Savage, 1998). Rather, the problem is reliance on poor organizational strategies, which is consistent with impairment in executive functioning arising from a frontal–striatal dysfunction.

Poor Memory for Prior Actions

A number of researchers have investigated whether memory difficulties in compulsive checking might be specific to the recall of prior actions. In the typical memory for action experiment, participants engage in several obsessive–compulsive-neutral tasks and are then asked to describe briefly each of the tasks. In both analogue and clinical studies, participants with checking compulsions showed poorer recall of prior actions than non-checking participants (controls) (Ecker & Engelkamp, 1995; Rubenstein, Peynircioglu, Chambless, & Pigott, 1993; Sher, Frost, & Otto, 1983; Sher et al., 1989). Radomsky, Rachman, and Hammond (2001), however, found that patients with compulsive checking rituals actually remembered more threat-relevant information (e.g., how many times they touched the stove) than threat-irrelevant material in a high-responsibility condition. Constans, Foa, Franklin, and Mathews (1995) also found that compared with nonclinical individuals (controls), compulsive checkers did not show poorer memory for prior action in a low-anxiety condition, but instead, their recall was significantly better for actions rated as high anxiety.

Although there is evidence that compulsive checkers may exhibit poorer recall of prior actions, the latter studies suggest that recall may be enhanced when it comes to memory for obsessive–compulsive-relevant situations. Moreover, reduced memory for prior actions has obvious relevance to compulsive checking where symptoms of doubt and indecision are prominent. It is less certain that poor memory for actions would be evident in other OCD subtypes.

Impaired Reality Monitoring

Johnson and Raye (1981) defined reality monitoring as "the process of distinguishing a *past* perception from a *past* act of imagination, both of which resulted in memories" (p. 67, emphasis in original). This process may have particular relevance for obsessional checking where uncertainty and doubt over whether one has or has not performed an action is prominent. It may be that compulsive checking arises from the patient's difficulty in distinguishing "memories of doing from memories of imagined doing" (McNally, 2000, p. 110).

Some studies found evidence of impaired reality monitoring in compulsive checking (Ecker & Engelkamp, 1995), whereas others found no significant difference between those with and those without checking compulsions (Constans et al., 1995; Sher et al., 1983). In a study involving patients with OCD with checking compulsions, those with nonchecking compulsions, and a nonclinical control group, McNally and Kohlbeck (1993) found no significant differences between the two OCD groups and the nonclinical control group in the individuals' ability to recognize whether they had previously traced with a capped pen, imagined tracing, or merely looked at cards with written words or line drawings. Brown, Kosslyn, Breiter, Baer, and Jenike (1994) compared an OCD sample and a nonclinical control group on the ability to discriminate memories of visual percepts from memories of mental images (i.e., discriminating actions performed from actions imagined). Contrary to predictions, the OCD group was significantly better at discriminating a previously seen stimulus from a previously imagined item, as compared with the nonclinical group. More recent evidence indicates that individuals with compulsive repeating rituals did not differ from nonanxious individuals (controls) in their reality monitoring of neutral or obsessive–compulsive-relevant actions (Hermans, Martens, De Cort, Pieters, & Eelen, 2003). These generally negative findings raise serious doubts that compulsive checking is characterized by impairment in reality monitoring.

Reduced Confidence in Memory

Radomsky et al. (2001) suggested that lack of confidence in memory, rather than memory deficits per se, may be a contributing factor to the development and persistence of OCD. Findings from a number of studies indicate that individuals with OCD report significantly lower confidence in their memory judgments than nonclinical individuals (controls) (Ecker & Engelkamp, 1995; MacDonald et al., 1997; McNally & Kohlbeck, 1993; Tolin, Abramowitz, Brigidi, et al., 2001).

Radomsky et al. (2001) found that their sample of patients with OCD had significantly lower confidence ratings in memory performance, but only for threat-relevant material under a high-responsibility condition. However, Hermans et al. (2003) reported contrary results, with the sample of patients with OCD producing lower confidence ratings only in their recall of neutral actions, and not for obsessive–compulsive-relevant actions. Constans et al. (1995) noted that individuals with compulsive checking may require a higher level of memory vividness in order to feel satisfied with their recall of prior actions. Dar, Rish, Hermesh, Taub, and Fux (2000) found that patients with compulsive checking were significantly less confident in their performance on a general knowledge questionnaire relative to nonclinical individuals (controls), even though there was no difference in their actual performance. This raises the possibility that lack of confidence in compulsive checking may not be unique to memory, but instead may be applicable to a broader range of performance.

Tolin, Abramowitz, Brigidi, et al. (2001) exposed individuals with OCD and anxious and nonanxious individuals (controls) to a set of objects that were previously identified as safe, unsafe, or neutral by those in the OCD group. The safe, unsafe, and neutral objects were arranged randomly on a table, and participants were given 10 seconds to look at the table (learn phase). They were then asked to recall what they had just seen and to provide confidence ratings of their recall accuracy. This learn-recall-confidence sequence was repeated five times. Between-group analyses revealed that those in the OC group did not have poorer recall for safe and neutral objects, nor did they show superior recall of unsafe objects. However, those in the OCD group did exhibit significantly greater decrease in memory confidence for unsafe objects over time, although lower confidence in memory for unsafe objects was related only to checking behavior at a follow-up assessment conducted 1 week after the experiment.

Despite considerable research on memory functioning in OCD, evidence of a general memory deficit, even in compulsive checking, is not convincing. There is some evidence that individuals with OCD may have impaired immediate recall of nonverbal material, but this may be due to difficulties in organizational strategies rather than to a primary memory (i.e., storage) deficit. Another likely reason for memory deficit is poorer recall of prior actions, but, again, it is apparent that individuals with OCD have a particularly good memory for obsessive–compulsive-relevant actions and situations. The most reliable conclusion that can be drawn from the research on memory is that individuals with compulsive checking rituals do not have a primary deficit in their memory ability. Instead, it is clear that they have significantly less confidence in the accuracy of their memory judgments.

At this point our conclusions about memory functioning in OCD must be tentative. Some studies used nonclinical analogue groups or mixed clinical samples of individuals with OCD that limit the generalizability and sensitivity of experimental manipulations. Even studies that reported significant group differences often failed to show a relation between memory impairment and obsessive–compulsive symptom severity. Most studies lacked clinical controls, so specificity of impairment to OCD can not be determined. There is also no standardization of memory tasks, so comparison across studies is difficult (see Tallis, 1997). Tallis commented that the general memory deficit hypothesis cannot explain the highly restricted range of checking rituals (i.e., individuals appear to doubt and repeatedly check only certain actions but not others). Finally, even when stronger results are reported, inconsistencies abound. For example, one study found lower memory confidence ratings only for obsessive–compulsive-relevant material (Radomsky et al., 2001), whereas another study obtained a completely opposite effect (Hermans et al., 2003). It may be that subtle differences in experimental design affect individuals' confidence ratings, or that individuals' evaluations of their memory judgments are highly situational.

Directed Forgetting and Cognitive Inhibition

The ability to respond effectively and recall prior actions depends, in part, on the capacity to ignore or inhibit irrelevant information and to focus on the task at hand. Reduced memory performance in OCD may be due to interference effects resulting from a failure to inhibit irrelevant or distracting material. Moreover, the repeated intrusion of unwanted obsessions that is so characteristic of OCD may reflect a failure in cognitive inhibitory processes. Based on research from experimental cognitive psychology, two inhibitory mechanisms have been investigated; directed forgetting and cognitive inhibition.

Directed Forgetting

The ability to intentionally dispel certain highly relevant thoughts, like obsessional ruminations, has been investigated using a "directed forgetting" experimental paradigm. It is unclear whether the problem in controlling obsessions is due to a highly elaborate encoding of threat information or a dysfunction in the mechanism of forgetting (McNally, 2000). Wilhem, McNally, Baer, and Florin (1996) compared patients with OCD and nonclinical individuals (controls) on their ability to forget or remember a list of threat words, positive words, and neutral words. The OCD group, but not the control group, had greater difficulty forgetting threat words relative to positive or neutral words, as evidenced by significantly greater recall and recognition of the threatening "forget" words. Furthermore, the difficulty in forgetting threat words resulted from greater allocation of attentional resources and deeper encoding of threat words in the encoding phase (see Maki, O'Neill, & O'Neill, 1994, for contrary results with an analogue sample).

Reduced Cognitive Inhibition

Individuals with OCD may exhibit enhanced processing of threatening stimuli because of a reduced ability to inhibit irrelevant information (McNally, 2000). A negative priming experiment has been used to investigate reduction in preconscious cognitive inhibition in OCD. In this experiment, participants are simultaneously shown two stimuli printed in different colors and told to name one stimulus (i.e., target word) and ignore the other stimulus. If the ignored word on the first trial then becomes the target word on a second trial, the participant will take longer to read the word because of active inhibition of the word as a distracter on the first trial (i.e., negative priming effect). Thus, active inhibition of the distracter delays its subsequent identification (McNally, 2000).

In a series of studies, Enright and Beech (1990, 1993a, 1993b) showed that individuals with OCD had reduced ability to inhibit the processing of distracting information relative to participants with other anxiety disorders. Individuals with other anxiety disorders and nonclinical individuals (controls) showed the standard negative priming effects as a result of actively inhibiting the distracter stimuli from a previous trial. This differential effect was obtained with a Stroop-like negative priming task and a semantic negative priming task. In a study by Enright and Beech (1993b), individuals in the OCD group had significantly less negative priming than those in all other anxiety groups except those with panic disorder and specific phobia. The researchers concluded that as the complexity of a cognitive task increases, the greater the deficit in cognitive inhibition of individuals with OCD relative to those with other anxiety disorders. They suggest that a central deficit of cognitive inhibition indicates that OCD is different from other anxiety disorders and, in this regard, individuals with OCD resemble highly schizotypal individuals.

Other cognitive clinical researchers have not been able to replicate Enright and Beech's findings. McNally, Wilhem, Buhlmann, and Shin (2001) reported that 26 patients with OCD with checking compulsions did not show less negative priming for threat or neutral targets, nor did they exhibit disproportionately defective inhibition for threat words, as compared with nonclinical individuals (controls) (see also MacDonald, Antony, MacLeod, & Swinson, 1999; Maki et al., 1994, for nonsignificant results). Finally, Clayton, Richards, and Edwards (1999) found that individuals with OCD performed less well than those with panic disorder and nonclinical groups of individuals on three out of four tests of selective attention, with difficulties evident in ability to rapidly switch attention and sustain attention. The authors concluded that OCD may be characterized by reduced ability to ignore unimportant external (sensory) or internal (cognitive) stimuli.

At this time, the research on directed forgetting and reduced cognitive inhibition is too preliminary and the findings too inconsistent to conclude that OCD is characterized by a general deficit in cognitive inhibitory processes. It is likely that if reduced inhibition is present, it will be specific to obsessive–compulsive-relevant stimuli (e.g., threat of dirt, contamination, injury, etc.). Moreover, the possibility of a deficit in inhibitory mechanisms, whether general or selective in nature, links well with the literature on the paradoxical effects of thought suppression and the intrusiveness and uncontrollability of obsessions (see Chapter 2). Reduction in cognitive inhibition and forgetting may also contribute to a selective attention and memory bias for obsessive–compulsive-relevant threat stimuli. Whatever the case, more research is needed before it can be concluded that individuals with OCD have a lesser ability to inhibit the processing of irrelevant information (see review by McNally, 2000).

Memory Deficits in Compulsive Checking

The clinical presentation in compulsive checking suggests that this sub-type of OCD may be characterized by memory deficits. When confronted with certain situations, the person with compulsive checking feels an urge to check (e.g., "Did I lock the door, turn off the stove, leave the lights on?"). However, checking behavior is repetitive to the point where one check is rarely enough. So why do individuals continue to doubt after they have checked, leading them to check over and over again? Many of the studies cited previously focused on compulsive checking. It was assumed that poor memory for prior actions, impaired reality monitoring, or low-ered memory confidence might explain the persistence of doubt and the repetitive nature of checking compulsions. After all, if a person has diffi-culty remembering prior actions, then he or she is more likely to repeat the checking.

As previously noted, it is not clear that individuals with compulsive checking suffer from a general memory deficit (see also the review by van den Hout & Kindt, 2003a). Differences between individuals with compul-sive checking and those of nonclinical groups on memory tests have not been consistent, and the correlations between memory performance and severity of checking symptoms have not been strong. However, there is more consistent evidence for reduced memory confidence in compulsive checking. Van den Hout and Kindt (2003a) proposed that checking behavior persists because "repeated checking causes memory distrust" (p. 303). Repeated checking increases familiarity but reduces the vividness and detail of a person's recollection of situations because it causes seman-tic processing to be prioritized at the expense of perceptual processing. As a result, repeated checking, ironically, leads to increased doubt and re-duced confidence. In two experiments involving an interactive computer animation, students were randomly assigned to engage in relevant or ir-relevant checking on whether they turned off a virtual gas stove (van den Hout & Kindt, 2003a). Comparisons revealed that members of the group who engaged in repeated relevant checking reported significantly reduced vividness and detail in their recollections of checking behavior and less confidence in their memory. These findings emerged in spite of no differ-ence between groups in the accuracy of their memory of their prior checking responses. These results were replicated in a third experiment by van den Hout and Kindt (2003b), who also found that individuals' re-peated checking induced a sense of ambivalence about their memory of checking.

Van den Hout and Kindt (2003a, 2003b) have introduced a novel per-spective on the role of memory difficulties in the persistence of compul-sive checking. As discussed in their second paper, the domain-specificity of doubting that characterizes compulsive checking is difficult to reconcile with the idea of a general memory deficit. If individuals with compulsive checking have a general memory deficit, should not doubt and uncertainty be present in most situations? Why memory impairment would manifest itself only in a highly restrictive range of circumstances is hard to explain by those who propose that compulsive checking is caused by a general memory deficit. However, if the primary memory problem in compulsive checking is reduced confidence, than this would occur only under certain circumstances when uncertainty is activated (van den Hout & Kindt, 2003b).

The more recent research on memory bias and reduced confidence in OCD offers fresh insights into the role of memory in the persistence of obsessive–compulsive symptoms, especially compulsive checking. Because it is much more closely tied to the phenomenology of the disorder, it may have greater relevance for treatment than the earlier neuropsychological research based on standard memory tests.

Critique of Neuropsychological Research

Table 4.1 presents a summary of the cognitive impairments that have been implicated in OCD. These conclusions are very tentative because most of the cognitive processes listed in the table have not been sufficiently researched. However, the most consistent finding is that OCD may be characterized by a decline in executive function (i.e., poor organizational strategies), poor immediate recall of nonverbal material, reduced memory confidence, and possibly reduced memory for prior actions. The latter two impairments may be seen only in compulsive checking.

Despite some encouraging findings, there are a number of limitations with neuropsychological research on OCD (for reviews see Greisberg & McKay, 2003; Tallis, 1995). The research on most cognitive processes is not well developed, and the few neuropsychological studies that have been done tend to use small samples and different test instruments or variations in experimental methodology. Significant test performance differences are often not replicated, or they emerge within a number of analyses showing no significant differences (Amir & Kozak, 2002). Frequently, test performance deficits show, at best, a weak association with symptom severity, which calls into question the functional significance of the finding (e.g., Bolton, Raven, Madronal-Luque, & Marks, 2000; Savage et al., 1999; Tallis et al., 1999). Performance on neuropsychological tests may have minimal treatment implications (Bolton et al., 2000). Given the complexity of most neuropsychological tests, poor performance could also be due to a number of different cognitive deficits.

Most studies fail to include comparison groups with other clinical disorders, so it is unclear whether poor performance is specific to OCD. Furthermore, without controlling for depression and other comorbid condi-

TABLE 4.1. Summary of General Cognitive Deficits in OCD

Cognitive impairment	Predicted difference	Empirical status
General intelligence	Superior intelligence	Slightly higher
Executive functioning	Lower performance on shifting cognitive set, planning, verbal fluency, directional orientation, concept formation, making attentional shifts, and time estimation	Inconsistent findings, with the possible exception of lower ability to shift cognitive set and greater interference effects
General memory ability	Superior recall in OCD	Inconsistent findings
Memory for prior actions	Lower recall and recognition performance for prior actions in compulsive checking	Some evidence that compulsive checking is characterized by poorer memory that is specific to a person's prior actions
Reality monitoring	Compulsive checking is associated with lower ability to discriminate between memories of doing (visual percepts) versus memories of imaging (mental images)	Weak and inconsistent evidence
Memory confidence	Individuals with OCD, especially with checking compulsions, have less confidence in their memory performance	Strong evidence of reduced confidence in memory functioning
Directed forgetting	Reduced ability to intentionally dispel highly relevant thoughts	Too little research to draw conclusion; may be specific to current concerns of the patient
Cognitive inhibition	A general deficit in ability to inhibit irrelevant information	Inconsistent findings on general deficit in cognitive inhibitory processes

tions, it may be that poor cognitive performance is due to symptoms other than the presence of obsessions or compulsions. For example, Moritz et al. (2001) provide evidence that the deficits in executive functioning found in OCD may be due to comorbid depression rather than the obsessional state itself.

Tallis (1995) noted that the connection between a specific cognitive deficit, like general set shifting, and actual obsessive–compulsive symptom expression, such as compulsive washing and checking, is not at all clear. Salkovskis (1996a) noted that general deficit theories have difficulty explaining why patients with OCD exhibit memory problems only in situations linked to their obsessional problems. This last criticism has been addressed to some extent by the recent research on memory, which is more closely connected to OCD phenomenology. Moreover, a neuropsychological model, such as the one proposed by Savage (1998), does highlight the connections between brain dysfunction, neuropsychological impairment, and clinical presentation. Nevertheless, the ecological validity of neuropsychological test results can also be questioned, given that the cognitive deficits found on standardized tests or in the laboratory do not lead to the serious impairment in daily functioning seen with patients suffering other neuropsychiatric conditions (Greisberg & McKay, 2003).

Finally, the most serious concern is that poor neuropsychological test performance may be confounded by the clinical presentation of OCD. For example, the impairment in executive function could be due to a pathological response style adopted by individuals with OCD who suffer from excessive slowness, doubt, and meticulousness (Greisberg & McKay, 2003). Purcell et al. (1998), for example, noted that significant response slowing was evident on some tests of executive function. In sum, the causal status of neuropsycholgical test performance is unknown. Whether reduced cognitive ability is a cause or a consequence of the obsessive–compulsive symptoms has not been addressed by the current research. At this time, the role of general cognitive deficits in the etiology and persistence of OCD remains unknown.

INFORMATION-PROCESSING BIAS IN OCD

Over the last 20 years extensive experimental research has adapted the methods and procedures of experimental cognitive psychology to explore the nature of the information-processing bias in anxiety disorders. This perspective views the cognitive nature of psychopathology in terms of a biased or selective information-processing system, in which a particular class of stimuli are attended to, interpreted, and remembered more than others because certain underlying schemas are activated that allocate processing priority to this type of information (Clark & Beck, 1999; Gotlib & Neubauer, 2000). A basic premise of the cognitive perspective is that the central function of anxiety is "to facilitate the detection of danger or threat in potentially threatening environments" (M. W. Eysenck, 1992, p. 4). In anxiety disorders the danger detection processes become hypervigilant, so that the number and severity of threatening or dangerous events in the environment becomes exaggerated (M. W. Eysenck, 1992). A number of theoretical papers and empirical critical reviews have elaborated on the maladaptive information-processing style evident in anxiety disorders (Barlow, 2002; Beck & D. A. Clark, 1997; D. M. Clark, 1999;

Dalgleish & Watts, 1990; M. W. Eysenck, 1992; Mathews, 1997; Mathews & MacLeod, 1994; Mineka & Sutton, 1992; Wells & Matthews, 1994; Williams et al., 1997).

A number of experiments have investigated attentional bias in OCD. Based on a dichotic listening task involving obsessive–compulsive-relevant threat and neutral words, Foa and McNally (1986) found that participants with OCD detected significantly more fear-relevant than neutral target words in the unattended channel as indicated by number of button presses and magnitude of skin conductance response. After treatment, this differential response to fear-relevant stimuli disappeared. Summerfeldt and Endler (1998) are critical of this study because individuals with washing compulsions were overrepresented in the OCD sample.

The emotional Stroop task is the experimental paradigm most often used to investigate attentional processing bias in OCD. Participants are shown words of varying emotional significance (i.e., neutral, specific threat words, general threat words, nonthreat words) that are printed in different colors. Individuals are told to ignore the meaning of the words and to name the color of the printed word as quickly as possible. The extent to which color naming is delayed reflects the degree to which the person's attention was diverted to the meaning of the word. Thus, the longer the delay in color naming a word, the more that attention has been selectively shifted to the meaning of the word. Color-naming interference, then, becomes the index of attentional bias (McNally, 2000).

Foa, Ilai, McCarthy, Shoyer, and Murdock (1993) had patients with OCD, with or without washing compulsions, and nonclinical individuals (controls) color name contamination, general threat, and neutral words, as well as nonwords, in an emotional Stroop priming task. Analyses of color-naming latencies revealed that individuals in the obsessive–compulsive washer group took significantly longer to color name contamination words than neutral words, but not general threat words or nonwords. Moreover, compulsive washers took significantly longer in color naming contamination words than the normal group but did not differ significantly from those in the nonwasher OCD sample. The authors concluded that a processing bias for personally threatening material was evident among those in the OCD group with washing compulsions. However, these results are fragile at best. A number of the response latency comparisons that would indicate specificity were not statistically significant, and the Stroop interference scores did not correlate with symptom severity, which calls into question the clinical relevance of the findings (Summerfeldt & Endler, 1998).

In a second emotional Stroop study, Calamari et al. (1993) failed to find that patients with OCD showed greater interference to obsessive–compulsive-relevant threat words as compared with general threat words, threat words relevant to other anxiety disorders, or words representing positive or negative life concerns. Overall, these results fail to support a specific attentional bias for personally threatening material in OCD. McNally et al. (1994) also failed to find that those in their OCD clinical control group had significantly greater interference for panic or general threat words, a finding that Summerfeldt and Endler (1998) note is surprising, because many of these words contain somatic, contamination, and violence themes that are relevant to OCD.

Some researchers have found evidence of an attentional bias in OCD that is specific to obsessive–compulsive concerns (i.e., disorder specific). Lavy, van Oppen, and van den Hout (1994) used an emotional Stroop task to show that patients with OCD with washing or checking compulsions had significantly greater interference effects only for negative obsessive–compulsive-relevant words and not for positive obsessive–compulsive-relevant words or general positive or negative emotional words.

Kyrios and Iob (1998) employed both masked and unmasked presentations of neutral, obsessive–compulsive-relevant threat words and general threat words to 15 patients with OCD and 15 nonclinical individuals (controls). Interference effects on the masked trials are interpreted as evidence of an automatic, preconscious attentional bias, whereas interference on unmasked trials suggests attentional bias at a later conscious and effortful stage of information processing. Contrary to prediction, in the unmasked presentation (supraliminal) the patients with OCD were actually faster at color naming obsessive–compulsive threat-related words as compared with neutral words. However, on the masked trials (subliminal), the patients with OCD showed significantly slower color naming for the obsessive–compulsive threat-related words.

These results appear to suggest that patients with OCD have an attentional bias for threat cues that are specific to their diagnostic concerns and that this bias operates at the automatic but not the strategic level of information processing. However, other emotional Stroop studies failed to find any evidence that OCD is characterized by a disorder-specific attentional threat bias at either the subliminal or the supraliminal level of consciousness (Freeston, Ladouceur, Letarte, et al., 1992; Kampman, Keijsers, Verbraak, Naring, & Hoogduin, 2002).

Tata, Leibowitz, Prunty, Cameron, and Pickering (1996) used a modified dot-probe task to compare attentional bias for neutral, contamination, and social threat words in 13 patients with OCD with washing compulsions and 18 high-trait anxious nonclinical individuals (controls). Analysis revealed that the patients with OCD were significantly faster at detecting probes preceded by contamination threat words, but not social threat words. Those in the high-trait anxious group had significant vigilance for the social threat words, but not the contamination words. These results provide fairly strong evidence of an attentional bias for obsessive–compulsive-relevant threat stimuli that may be operating at the preconscious, automatic processing level. However, Summerfeldt and Endler (1998) are critical of this experiment, noting that many outlying scores were excluded from the OCD group and multiple *t* tests were performed without adjustment for an inflated Type I error rate.

McNally (2000) concluded that there is evidence that OCD is characterized by an attentional bias for threatening stimuli, but unlike such a bias in other anxiety disorders, it is specific to the person's primary symptom concerns. Summerfeldt and Endler (1998), however, concluded that evidence of a processing bias for threat stimuli in OCD is not as robust as seen in other anxiety disorders. They indicate that too few studies have investigated information processing in OCD, the studies that have been done have serious methodological shortcomings, and the results that are reported are quite inconsistent. Furthermore, there is emerging evidence that OCD is a heterogeneous syndrome that may make generalization difficult. Thus, an attentional bias for personally threatening stimuli may be evident only among those with OCD washing compulsions.

It may be that an information-processing bias in OCD is more apparent in memory than in attentional processes. Radomsky and Rachman (1999), for example, found that patients with OCD, but not nonobsessional anxious or nonclinical individuals (controls), had significantly better memory for contaminated objects than for clean objects, even though general memory functioning did not differ between groups. However, other studies have not found enhanced memory bias for contaminated objects in patients with compulsive washing rituals (Ceschi, van der Linden, Dunker, Perroud, & Brédart, 2003). Clearly, more research is needed to determine whether there is a biased threat-related processing style that is evident across the various subtypes of obsessional states. The varied clinical presentations evident in OCD will make it more difficult to find a common attentional bias across all OCD subtypes. As compared with those with other anxiety disorders, individuals with OCD may selectively process a much narrower range of stimuli that are directly connected to their obsessional concerns. Amir and Kozak (2002) concluded in their review that it is not clear whether the attentional bias for threat in OCD is disorder specific or content specific. At the very least, the failure to find a consistent processing bias for disorder-specific threat raises doubts about whether anxiety has the same status in OCD as seen in other anxiety disorders (Summerfeldt & Endler, 1998).

SUMMARY AND CONCLUSION

The presence of doubt, repetitive checking, and slowness has led researchers to investigate whether individuals with OCD have a deficit in certain general cognitive processes. Neuropsychological research suggests that deficits in executive function, nonverbal memory, and confidence in memory judgments may characterize OCD. These findings are consistent with neurophysiology studies indicating that OCD may involve dysfunction in the frontal–striatal system. If these neuropsychological deficits are present in OCD, they would probably interact with environmental learning consequences to create the clinical dysfunction we see in OCD (Greisberg & McKay, 2003). Some type of training in the use of more efficient organizational strategies or memory skills could be added to conventional treatment regimens to improve the effectiveness of therapy (Greisberg & McKay, 2003). However, the shortcomings previously noted in the neuropsychological research on OCD would make such treatment applications premature. The role of general cognitive deficits in OCD remains to be determined.

Research on information-processing bias in OCD has failed to establish the presence of a disorder-specific bias for threat (Amir & Kozak, 2002). The most cogent conclusion is that any attentional bias in obsessional states is specific to the current symptom concerns of the individual under investigation. This suggests that the information-processing apparatus in OCD may be quite different from that in other anxiety disorders where a more pervasive attentional bias for threat has been established. This would support the need for a more varied treatment approach that can be tailored to the unique cognitive biases of individual patients. The cognitive strategies described in later chapters could potentially be adapted to the particular cognitive dysfunction associated with the idiographic symptom concerns of each individual with OCD.

CHAPTER 5

Cognitive Appraisal Theories of OCD

Theory, research, and treatment within the cognitive-clinical stream of psychology focuses on the thoughts, appraisals, and belief content that characterize psychopathological conditions (McNally, 2001a). This perspective is rooted in clinical theorists like Beck and Ellis, and it relies on both experimental and self-report methods of investigation. The "appraisal" perspective dominates cognitive-behavioral theory, research, and practice in OCD. As evident in the chapters to follow, this perspective has had a much greater impact on the treatment of OCD than the neuropsychological or information-processing research discussed in the previous chapter.

A central tenet of any appraisal-based theory is that normal and abnormal emotional states are based on "a person's subjective evaluation or appraisal of the personal significance of a situation, object, or event on a number of dimensions or criteria (Scherer, 1999, p. 637). Consequently, appraisal theories in clinical psychology consider the content and product of the dysfunctional information-processing system in clinical disorders, the conceptual level most important in understanding the etiology and persistence of psychopathology. Here the focus is on *what* one thinks rather than on *how* one thinks. Although criticisms have been raised about the appraisal perspective in cognitive-clinical psychology (MacLeod, 1993), a vigorous defense of its validity has been offered, citing various factors, not the least being its significant contribution to improved treatment of clinical disorders (McNally, 2001a).

This chapter examines the dominant cognitive appraisal theories of OCD. The key features of each model are discussed, and a critical review of the supporting research is offered. Because cognitive-behavioral therapy of OCD adopts a theory-driven approach to treatment, it is important to evaluate the theoretical and empirical foundations of the treatment.

The chapter begins with a discussion of early contributions to the cognitive-clinical perspective on OCD. However, the bulk of the chapter focuses on cognitive-behavioral models of OCD advanced by Salkovskis, Rachman, and the Obsessive Compulsive Cognitions Working Group (OCCWG).

EARLY COGNITIVE APPRAISAL THEORIES OF OCD

Cognitive theory and therapy were not considered relevant for OCD until the publication of Salkovskis's (1985) article on cognitive-behavioral analysis of obsessions and compulsions. Beck's (1967, 1976) early writings on his cognitive formulation of emotional disorders barely made reference to obsessional states. Beck and Emery (1985) did not offer a cognitive therapy and treatment of OCD. As recently as 1986, Hollon and Beck concluded that the most effective treatment for OCD was ERP and that "it also remains possible that explicit cognitive interventions have little to offer this disorder" (p. 467).

Carr (1974) proposed one of the first cognitive theories of OCD in response to limitations with the anxiety reduction hypothesis of compulsive behavior that was widely accepted by behavioral psychologists of that day. The core tenet of his model is that obsessional states are characterized by an abnormally high subjective estimate of the probability that unfavorable outcomes will occur. In OCD, any situation that involves potential harm (i.e., high subjective cost) will result in a heightened threat or anxiety, because the individual generates an elevated estimate of the probability of occurrence of the undesired outcome. Compulsive rituals develop as threat-reducing activities that function to lower the subjective probability of an undesired outcome. The occurrence of obsessive–compulsive symptoms in a specific situation depends on the person perceiving high subjective cost (i.e., harm) and high subjective probability of the undesirable outcome. Cognitive compulsions will occur when an appropriate threat-reducing behavior is not available. Cognitive or behavioral compulsions become ritualistic because the person perceives that this is the most efficient way to reduce the probability of an unfavorable outcome. Carr admitted that the threat appraisal model does not explain what causes people to make high subjective probability estimates for unfavorable events in the first place. Moreover, it may be that overestimated threat appraisals may be more important in the pathogenesis of phobias and other anxiety disorders than they are in OCD (e.g., see Volans, 1976).

Based on Carr's (1974) formulation, McFall and Wollersheim (1979) proposed that patients with OCD make a faulty primary threat appraisal involving the overestimation of the probability of threat and its negative consequences. In addition, an erroneous secondary appraisal occurs in which patients underestimate their ability to cope with the threat. Both primary threat and secondary vulnerability appraisals are based on certain maladaptive preconscious beliefs such as (1) it is necessary to be perfect, (2) mistakes should be punished, (3) one has the power to prevent terrible outcomes by magical rituals or ruminative thinking, (4) certain thoughts are very unacceptable because they can cause some catastrophe to occur, (5) it is easier and more effective to engage in neutralizing activity than to confront one's feelings, and (6) feelings of uncertainty and loss of control are intolerable. The faulty primary and secondary appraisals give rise to feelings of uncertainty, loss of control, and anxiety. Because obsessional individuals perceive that they cannot deal with this distress in a realistic or adaptive manner, they resort to magical rituals and compulsive strategies as the best option for reducing distress. Based on this model, McFall and Wollersheim (1979) recommend that behavioral exercises and cognitive restructuring, based on the rational-emotive (RET) perspective, be used to directly modify unrealistic primary threat and secondary vulnerability appraisals.

Salkovskis (1985) was critical of the McFall and Wollersheim formulation because of (1) their attempt to bridge the gap between behavioral and psychoanalytic theory, (2) their emphasis on preconscious and unconscious cognitions without elaborating on the direct cognitive and behavioral expression of these concepts, and (3) a failure to specify how the primary threat appraisals in OCD differ uniquely from the threat appraisals seen in other anxiety disorders. Although Salkovskis's critique of McFall and Wollersheim's model is warranted, it is interesting that contemporary cognitive models contain a number of key concepts that bear some similarity to ideas described in the model (e.g., inflated responsibility, thought–action fusion, and excessive concern with thought control).

CONTEMPORARY COGNITIVE-BEHAVIORAL THEORIES

In the last decade a number of different cognitive-behavioral models have been proposed to explain the role of cognition in the etiology and persistence of OCD. The models differ in which cognitive constructs are emphasized as most important in the pathogenesis of obsessions and compulsions. However, they all tend to ascribe to certain central tenets and fundamental assumptions about the role and function of maladaptive cognition in OCD. Figure 5.1 presents a general theoretical framework adopted by most cognitive-behavioral appraisal theories of OCD.

Most of these models consider the unwanted intrusive thoughts, images, and impulses first identified by Rachman and de Silva (1978) the ini-

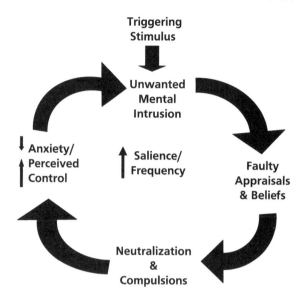

FIGURE 5.1. Basic outline of cognitive-behavioral appraisal theories of OCD.

tial starting point in the pathogenesis of obsessions. Usually these un-wanted, ego-dystonic mental intrusions are triggered by an identifiable external stimulus (Parkinson & Rachman, 1981a). An example is the per-son who feels an impulse to jump in front of a subway car but only when in a subway station, or the impulse to check the door but only when leav-ing the house. Once an unwanted intrusive thought occurs, whether or not it spirals into a clinical obsession depends on the way it is appraised or evaluated.

Although the cognitive-behavioral theories differ on which errone-ous appraisal or combination of appraisals is most pathonomic to obses-sions, they all agree that faulty appraisals are necessary, but not sufficient, for creating obsessions. The faulty appraisal of the mental intrusion will then lead to some attempt to control the thought or neutralize the distress or anticipated negative consequences associated with the thought, image, or impulse. Together, faulty appraisals and the use of neutralization, com-pulsions, or other control strategies are the two main processes resulting in the escalation of unwanted intrusions into obsessions. In the short term, the compulsion will result in a reduction in anxiety or distress and a rise in the person's perceived control over the obsession. However, in the long term, the faulty appraisals and control strategies will both heighten the salience of the mental intrusion and cause an increase in its fre-quency.

SALKOVSKIS'S INFLATED RESPONSIBILITY MODEL

Description of the Model

Unwanted Intrusive Thoughts

Salkovskis's inflated responsibility model posits that obsessional thinking has its origins in the unwanted and unacceptable intrusive thoughts, images, and impulses that are experienced by the majority of individuals (Salkovskis, 1985, 1989a, 1996a, 1996b, 1998, 1999). These unwanted cognitive intrusions, which are very similar in form and content to clinical obsessions, reflect individuals' current concerns and interests and may represent an aspect of active problem solving (Salkovskis, 1996a). Problem solving involves the generation of ideas, so intrusive thoughts may be seen as the product of an "idea generator." To be useful in problem solving, these thoughts must be subjected to further evaluation and analysis. If an evaluation of a thought suggests that some action is required, then processing priority will be very high and the thought will be experienced as quite compelling (Salkovskis & Freeston, 2001). That is, cognitive intrusions perceived as having an important implication for the individual's current concerns will be given processing priority. If the intrusive thought, image, or impulse is perceived to be useless or irrelevant to current concerns, then it is ignored.

Inflated Responsibility

The difference between a normal intrusive thought and an obsession does not lie in its occurrence, content, or even uncontrollability. Instead, it is the manner in which the intrusive thought is appraised or interpreted that determines its pathological significance (Salkovskis, 1999). Intrusive cognitions are emotionally neutral when they first occur but take on positive, negative, or neutral emotional significance, depending on a person's prior experience and the context of the thought (Salkovskis, Richards, & Forrester, 1995). Any thought has the potential to become obsessional if it is interpreted as implying high personal responsibility and significance.

Two processes are considered critical to the pathogenesis of obsessions, *appraisals of responsibility* and the occurrence of *neutralizing activities*. A key assumption of this model is that the obsession per se is not the problem, but rather the meaning that is attached to it. Salkovskis and colleagues define responsibility as

> The belief that one has power which is pivotal to bring about or prevent subjectively crucial negative outcomes. These outcomes may be actual, that is, having consequences in the real world, and/or at a moral level. (cited in Salkovskis, 1998, p. 40)

Responsibility is conceptualized on two levels, according to Salkovskis (1985, 1989a, 1996a, 1996b, 1998). High-risk individuals possess particular *responsibility beliefs* that lead to a tendency to misinterpret their mental activities as indications of personal responsibility. At a secondary level, these vulnerable individuals generate *responsibility appraisals* or interpretations of their intrusive thoughts. Once an obsessional thought, image, or impulse is misinterpreted as signifying increased personal responsibility, certain processes follow (Salkovskis & Wahl, 2003).

- The intrusion is associated with increased discomfort, anxiety, and depression.
- The intrusion and related thoughts achieve greater accessibility or salience.
- Increased focused attention is shifted onto the intrusion and its environmental trigger.
- Neutralizing responses are initiated in an effort to escape or avoid responsibility.

The inflated responsibility appraisals can focus either on the occurrence or on the content of the intrusive thought (Salkovskis & Wahl, 2003). For example, a patient with multiple obsessions might misinterpret his failure to dismiss intrusive thoughts as a sign that he is losing control and could be responsible for committing some horrendous act of violence. In this case the responsibility appraisal is associated with the occurrence of any unwanted cognitive intrusion. However, if the content of an intrusive thought suggests a specific reaction, then control processes (e.g., compulsions) will occur to limit the person's experience of the obsession. A patient with the obsession "I might get sick and vomit" interpreted this thought as a sign that she must take responsibility for her health and ensure that she does not get sick. Here we see a controlled processing response to the content of the intrusion, rather than to its mere occurrence.

Salkovskis (1989a, 1998) argues that appraisals of responsibility for harm are specific to obsessional thinking. What distinguishes obsessions from other forms of anxious and depressive thinking is their association with appraisals of responsibility. If a thought results only in harm or danger appraisals, then the emotional response will be anxiety, whereas appraisals of loss will be associated with depression (Salkovskis, 1999). It is further argued that the inflated responsibility misinterpretation is necessary for an intrusion to become pathological; "without appraisal of responsibility, an obsessional episode would not result" (Salkovskis, 1989a, p. 678). The adverse mood (e.g., discomfort, guilt, anxiety) associated with an obsession arises from misinterpretations of responsibility (Salkovskis, 1999).

It is evident from the definition that responsibility is closely tied with appraisals of threat and danger. The excessive responsibility that characterizes obsessional thinking has less to do with perceiving that one is responsible for having such thoughts and more to do with being responsible to prevent the perceived negative or threatening consequences that *might* occur as a result of thinking violent or other harmful thoughts (Salkovskis & Wahl, 2003). Appraisals involving threat evaluations will lead to anxiety and attempts to achieve safety. O'Connor and Robillard (1995) take this one step further by pointing out that in OCD the perceived fear or negative outcome is construed in terms of preventing a highly improbable, possibly even completely fictitious, threatening outcome. For example, a woman with OCD felt compelled to check her freezer every time she walked by it because of a concern that someone might be trapped inside. According to a "responsibility formulation," the checking compulsion did not result from a desire to rescue a person trapped inside the freezer, because the woman knew this was impossible, a nonsensical idea. Rather, she checked in order to alleviate an elevated sense of responsibility.

Neutralization

A second process considered important in the pathogenesis of OCD is the development of neutralizing responses. Neutralization is defined as "voluntarily initiated activity which is intended to have the effect of reducing the perceived responsibility and can be overt or covert (compulsive behavior or thought rituals)" (Salkovskis, 1989a, p. 678). The OCD-prone individual will revert to neutralizing responses in an effort to reduce a perceived sense of responsibility for the negative outcomes represented by the obsession. Once the neutralizing responses are established, individuals continue to engage in them because they perceive that the neutralizing response led to a reduction in responsibility and discomfort. Neutralizing will also prevent obsessive–compulsive individuals from processing any evidence that would disconfirm their inferences of responsibility for preventing highly improbable, frightening events. The avoidance of disaster can always be attributed to the performance of the neutralizing ritual. In the previous example, repeated freezer checking reassured the patient that she was not responsible for locking someone inside her refrigerator.

Overcontrol of Mental Activity

Another consequence of responsibility appraisals is that individuals with OCD will try too hard to exert control over their intrusive thoughts, images, and impulses (Salkovskis et al., 1995). Salkovskis (1998) argued that an increased effort to suppress unwanted intrusive thoughts will inadvertently heighten the distress associated with obsessions because (1) it will change the contents of conscious thought, (2) it will result in failure and

possibly increased frequency of the intrusion, (3) it will increase the salience and accessibility of thoughts dealing with harm, and (4) it prevents
disconfirmation of the belief that harm must be prevented. Thus, "obsessional problems are a result of sensitive individuals *trying too hard* to be
certain that they have not caused harm" (Salkovskis, 1999, p. S34, emphasis in original). OCD is caused by inflated responsibility, and it is maintained by trying too hard to control obsessions (Salkovskis & Wahl, 2003).
Salkovskis and Freeston (2001) note that there is an internal logic (reasonableness) to the patient's exaggerated attempts to control the obsession,
given the person's faulty assumptions and beliefs that result in exaggerated threat being attached to the obsession.

Biased Cognitive Processing

Salkovskis (1996a, 1998; Salkovskis & Wahl, 2003) also proposes that certain cognitive errors are evident in the thinking of obsessional patients.
These errors are a product of preexisting OCD beliefs. Moreover, com-
mission of the errors increases the probability of misinterpretations of responsibility. The errors most characteristic of OCD include the following:

1. *Responsibility bias.* The individual tends to equate any personal influence over negative outcome with responsibility for that outcome.
2. *Absence of omission bias.* Most individuals believe their responsibility for negative consequences is diminished when "failing to act"
   (omission) is involved, as opposed to situations where the commis-
   sion of a specific act could bring about a negative outcome. For
   example, we feel less responsible for causing injury to someone if
   we fail to pick up a board with nails in it, as compared with drop-
   ping the nailed board on a pathway. Individuals with OCD, however, do not show this bias in relation to their obsessional concerns.
3. *Misperceptions of personal agency.* Individuals with OCD often mis-
   takenly assume that they can foresee possible harmful outcomes
   (i.e., premonition). Not acting when we can foresee possible harmful outcomes leaves us with an inflated sense of responsibility because by choosing not to act, we increase the chances of the negative consequences.
4. *Thought–action fusion.* Although not directly stated, thought–
   action fusion (i.e., thought is perceived as equivalent to action)
   would be considered a cognitive error that is directly connected
   with inflated responsibility appraisals.
5. *Errors of decision making.* Individuals with OCD have particular difficulty in deciding when to stop a compulsion or neutralizing ac-

tivity. The criteria for knowing when the ritual is complete may be vague, highly subjective, and open to considerable variation across situations.

Dysfunctional Assumptions

Salkovskis (1985, 1996a, 1998) views vulnerability to OCD in terms of pre-existing assumptions or beliefs that are triggered by the occurrence of unwanted intrusive thoughts and give rise to the cognitive biases and appraisals of responsibility described previously. These enduring beliefs are learned over long periods of time or as a result of unusual or critical events (Salkovskis, 1998; Salkovskis & Freeston, 2001; Salkovskis & Wahl, 2003). All of the dysfunctional assumptions described by Salkovskis are related to the theme of responsibility:

1. *Responsibility beliefs* (e.g., not trying to prevent harm to self or others is equivalent to causing the harm)
2. *Thought–action fusion beliefs* (e.g., having a thought is like performing the action)
3. *Thought control beliefs* (e.g., one can and should exercise control of his or her mental activity)
4. *Neutralization beliefs* (e.g., one should neutralize in order to prevent possible harm from occurring to others)

Salkovskis, Shafran, Rachman, and Freeston (1999) postulate five pathways that may lead to the development of maladaptive responsibility beliefs in persons predisposed to OCD.

- A generalized sense of responsibility for preventing threat that is deliberately or implicitly encouraged or promoted in childhood (i.e., given too much responsibility),
- Exposure to rigid and extreme codes of conduct and duty,
- Childhood experiences, such as overindulgence, which shield him or her from assuming responsibility. What is implied is that the child is incompetent, which leads to increased sensitivity to ideas of responsibility (i.e., given too little responsibility),
- Incident(s) involving action or inaction that significantly contributed to serious misfortune to self or others, or
- Incident(s) in which the person erroneously assumes that his or her thoughts, actions, or inactions contributed to a serious misfortune.

In addition to these distal contributors, certain proximal factors may be involved in the etiology of inflated responsibility, like an experience of systematic criticism and/or scapegoating, a situational increase in responsibility, or a specific critical incident involving real or perceived responsibility (blame) for causing harm or near misses (Salkovskis et al., 1999). At this point, there is no empirical evidence to support these speculations on the origins of inflated responsibility. Salkovskis et al. (1999) provide only anecdotal support based on illustrative case histories. Although they conclude with some suggestions for researching the etiology of maladaptive responsibility beliefs, Salkovskis and colleagues caution that more is gained clinically from emphasizing the maintenance than the etiological factors of inflated responsibility.

Empirical Status

Inflated responsibility is one of the most extensively researched of the cognitive constructs of obsessional states. Support for Salkovskis's formulation depends on evidence that inflated responsibility for averting harm is a necessary factor in the maintenance of obsessions. This assertion is tested by four main hypotheses, which are summarized in Table 5.1.

Hypothesis 1

Salkovskis's model hypothesizes that inflated responsibility appraisals and beliefs are core features of all obsessional thinking. Evidence of obsessionality without inflated responsibility would be difficult to reconcile with the model. In many studies measures of responsibility appraisals and beliefs correlated significantly with self-report measures of obsessive and compulsive symptoms (OCCWG, 2001, 2003a; Rhéaume, Freeston, Dugas, Letarte, & Ladouceur, 1995; Rhéaume, Ladouceur, Freeston, & Letarte, 1994; Salkovskis et al., 2000; Smári & Hólmsteinsson, 2001; Steketee, Frost, & Cohen, 1998; Wilson & Chambless, 1999). Further-

TABLE 5.1. Key Hypotheses in Salkovskis's Responsibility Theory of OCD

Responsibility hypotheses	Empirical status
Inflated responsibility appraisals and beliefs are central characteristics of OCD.	Partial support
Inflated responsibility for harm is specific to obsessional thinking.	Limited support
Elevated perceived responsibility will cause an increased urge to neutralize, greater discomfort, and increased frequency and salience of the obsession.	Consistent evidence for checking, at least
Neutralization will increase the frequency, salience, and subjective discomfort of obsessions.	Emerging support

more, there is evidence that individuals with OCD score significantly higher on measures of perceived responsibility for harm than those in nonobsessional clinical and nonclinical control groups (OCCWG, 2001, 2003a; Salkovskis et al., 2000; Steketee, Frost, & Cohen, 1998). Yet, perceived responsibility may account for only a small, albeit significant, amount of variance in specific obsessional symptoms (Emmelkamp & Aardema, 1999; Wilson & Chambless, 1999).

Inflated responsibility may not be a stable personality trait, but instead may be more idiosyncratic and situationally determined than originally formulated (Rachman, Thordarson, Shafran, & Woody, 1995). Rachman and Shafran (1998) concluded that inflated responsibility was common in obsessional checking and doubting, but less apparent in compulsive cleaning (see also Menzies, Harris, Cumming, & Einstein, 2000). However, Lee and Kwon (2003) found that Korean students rated responsibility appraisals significantly higher for dirt/contamination intrusions than for unwanted sex and aggression intrusive thoughts. Moreover, there appear to be sharp boundaries to inflated responsibility, with obsessional patients having exaggerated responsibility in one setting but not another, or feeling unduly responsible for certain negative events but normal levels of responsibility for positive events (Rachman & Shafran, 1998).

Overall, the first hypothesis is only partially supported. OCD groups have elevated scores on measures of inflated responsibility for harm, and these measures correlate with obsessive–compulsive symptom measures. However, inflated responsibility appears to account for much less variance in obsessional symptoms than might be expected, there is considerable instability, idiosyncrasy, and situational specificity in the construct, and it may be that the concept is applicable to a narrower set of obsessive–compulsive symptoms or subtypes than assumed by Salkovskis.

Hypothesis 2

The model hypothesizes that inflated responsibility for harm is a distinct cognitive construct that is specific to obsessional thinking. In support of the hypothesis, various correlational studies that included multiple self-report measures of different cognitive constructs found that responsibility correlates highly with other cognitive concepts considered relevant to OCD (OCCWG, 2001, 2003a, 2003b; Steketee, Frost, & Cohen, 1998).

Strong support for the specificity of responsibility was reported by Salkovskis et al. (2000), who found that responsibility appraisals and beliefs were uniquely related to obsessional symptoms but not to anxiety or depression (see also positive findings by Smári, Glyfadóttir, & Halldórsdóttir, 2003) . In partial support for the model, Foa, Amir, Bogert, Molnar, and Przeworski (2001) found that their OCD sample evidenced significantly higher responsibility ratings for low-risk and obsessive–compulsive-relevant hypothetical situations than the anxious and nonclinical controls. However, in a replication study, the heightened ratings of responsibility and urge to rectify the situation were entirely associated with compulsive checking and were not present in an obsessive–compulsive nonchecking group (Foa, Sacks, Tolin, Przeworski, & Amir, 2002). The authors concluded that inflated responsibility might be a critical factor only for compulsive checking. Contrary to the model, responsibility appraisals may not be a critical feature of other OCD subtypes.

The obsessive–compulsive specificity of responsibility has not always been achieved in other correlational studies. In the OCCWG Stage III study (OCCWG, 2003a) responsibility had significant correlations with measures of worry and other negative affect states even after controlling for obsessive–compulsive symptoms. In a subsequent regression analysis, responsibility beliefs significantly predicted harming obsessions, but no other obsessive–compulsive symptoms after controlling for anxious and depressive symptoms (OCCWG, 2003b). Foa et al. (2001) found that a social anxiety group also exhibited inflated responsibility, albeit at a lower level than individuals with OCD. Furthermore, the OCD and socially anxious groups did not differ from nonclinical controls on the high-risk situations, indicating that responsibility may vary with the content of situations.

At present it remains to be determined how well the construct of inflated responsibility can be differentiated from other cognitive features of OCD. In the OCCWG research, responsibility appraisals and beliefs were very highly correlated with other obsessive–compulsive-relevant cognitive constructs (OCCWG, 2003a, 2003b). Moreover, inflated responsibility for harm may not be as specific or unique to obsessional thinking as assumed by Salkovskis's model (Rachman & Shafran, 1998), or its relevance may be limited to compulsive checking.

Hypothesis 3

It is hypothesized that higher perceived responsibility will lead to an increased urge to neutralize, heightened discomfort, and, in the end, increased frequency and salience of obsessions. A number of experimental studies have manipulated the level of perceived responsibility to assess temporary changes in obsessive and compulsive behavior. These studies are particularly important because they can determine whether inflated responsibility for harm has a causal impact on obsessive–compulsive symptoms.

Lopatka and Rachman (1995) reported the first responsibility manipulation experiment. Individuals exposed to a low perceived responsibility manipulation evidenced significant decreases in perceived discomfort, urge to check, and estimates of harm and criticism, as compared with the control condition. There was a nonsignificant trend for the high perceived responsibility condition to cause increases in perceived discomfort, urge to check, and severity of anticipated criticism. However, the researchers reported that it was difficult to manipulate perceived responsibility for compulsive cleaners, which calls into question the relevance of inflated responsibility for this OCD subtype.

Ladouceur, Rhéaume, et al. (1995) reported two studies in which nonclinical individuals were randomly assigned to a high or low responsibility condition. In the first study there was no significant difference between the two groups in checking behavior. In the second study the high responsibility group exhibited significantly more hesitations and checking behavior and reported more anxiety and preoccupation with avoiding errors during a task classification than the low responsibility group. However, findings by Bouchard, Rhéaume, and Ladouceur (1999) indicate that presence of perfectionism will cause people to overestimate their personal responsibility for negative events. Shafran (1997) also found that ratings of urge to neutralize, subjective discomfort/anxiety, and estimates of threat probability were significantly higher under a high responsibility ERP treatment condition than under a low responsibility treatment condition.

Generally, there is support for Salkovskis's contention that high personal responsibility for harm will increase subjective discomfort and urge to engage in compulsive rituals and other neutralization strategies. What is unclear at this time is whether this effect is apparent in all forms of compulsion, such as cleaning rituals, and whether other cognitive variables like perfectionism or degree of threat estimation might be as important in the promotion of compulsive urges. Moreover, some findings are not consistent with the model. For example, there is little association between ratings of perceived responsibility and estimates of control (Shafran, 1997), and some studies did not find a significant increase in compulsive urges or checking behavior under high responsibility conditions (Kyrios & Bhar, 1997; Lopatka & Rachman, 1995).

Hypothesis 4

The model predicts that neutralization of an obsession will result in an increase in the frequency and salience of the obsession, as well as in subjective discomfort. Rachman et al. (1996) investigated the effects of neutralization in students who exhibited a thought–action fusion bias. After completing a task that provoked unwanted harming thoughts, individuals allowed to neutralize reported significant reductions in guilt, estimates of the probability of threat, responsibility for the threat, judgments of immorality, and urge to neutralize. The authors concluded that neutralization has a functional similarity to overt compulsions.

Although neutralization may lead to an immediate reduction in discomfort and other negative appraisals, over the longer term it is associated with an increase in distress and urge to neutralize. In an experiment involving students exposed to an audiotape of their unwanted intrusive thoughts, those who neutralized experienced more discomfort during subsequent presentations of the intrusion, a greater urge to neutralize, and an increased rate of actual neutralizing activity (Salkovskis et al., 1997).

Summary

There can be little doubt that Salkovskis's theory and research on the cognitive basis of obsessions has reignited interest in OCD. The two key constructs of his model, appraisals/beliefs of responsibility and neutralization, are clearly core elements in the persistence of obsessions. However, many questions remain. The critical defining elements of inflated responsibility for harm are still not well understood, the contextual or situational aspects of the construct need further investigation, its specificity and sensitivity to all subtypes of OCD are in question, and its role and function in the persistence of obsessive and compulsive symptoms require more research. Although inflated responsibility is often apparent in obsessional states, it is evident that its significance may be overstated in Salkovskis's formulation. This has led cognitive-behavioral researchers to consider other cognitive constructs that may be even more robust in obsessional conditions.

RACHMAN'S MISINTERPRETATION OF SIGNIFICANCE THEORY

Description of the Model

Rachman (1997, 1998, 2003) proposed a cognitive theory of obsessions that is a refinement and reformulation of an earlier, more behavioral account presented in *Obsessions and Compulsions* (Rachman & Hodgson, 1980). On the basis of D. M. Clark's (1986) cognitive theory of panic and Salkovskis's (1985) cognitive-behavioral formulation of obsessions, Rachman asserts that normal unwanted intrusive thoughts escalate into obsessions when a person misinterprets the intrusive thought as a personally important and threatening phenomenon. Like the inflated responsibility model, Rachman's cognitive theory starts with the premise that unwanted intrusive thoughts, images, or impulses are universally experienced. These naturally occurring unwanted thoughts become the basis of obsessions when individuals misinterpret their mental intrusions in a personally significant and threatening manner (Rachman, 2003). Rachman proposes that a number of key cognitive concepts and processes are involved in the escalation of "normal" unwanted intrusive thoughts into highly persistent clinical obsessions.

Misinterpretations of Significance

The central tenet of Rachman's cognitive theory is that obsessions are caused by a "catastrophic misinterpretation of the significance of one's intrusive thoughts/images/impulses" (Rachman, 1998, p. 385). Obsessions persist as long as the misinterpretations of significance continue but will decrease when the misinterpretations are weakened or eliminated (Rachman, 1997, 2003). Misinterpretations of significance involve the erroneous view that an intrusive thought is a sign or indication of something meaningful about one's character. The meaning attached to the intrusive thought is important, because it signifies something about the person that could lead to very serious negative consequences. Often the feared negative consequences involve losing control, harming others, acting violent or unpredictable, making mistakes, or causing accidents, sickness, or injury. An example of a catastrophic misinterpretation of significance is evident in a female day care worker who complained of very upsetting, repetitive intrusive thoughts that she might have inappropriately touched a child in her care. She found these unwanted intrusive thoughts extremely distressing because she worried that the thoughts meant she had latent desires to molest children. Her great fear was that she might snap, lose control, and then actually cause harm to a child. As a result, she tried to avoid any physical contact with children and was deciding on whether she should quit her job. Interestingly, she did not develop any overt or covert compulsions or neutralization strategies but instead relied on avoidance to limit her obsessional ruminations.

Rachman (1997, 2003) defined misinterpretations of significance in terms of the following five dimensions:

- *Importance.* The cognitive intrusion is viewed as meaningful, not trivial, because it reveals something about the person.
- *Personalized.* The significance of the intrusive thought is personal in that it is "my own thought of particular importance to me."
- *Ego-alien.* The content or theme of the intrusion is "unlike me, uncharacteristic of me."
- *Potential consequences.* The cognitive intrusion is viewed as having potential consequences, no matter how unlikely.
- *Serious consequences.* The perceived consequences associated with the intrusion are considered serious, usually involving some intolerable degree of threat, harm, or danger.

Rachman (1998) states that an unwanted intrusive thought can escalate into a persistent obsession only if it is misinterpreted as *personally significant* and as *signifying a threat.* Furthermore, which intrusive thought becomes obsessional depends on whether it is "important in the patient's system of values" (Rachman, 1998, p. 390). For example, if a person strongly values being courteous and nonviolent, then the emergence of intrusive thoughts, images, or impulses of perpetrating aggressive actions against others will be particularly unwelcome and distressing. The content of the intrusion, then, determines which thoughts will become obsessive and which neutral cues will be converted into threat stimuli (Rachman, 2003).

Vulnerable individuals are most likely to attach excessive importance to ego-dystonic intrusive thoughts involving unacceptable sexuality, harmful or aggressive impulses, bizarre and puzzling content, or shocking or extremist themes, which will then be interpreted as immoral, dangerous, or a sign of insanity or an antisocial character, respectively (Rachman, 1998, 2003). Of course, which of these thoughts is misinterpreted as significant depends on the value system, current concerns, and mood state of the individual. In this regard, O'Connor (2002; O'Connor & Robillard, 1995) argues that a faulty inferential reasoning process underlies obsessional thinking, so the person can construct a completely fictional threatening narrative based on the remotest of possibilities. In addition, people are also more likely to make catastrophic misinterpretations of the significance of their intrusive thoughts when they are depressed.

Frequency and Persistence of Obsessions

Rachman (1998) argues that two processes are primarily responsible for an increase in the frequency of unwanted, ego-dystonic cognitive intrusions. First, interpreting a thought as personally significant can increase the range and seriousness of potentially threatening stimuli. A wider range of neutral stimuli are thereby converted into a potential threat because they trigger the intrusive thought. This leads to an increase in situations that will provoke the obsessive intrusive thought, and so an increase in its frequency. Second, internal sensations of anxiety (e.g., trembling, sweating, etc.) can be misinterpreted as signs that one is losing control. The avoidance of such stimuli and the consequent reduction in anxiety will further reinforce this belief. "Hence, the catastrophic misinterpretation of one's anxiety can interact to increase the catastrophic misinterpretation of the intrusion" (Rachman, 1998, p. 386). Both internal signs of anxiety and external provocation cues for the obsession become signs of potential threat that lead to avoidance, which prevents exposure to any disconfirming evidence against the person's belief in the potential danger in his or her thoughts. Because more frequent intrusive thoughts are more salient and more difficult to control, a vicious cycle ensues, producing increasingly more frequent unwanted intrusive thoughts.

Obsessions are persistent because neutralization responses and avoidance behavior prevent disconfirmation that there is no catastrophic consequence to the obsession (Rachman, 1998, 2003). Moreover, the occurrence of bodily sensations (i.e., anxiety) is interpreted as a sign that danger is imminent and so confers great importance to the intrusive thought. Lack of control over the obsession despite repeated efforts is interpreted as a lack of control over one's impulses. Thus, an increase in the frequency of the unwanted ego-dystonic intrusive thought is taken as further proof of its significance.

Other Cognitive Processes

Rachman (1997, 1998, 2003) recognizes that there are a number of other cognitive processes involved in the pathogenesis of obsessions that contribute to the catastrophic misinterpretation of personal significance. He first proposed the concept *thought–action fusion* (TAF) to refer to the tendency of obsession- prone individuals to equate thoughts with actions (Rachman, 1993). TAF is defined as "the psychological phenomenon in which the patient appears to regard the obsessional thought and the forbidden action as being morally equivalent and/or feeling that the obsessional thought increases the probability of the feared event" (Rachman & Shafran, 1998, p. 72).

Two types of TAF are evident in OCD. Likelihood (Probability) TAF refers to the belief that thinking about a disturbing event will make the event more probable or likely to happen (e.g., "if I think about an accident it is more likely to happen"), whereas Moral TAF is the belief that having obsessional thoughts is morally equivalent to engaging in forbidden actions (e.g., "thinking about exposing one's self is as bad as actually doing it") (Rachman & Shafran, 1998; Shafran, Thordarson, & Rachman, 1996). Both types of TAF are considered cognitive biases that constitute a vulnerability for obsessionality. Individuals who show such TAF bias are more likely to make misinterpretations of personal significance and appraisals of excessive responsibility in response to their unwanted ego-dystonic cognitive intrusions.

Rachman (1997, 2003) acknowledges that *inflated responsibility* can take the form of either an appraisal of the intrusive thought or a particular type of belief. Responsibility beliefs may contribute to making catastrophic misinterpretations of significance for unwanted intrusive thoughts. Moreover, inflated responsibility may be both a cause and an effect of the TAF bias. However, appraisals of personal responsibility associated with unwanted cognitive intrusions will lead to feelings of blame and guilt for having such horrible, disgusting intrusive thoughts, images, or impulses.

Neutralization

Neutralization, defined as "an attempt to 'put right' the obsession, to cancel its effects, or prevent a feared outcome" (Rachman & Shafran, 1998, p. 53), persists because it is partly successful. It brings temporary relief (i.e., significant reductions in anxiety/discomfort), but it indirectly preserves the causal misinterpretations and anticipated consequences of the intrusive thought (Rachman, 1997, 2003). "Successful" neutralization reinforces the patient's belief that the neutralization response was responsible for preventing a feared event from occurring, or that the discomfort caused by the obsession would persist without the person's having engaged in neutralization (Rachman, 1998). Thus, neutralization is caused by, and then reinforces, the catastrophic misinterpretation of unwanted intrusions.

The role of neutralization is summed up in the following hypothesis: "The significance attached to an obsession will remain unchanged, or increase slightly, after repeated instances in which the obsession is followed by neutralization" (Rachman, 1998, p. 393). Temporary relief resulting from neutralization will confirm the patient's erroneous belief that the unwanted intrusive thought or obsession was dangerous and that neutralization was a necessary and effective way to deal with the upsetting obsession (Rachman, 2003). In this way neutralization contributes to the vicious escalating cycle of the obsession.

Rachman (1998) also recognized that *excessive thought control* is a consequence of catastrophic misinterpretations of significance. As the perceived significance or importance of an intrusion increases, the individual will engage in ever more vigorous attempts to suppress or control such thoughts. However, these control efforts are bound to fail, thereby, paradoxically, resulting in an increase in the frequency of the intrusion, which in turn will increase the significance ascribed to the thought (Rachman, 2003).

Cognitive Vulnerability

Rachman (1993, 1997, 2003) noted that certain people may show a vulnerability or tendency toward making catastrophic misinterpretations of significance when they experience unwanted ego-dystonic intrusive thoughts, images, or impulses. Four possible vulnerability pathways to obsessions were highlighted:

1. *Moral perfectionism.* Individuals may be taught that all of their value-laden thoughts are of great significance and so strive to be moral in all thought and action.

2. *Preexisting cognitive beliefs and biases.* Individuals may have inflated responsibility beliefs and TAF biases (e.g., "Immoral thoughts are as bad as immoral actions"; "It is my responsibility not to think such evil thoughts").

3. *Depression.* This may increase the tendency to interpret an individual's cognitive intrusions in a negative way because of the activation of depressogenic schemas.

4. *Anxiety proneness (high-trait anxiety).* Individuals who react with anxiety to a wide range of stimuli will experience more intrusive thoughts in response to stressors.

Cognitive Theory of Compulsive Checking

Rachman (2002) proposed a specific application of cognitive theory to explain the persistence of compulsive checking. The central feature of this proposal is that compulsive checking occurs when individuals perceive heightened responsibility to prevent harm but feel unsure as to whether they have adequately reduced or removed the harm. To be certain that the harmful event will not occur, they repeatedly check for safety. Although checking may provide temporary reduction in anxiety/distress, it is also associated with a number of other adverse effects that will paradoxically ensure continued repetition of the checking behavior.

Checking for safety can never provide the desired level of certainty that the likelihood of future harm to self or others has been eliminated, because such certainty for future events is elusive. This ensures that the compulsive checking will continue indefinitely. Second, repeated checking clouds individuals' memory of their checking behavior because of the interfering effects of anxious arousal. They are so intently focused on the threat and their emotional reactions that they fail to recall specific details of their checking. Low confidence in their memory of their checking behavior will reduce certainty that safety is established and so increase the likelihood that checking is repeated. Furthermore, negative or catastrophic misinterpretations about the importance of "not remembering" will contribute to an escalation in the checking behavior (e.g., "I must be really stupid or irresponsible because I'm not sure I completely locked the door").

Third, for individuals with inflated responsibility, checking will increase the perceived probability of the harmful consequence. Finally, checking behavior will increase an individual's sense of personal responsibility after a check for safety is completed. Because of the adverse effects of checking for safety, a self-perpetuating cycle is established that ensures that "one check is never enough."

The cognitive basis of compulsive checking centers on two key concepts (Rachman, 2002). The belief that one has special inflated responsibility to protect self or others from harm is a critical cognitive factor in compulsive checking. Second, the maladaptive misinterpretation of the significance of one's out-of-control, repetitive checking and poor memory will also contribute to a conviction that further checking is needed. On the basis of this cognitive formulation, Rachman (2002) proposed that cognitive-behavioral treatment of compulsive checking must include:

- Modification of the belief that one has special responsibility to protect self or others from harm
- Change in the misinterpretation of one's checking behavior and low confidence in memory
- Use of response prevention to challenge beliefs about the need to ensure safety and the elimination of potential harm

Rachman's formulation is an example of how cognitive models can be tailored to the unique phenomenology of different subtypes of OCD. Because this is a very recent proposal, Rachman's predictions about the cognitive mechanisms of compulsive checking have not yet been empirically tested.

Empirical Status

Hypothesis 1

A key hypothesis of Rachman's model is that obsessions are characterized by a catastrophic misinterpretation of personal importance or significance involving threat. Clinical observation confirms that individuals with OCD usually place exaggerated importance on their obsessions (see review by Thordarson & Shafran, 2002). However, a specific prediction of this hypothesis is that obsessional thoughts will be evaluated as more personally significant than nonobsessional intrusive cognitions, and that individuals with OCD will be more likely to misinterpret their ego-dystonic intrusive thoughts as personally significant as compared with nonclinical individuals.

There is empirical evidence that individuals with OCD appraise their obsessions as more important or significant than nonclinical individuals (controls), and that frequent obsessive-like intrusive thoughts are characterized by heightened personal significance as indicated by higher ratings of importance, unacceptability, or self-referent meaningfulness (e.g., Clark & Claybourn, 1997; Freeston et al., 1991; Freeston & Ladouceur,

1993; Parkinson & Rachman, 1981a; Rachman & de Silva, 1978; see also findings from the thought suppression experiments of Janeck & Calamari, 1999; Purdon, 2001). Rowa and Purdon (2003) found that students rated certain intrusive thoughts more upsetting because they contradicted important and valued aspects of the self. In two studies conducted by the OCCWG, the OCD group scored significantly higher on the Interpretations of Intrusions Inventory (III) Importance of Thoughts subscale than nonobsessional anxious and nonclinical control groups (OCCWG, 2001, 2003a). The III Importance subscale includes items that assess thought–action fusion, significance of the intrusion for the self, and significance attached to the mere occurrence of the intrusion (OCCWG, 1997). Together these findings support Rachman's assertion that obsessions are characterized by misinterpretations of personal significance and that the significance and distress of an intrusive thought may be greater for thoughts that are contrary to valued aspects of the self.

Rachman's formulation of a catastrophic misinterpretation of unwanted ego-dystonic intrusions includes not only the element of personal significance but also the element of exaggerated threat estimation. The person considers the intrusive thought important because it is interpreted as a sign (1) that something negative or threatening might happen, (2) that somehow the occurrence of the obsession will make this negative consequence more likely, and/or (3) that one is more likely to lose control because of the thought intrusion (see Purdon, 2002). Other researchers have also commented that OCD is characterized by an overestimation of the probability and severity of future harm or threat (Carr, 1974; Kozak, Foa, & McCathy, 1988; Steketee, Frost, Rhéaume, & Wilhelm, 1998; Sookman & Pinard, 2002).

There is empirical evidence that individuals with OCD overestimate the probability and severity of threat and are thus generally less risk taking. Individuals with OCD provide significantly lower risk taking scores, even for everyday activities, than nonclinical subjects (Steiner, 1972; Steketee & Frost, 1994). Foa et al. (2001) found that individuals with OCD overestimated harm and their responsibility to prevent that harm, particularly in low-risk (i.e., benign) situations, significantly more than those in generalized social phobia and nonclinical control groups. Jones and Menzies (1997) found that danger expectancies, as indicated by ratings of likelihood and severity of catching a disease after exposure to dirt/contamination, were the only variables to significantly predict level of anxiety, urge to wash, and time spent washing hands (see also Menzies et al., 2000).

Some inconsistencies have emerged in the literature. Woods, Frost, and Steketee (2002) found that perceived coping ability, but not estimates of the probability or severity of threatening obsessive–compulsive-relevant future events, predicted obsessive–compulsive symptoms as measured by the Padua Inventory. Elevated threat estimates have not always been associated with other obsessive–compulsive-relevant constructs such as inflated responsibility (Lopataka & Rachman, 1995). Overestimation of threat is also characteristic of other forms of anxiety such as worry (Constans, 2001; Suarez & Bell-Dolan, 2001).

Overall, we can conclude that there is evidence that individuals with OCD misinterpret the significance of their obsessions and overestimate the probability and severity of obsessive–compulsive-relevant negative consequences. However, it is also clear that these processes are evident in other forms of anxiety, especially worry. What is unknown is whether there are particular features of personal significance and threat interpretations in OCD (e.g., their ego-dystonic relation to core personal values) that distinguish these constructs from their role in other anxiety states.

Hypothesis 2

Rachman (2003) hypothesized that certain cognitive bias, like inflated responsibility and TAF, are associated with vulnerability to obsessions. One of the more promising constructs in Rachman's reformulation of obsessions is his proposal that the cognitive bias, thought–action fusion (TAF), can serve to inflate the significance of obsessional thinking (Rachman & Shafran, 1999; see also Thordarson & Shafran, 2002). Both types of TAF, Probability and Morality, are closely connected with inflated responsibility.

There is evidence that individuals with OCD score significantly higher on measures of TAF Probability than nonclinical individuals (controls), although findings are very inconsistent for TAF Morality (Shafran et al., 1996; Rassin, Merckelbach, Muris, & Schmidt, 2001). The latter TAF construct appears to have a strong relationship with religiosity (Rassin & Koster, 2003). In other studies nonobsessional anxious and OCD patient groups did not differ significantly in their levels of TAF bias (Rassin, Diepstraten, Merckelbach, & Muris, 2001; Rassin, Merckelbach, et al., 2001). There is further evidence that TAF may be *more* specific to at least some obsessional symptoms than to depression or worry (Coles et al., 2001; Emmelkamp & Aardema, 1999; Rachman, Thordarson, & Radomsky, 1995; Rassin, Merckelbach, et al., 2001). Yet other studies suggest that TAF also correlates with measures of other anxious symptoms (e.g., pathological worry) and possibly even depression, although its relation to obsessional symptoms tends to be stronger (Hazlett-Stevens, Zucker, & Craske, 2002; Muris, Meesters, Rasssin, Merckelbach, & Campbell, 2001). Furthermore, TAF does appear to be a significant correlate of the frequency, emotional intensity, and perceived control of obsessions in clinical and nonclinical samples (Clark et al., 2000; Purdon & Clark, 1994a, 1994b; Smári & Hólmsteinsson, 2001). It may be that TAF Probability, especially the likelihood of negative events happening to a friend/relative, has a closer and more specific relationship with obsessionality than TAF Morality (Clark et al., 2000; Shafran et al., 1996).

Given that TAF bias contributes to inflated interpretations of significance, an interaction between TAF and thought suppression might be expected. In a nonclinical correlational study, Rassin, Muris, Schmidt, and Merckelbach (2000) found evidence that TAF bias may lead to suppression effects and that suppression in turn results in obsessive–compulsive symptoms. However, the connection between TAF and thought suppression was not confirmed in a later clinical study (Rassin, Diepstraten, et al., 2001). TAF bias and tendency to engage in thought suppression were uncorrelated, and both constructs showed significant reductions with treatment. Moreover, high pretreatment TAF and thought suppression did not influence treatment response in either individuals with OCD or subjects with other anxiety disorders.

Amir, Freshman, Ramsey, Neary, and Brigidi (2001) investigated whether a TAF bias might also be present with positive events (i.e., "by thinking about a positive event, it is more likely to happen"). They found that students who scored high on the Obsessive–Compulsive Inventory had higher TAF Likelihood for both positive and negative events than the low-scoring group. Amir and colleagues concluded that TAF may be a more general form of "magical" thinking that is evident even outside obsessive–compulsive-relevant situations.

There is some experimental evidence that TAF bias may be a causal factor in the pathogenesis of obsessions. In the first published experiment involving a TAF manipulation, Rachman et al. (1996) reported that students preselected for a tendency to engage in TAF bias showed significant increases in anxiety, guilt, and opportunity to neutralize subsequent to the TAF manipulation (Rachman et al., 1996). Rassin, Merckelbach, Muris, and Spaan (1999) investigated the causal relationship between TAF, responsibility, and obsessive intrusions in a bogus EEG experiment involving 45 nonclinical participants who were assigned to either an experimental or control condition. The experimental condition, which constituted a TAF manipulation (i.e., thinking of "apple" causes harm to a confederate), resulted in significantly more "apple" thought intrusions, more discomfort, and greater effort to avoid thinking of apple than the control condition. These results, then, indicate that experimentally induced TAF does result in more thought intrusions, discomfort, resistance, and neutralization responses to about 50% of participants' intrusions.

Rassin (2001) exposed 40 students to a TAF manipulation in which they wrote a sentence stating that they hoped a close friend/family member would have a car accident. Half the group were then told *to suppress* any thought of the accident, and the other half were told to think anything they like and *not to suppress* thoughts about the accident. Contrary to prediction, active thought suppression appeared to actually relieve the discomfort caused by the TAF manipulation and to reduce the amount of time spent thinking about the accident. Rassin concluded that intentional thought suppression might actually be an effective strategy for reducing the stress caused by TAF, at least in the short term.

Summary

Research on the key predictions of the misinterpretation of significance theory of obsessions is still in its infancy. However, there is already empirical support for the some of the main tenets of the model. Inflated misinterpretations of significance, especially TAF bias, and possibly overestimations of threat are involved in the pathogenesis of clinical and nonclinical obsessive intrusive thoughts. Furthermore, experimental manipulations of significance, by inflating either TAF or personal responsibility, have resulted in increased unwanted intrusions, greater discomfort, and neutralization, which suggests that TAF, in particular, may have a causal influence on obsessions.

It is also clear that misinterpretations of significance, including TAF bias, are not specific or unique to OCD. Currently, evidence is lacking as to whether TAF bias, inflated responsibility, and other appraisals of significance are true vulnerability constructs that play a critical role in the etiology of obsessions. Which particular features of these constructs make them pathological is still not clear. For example, TAF Likelihood for Others may be more relevant to OCD than TAF Likelihood for Self, and TAF Morality may be more common and less pathological than originally postulated (Rachman et al., 1996). TAF bias may be related to a broader form of "magical thinking" that is not confined to obsessive–compulsive-relevant contexts. Thus, individuals may evidence TAF cognitive bias to positive events as well as obsessive–compulsive-relevant negative or threatening circumstances. TAF Likelihood does appear to have greater relevance to obsessional thinking, but evidence of more moderate relationships with other anxiety phenomena, like worry, indicates that TAF bias is not entirely specific to OCD.

Finally, the relationship between significance appraisals (i.e., TAF bias) and active attempts to control unwanted intrusions and neutralize their deleterious effects may be more complicated than first anticipated. It appears that both neutralization and intentional thought suppression can mitigate, at least in the short term, the heightened discomfort caused by misinterpretations of significance (i.e., TAF). Although the empirical status of the model remains to be determined, Rachman (2003) proposed a new cognitive-behavioral treatment of obsessions that directly follows from the present cognitive formulation.

THE OBSESSIVE COMPULSIVE COGNITIONS WORKING GROUP

Description of the Model

At the World Congress of Behavioral and Cognitive Therapies in Denmark (July 1995), a small group of researchers interested in the cognitive basis of OCD agreed to collaborate in the development and evaluation of self-report measures and laboratory procedures on the cognitive basis of OCD. Called the Obsessive Compulsive Cognitions Working Group (OCCWG), the group has grown to 46 participants from nine countries. Under the leadership of Gail Steketee and Randy Frost, the group has sponsored several research meetings and has developed a self-report measure of obsessional beliefs called the Obsessive Beliefs Questionnaire (OBQ) and a measure of obsessional appraisals called the Interpretation of Intrusions Inventory (III).

At its third research meeting, the OCCWG issued a consensus statement on the primary and secondary belief domains of OCD (OCCWG, 1997). The working group also clarified the three levels of conceptualization that constitute the cognitive basis of OCD.

- *Intrusions.* Unwanted thoughts, images, or impulses that intrude into consciousness and are called obsessions when they attain clinical severity
- *Appraisals.* Expectations, interpretations, or evaluations of the meaning of particular phenomena such as unwanted intrusive thoughts
- *Assumptions (beliefs).* Relatively enduring ideas that are pan-situational and that may be specific to OCD or may be general assumptions about one's self, that are also relevant to other clinical disorders

Discussion of the relevant OCD literature and existing measures of obsessive–compulsive cognition resulted in the identification of 19 potential obsessive–compulsive belief domains (OCCWG, 1997). The OCCWG participants then rank ordered the 19 domains in terms of their specificity to OCD and etiologic importance. Six major belief domains were identified as having etiologic importance and probable specificity to OCD (see also Freeston, Rhéaume, & Ladouceur, 1996). Table 5.2 presents definitions of the six belief domains developed by the OCCWG (1997). Beliefs in the overimportance of mental control deserve special mention because a number of aspects of mental control relevant to obsessional thinking were identified. The maladaptive aspects of this belief domain focus on (1) the importance of monitoring and being hypervigilant for

TABLE 5.2. The Six Belief Domains of OCD Proposed by the OCCWG

Belief domain	Definition
Inflated responsibility	"the belief that one has power which is pivotal to bring about or prevent subjectively crucial negative outcomes" (OCCWG, 1997, p. 677)
Overimportance of thoughts	"beliefs that the mere presence of a thought indicates that it is important" (OCCWG, 1997, p. 678)
Overestimation of threat	"an exaggeration of the probability or severity of harm" (OCCWG, 1997, p. 678)
Importance of controlling thoughts	"the overvaluation of the importance of exerting complete control over intrusive thoughts, images and impulses, and the belief that this is both possible and desirable" (OCCWG, 1997, p. 678)
Intolerance of uncertainty	Beliefs about the necessity of being certain, the personal inability to cope with unpredictable change, and difficulty in functioning in ambiguous situations
Perfectionism	"the tendency to believe there is a perfect solution to every problem, that doing something perfectly (i.e., mistake free) is not only possible but also necessary, and that even minor mistakes will have serious consequences" (OCCWG, 1997, p. 678)

certain types of mental events, (2) the moral consequences of not control-ling thoughts, (3) the psychological and behavioral consequences of fail-ure to control thoughts, and (4) the efficiency of mental control (i.e., "One can achieve complete suppression of unwanted thoughts"). The first five belief domains were thought to be specific to OCD, whereas the sixth domain, perfectionism, was considered important but not exclusive to OCD (see also Taylor, 2002).

Empirical Status

Prior to the major research initiative of the OCCWG, a few studies investi-gated dysfunctional beliefs in OCD. Despite using different belief mea-sures, many of these studies reported that maladaptive beliefs concerning responsibility, threat estimation, intolerance of uncertainty, need for thought control, and/or importance of thoughts were significantly associ-ated with obsessive–compulsive symptom measures and that patients with OCD tended to score higher on the belief instruments than nonclinical control subjects (e.g., Clark, Purdon, & Wang, 2003; Freeston, Ladouceur, Gagnon, & Thibodeau, 1993; Sookman, Pinard, & Beck, 2001; Steketee, Frost, & Cohen, 1998). However, other studies found that certain obses-sion-relevant beliefs, like responsibility, perfectionism, and control of thoughts, did not have a significant unique relationship with obsessive–compulsive symptom measures (Emmelkamp & Aardema, 1999; Steketee, Frost, & Cohen, 1998; Wells & Papageorgiou, 1998). There was preliminary but inconsistent evidence that intolerance of uncertainty, and importance and control of thoughts (including TAF), might have some degree of specificity to obsessionality (Clark et al., 2003; Emmelkamp & Aardema, 1999; Steketee, Frost, & Cohen, 1998). However, need for certainty had minimal relationship to obsessional symptoms in a nonclinical Italian sample (Mancini, D'Olimpio, del Genio, Didonna, & Prunetti, 2002), whereas intolerance of uncertainty may be elevated only in compulsive checkers (Tolin, Abramowitz, Brigidi, & Foa, 2003).

The most authoritative investigation of dysfunctional beliefs in OCD was undertaken by the OCCWG (1997). This collaborative research effort enabled the development of more elaborated and finely tuned measures of obsessive–compulsive beliefs and appraisals, and it also allowed the group to generate large clinical and nonclinical databases by pooling across multiple treatment sites. Two studies were conducted. The first study, referred to as the Stage II data, included 101 individuals with OCD, 374 students, and 76 nonclinical community adults, who completed a battery of instruments that included an earlier 129-item version of the OBQ and a 43-item III (OCCWG, 2001). Psychometric analyses led to an item reduction of both measures. Thus, in a second Stage III study involving 248 patients with OCD, 105 people with other anxiety disorders, 87 nonclinical community control subjects, and 291 students, an 87-item OBQ and 31-item III were administered as part of the assessment battery (OCCWG, 2003a, 2003b).

A number of findings emerged from these large-scale studies. The six belief domains proposed by the OCCWG can be reliably measured by the self-report measures developed by the group. Three of the belief domains were highly relevant to OCD, as evidenced by substantial correlations with obsessive–compulsive symptom measures and the elevated scores of obsessive–compulsive patients over those of nonobsessional anxious and nonclinical control subjects (i.e., control of thoughts, importance of thoughts, and responsibility). However, all six belief domains were significantly related to other clinical phenomena such as worry, anxiety, and posttraumatic stress disorder (PTSD), although they may relate more strongly to obsessionality. In a further analysis of the Stage III data, OBQ Responsibility and Perfectionism/Intolerance of Uncertainty were the only significant predictors of obsessive–compulsive symptoms, although the OCD group did not score significantly higher than the anxious group on the latter OBQ subscale (OCCWG, 2003b). In a study of the OBQ and the III in an Italian clinical sample, Intolerance of Uncertainty, Control of Thoughts, and Perfectionism were quite specific to OCD, whereas Importance of Thoughts and Responsibility barely discriminated between patients with OCD and nonclinical control subjects (Sica et al., in press). Finally, a tendency to monitor and reflect on one's thought processes, which may have relevance to overimportance and control of thoughts, emerged as a specific characteristic of OCD (Janeck, Calamari, Riemann, & Heffelfinger, 2003).

Summary

Research on the specific cognitive appraisals and beliefs of OCD is still preliminary. Until recently, work in this area has been hampered by the lack of reliable and valid measures of obsessive–compulsive-specific beliefs and appraisals. The work of the OCCWG has resulted in the most comprehensive and accurate self-report measures of obsessive–compulsive appraisals and beliefs. The consensus among researchers and the investigation of their psychometric properties on two large international data sets is a feat in itself. In addition, it is now evident that appraisals and beliefs of inflated responsibility, overimportance of thoughts, control of thoughts, overestimation of threat, intolerance of uncertainty, and perfectionism constitute a cognitive profile of OCD. The implication of these cognitive constructs for treatment response or their etiological status remains to be determined.

There are also a number of conceptual problems that plague this research. There is a very high correlation between the III and the OBQ, suggesting that the distinction between beliefs and appraisals may be more difficult to delineate, at least with self-report measures (OCCWG, 2001, 2003a, 2003b; Sica et al., in press). In addition, the six belief domains were highly intercorrelated, which calls into question whether they assess distinct cognitive constructs. It is clear that certain beliefs, like responsibility, overimportance of thoughts, control of thoughts, and intolerance of uncertainty, may be specific to OCD, whereas overestimation of threat and perfectionism are nonspecific factors. However, even this statement must be accepted with caution because of the inconsistent findings across studies. An edited volume by the OCCWG provides a more detailed review of the theoretical and empirical status of the six belief domains; importance of thoughts (Thordarson & Shafran, 2002), control of thoughts (Purdon & Clark, 2002), responsibility (Salkovskis & Forrester, 2002), overestimation of threat and intolerance of uncertainty (Sookman & Pinard, 2002), and perfectionism (Frost, Novara, & Rhéaume, 2002).

SUMMARY AND CONCLUSION

The three cognitive appraisal theories of OCD presented in this chapter all assume that faulty appraisals of unwanted intrusive thoughts, images, or impulses and the subsequent attempts to neutralize the unwanted intrusions are the two key processes involved in the etiology and persistence of obsessions. However, unwanted intrusions will escalate into clinical obsessions for only a small number of highly vulnerable individuals. This predisposition to obsessional thinking is characterized by endorsement of certain enduring maladaptive beliefs, the presence of cognitive biases like TAF, and reliance on excessive and dysfunctional thought control strategies (i.e., neutralization, compulsions, thought suppression). Although the appraisal models differ in the relative emphasis placed on certain cognitive constructs, most cognitive-clinical researchers of OCD are convinced that inflated responsibility, TAF, misinterpretations of significance, overestimated threat, overimportance of thought, control of thoughts, intolerance of uncertainty, and perfectionism are highly relevant cognitive features of OCD.

Empirical investigations of the new appraisal theories of OCD are very recent and thus much work remains to be done. At this point we can conclude that inflated responsibility, TAF Likelihood bias, intolerance of uncertainty, overimportance of thought, and control of thought may be highly relevant and possibly specific cognitive features of OCD. Moreover, there is evidence that the faulty appraisal of unwanted intrusive thoughts (or obsessions) along these dimensions will lead to an increase in the frequency of the intrusion, distress, and urge to neutralize. Yet there are many inconsistent findings that leave us with more questions than answers. The level of specificity of these variables to OCD has not been established. It may be that many of these appraisals are only relatively more evident in OCD. Their function in other clinical disorders like generalized anxiety disorder remains to be established. Furthermore, it may be that certain appraisals are evident only in a particular OCD subtype (e.g., inflated responsibility may be specific to compulsive checking). The high correlation between different appraisal constructs calls into question whether we are dealing with distinct or largely overlapping variables. Finally, the etiological status of these variables has not been investigated. It is entirely possible that the faulty appraisals and beliefs noted by Rachman, Salkovskis, and others is a consequence, rather than a cause, of obsessive–compulsive symptoms. Despite these many unanswered questions, cognitive-clinical researchers have been undeterred in crafting new treatment approaches to obsessions and compulsions derived from the models presented in this chapter.

CHAPTER 6

Thought Suppression and Obsessions

Issues of control are paramount in obsessional states. This is evident in the excessive efforts to exert mental control over an obsession and to resist powerful compulsive urges. Yet the manifestation of control in OCD takes a paradoxical form. On the one hand, the obsessional person struggles valiantly to prevent or suppress the upsetting obsession. As Salkovskis et al. (1995) noted, individuals with OCD "try too hard to exert control over their own cognitive function" (p. 284). They resort to counterproductive strategies such as compulsive rituals, avoidance, reassurance seeking, and rationalization in an effort to reestablish a sense of control over their minds. Yet, on the other hand, despite such efforts, one is struck with how little control such persons have over their obsessions and compulsions. Individuals with severe OCD will report almost continuous preoccupation with an obsessive thought. Any success in dismissing an obsession may be measured only in seconds or minutes, as the obsession reemerges into consciousness with even greater emotional intensity and strength. No wonder the person with OCD is left with the feeling of a complete breakdown of mental control.

This chapter focuses on the theory and research of intentional mental control proposed by Daniel Wegner (1994a). Wegner and colleagues found that the deliberate attempt to suppress unwanted thoughts leads to a paradoxical increase in the frequency and distressing quality of the unwanted thoughts, either immediately, or as soon as suppression efforts cease. The relevance of this research for the persistence of obsessions is obvious. Individuals with OCD exert enormous effort to prevent obsessions from entering conscious awareness or to dismiss the obsessions once they occur. And yet the person with OCD suffers from high rates of obsessional intrusive thoughts.

Could the paradoxical recurrence of obsessions be a product of the obsessional person's excessive thought control efforts? If individuals with OCD cease intentional mental control over the obsession, will its frequency and salience decline? Do individuals with OCD have a general deficit in their ability to suppress any thought (Wenzlaff & Wegner, 2000)? As will be evident in the following review, the role of the paradoxical effects of intentional thought suppression in the pathogenesis of obsession is not nearly as straightforward as first envisioned. Conceptual and methodological problems abound, results across studies are inconsistent, and some researchers are beginning to question whether thought suppression plays any appreciable role in the persistence of obsessions. A critical evaluation of the research on thought suppression is presented in the following discussion, and the chapter concludes with the consideration of an alternative experimental approach to the investigation of mental control in OCD.

THOUGHT SUPPRESSION EXPERIMENTS

It is readily apparent from introspection or clinical observation that human beings have poor mental control over unwanted, distressing thoughts and images, especially in dysphoric and anxious states (Rachman & Hodgson, 1980; Wegner, 1994a). Moreover, individuals with OCD have particular difficulties in ignoring or suppressing certain highly distressing, recurring obsessive thoughts (Likierman & Rachman, 1982; Rachman & de Silva, 1978). People also find it very difficult to suppress unwanted intrusive thoughts that are interpreted as highly significant, that tend to interrupt their thinking (i.e., highly intrusive, attention-grabbing cognitions), or that are highly distressing or personally unacceptable (Wegner, 1994a). Thus, at the best of times the ability to suppress unwanted thoughts is less than perfect. But the obsessions evident in OCD represent some of the worst conditions for thought suppression, and so it is not surprising that suppression does not achieve the desired end in OCD.

Salkovskis, Rachman, and others argue that it is the faulty appraisals of importance that are responsible for the persistence of obsessional thinking (see previous chapter). Daniel Wegner and his colleagues pose a different explanation for the persistence of recurring intrusive thoughts. They argue that the very act or process of engaging in thought suppression is primarily responsible for the persistence of recurring intrusive thoughts (Wenzlaff & Wegner, 2000). Wenzlaff and Wegner further state that suppression causes an escalation in the unwanted thought because the process of thought suppression increases the accessibility of the target thought.

Thought suppression, which refers to the intentional, conscious removal of a thought from attention, must be distinguished from *repression,* which is unintended, "unconscious" forgetting (Beevers, Wenzlaff, Hayes, & Scott, 1999). However, what is significant about Daniel Wegner's research is not the observation that mental control is limited. This is a self-evident truth, obvious to anyone who has tried in vain not to think about an annoying musical tune or a phrase that one continues to think over and over again. Instead, the significance of Wegner's research is his assertion that the intentional effortful suppression of unwanted intrusive thoughts will have the opposite effect—making the target thought even more frequent or accessible than if we either did nothing or purposefully expressed the thought (Wegner, 1994a; Wenzlaff & Wegner, 2000). That is, the harder we try to control or suppress an unwanted thought, the more likely we are to be preoccupied with the very thought we are trying to vanquish from our minds. In the concluding remarks of their review article, Wenzlaff and Wegner note that the problem with thought suppression is not that it is simply ineffective but, rather, that it is counterproductive, leading to an intensification of the very state of mind that a person attempts to avoid. Because of the paradoxical effects of thought suppression, Wenzlaff and Wegner (2000) conclude that thought suppression is an important causal factor in the etiology and maintenance of a number of psychological disorders, like posttraumatic stress disorder, OCD, and depression.

The paradoxical effect of thought suppression was first reported in a seminal study by Wegner, Schneider, Carter, and White (1987). In the first experiment involving a crossover design, students were randomly assigned to either suppress thoughts of a white bear for 5 minutes or to express white bear thoughts. In the second 5-minute interval participants were given opposite express-or-suppress instructions. During initial suppression students were unable to attain complete success, given that the white bear thought continued to occur more than once a minute. In addition, significantly more white bear intrusions occurred during expression following initial suppression ($M = 7.71$) than in an initial expression period ($M = 4.86$). The authors concluded that suppression paradoxically leads to a *rebound effect,* that is, a surge in the frequency of the target thought once suppression efforts cease. In a second experiment, the rebound effect was replicated (greater frequency of target thoughts when expression follows suppression), but an *immediate enhancement* effect was also found. Students in the initial suppression group had significantly more thought occurrences ($M = 9.17$) than individuals who initially expressed white bear thoughts ($M = 4.13$). The provision of a single distracter resulted in a weakening of the postsuppression rebound effect. Wegner et al. (1987) concluded that efforts to suppress a thought lead to both immediate and delayed tendencies to become consciously preoccupied with the to-be-suppressed cognition.

Ironic Process Theory

Why is the intentional suppression of an unwanted thought so counterproductive, leading to the very effects a person is trying to avoid? Wegner and colleagues (Wegner, 1994b; Wegner & Erber, 1992; Wenzlaff & Wegner, 2000) proposed the theory of ironic processes to explain the factors involved in the success or failure of mental control. Thought suppression, and its paradoxical effects, result from the interplay of two cognitive processes: an intentional operating process and an ironic monitoring process. The intentional operating process endeavors to create a desired state of mind (e.g., think anything but the to-be-suppressed thought) by seeking thoughts that will distract the person from the to-be-suppressed thought and so promote the desired state of mind. The operating process, however, is conscious and effortful and therefore demands considerable attentional resources. Once the operating process is successful, in that the person becomes attentionally focused on a distraction that is consistent with the desired state of mind, it will cease to function.

There is, however, a second cognitive process, called ironic monitoring, which is much more automatic and continuous, operating in the background of consciousness. This automatic monitoring process is ironic in that it searches for mental incidents that signal failure to achieve the desired mental state. In the case of thought suppression, the monitoring process remains vigilant for occurrences of the unwanted intrusive thought. When the monitoring process detects the unwanted thought, this is an indication of failure in mental control, and so it initiates the intentional operating process. Resurgence of the to-be-suppressed thought is more likely when suppression ceases (i.e., postsuppression rebound) or when a cognitive load disrupts the operating process, because the more automatic, effortless monitoring process will continue to search for the unwanted target thought long after the intentional search for distracters is terminated.

Wenzlaff and Wegner (2000) concluded that the ironic process theory offers the most complete account of thought suppression phenomena. Support for the model is provided by experiments showing that imposition of a cognitive load (e.g., count backward by 3's), while a person is trying to suppress an unwanted thought, actually enhances the paradoxical effects of thought suppression (for reviews see Wegner, 1994b; Wenzlaff & Wegner, 2000). However, the model does not specify when the automatic monitoring process ceases, nor does it include the influence of motivational factors on thought suppression (Wenzlaff & Wegner, 2000). Yet the greatest difficulty for the model may be the inconsistent evidence reported for immediate enhancement and rebound across a variety of studies.

Empirical Status of Thought Suppression

After more than a decade of research, it is uncertain whether the paradoxical effects of thought suppression are as robust as claimed by its progenitors. A number of critical reviews of this literature have been published (Abramowitz, Tolin, & Street, 2001; Purdon, 1999; Purdon & Clark, 2000; Rassin, Merckelbach, & Muris, 2000; Wenzlaff & Wegner, 2000).

Abramowitz et al. (2001) conducted a meta-analysis on 28 thought suppression experiments that met their inclusion criteria. There was no evidence of immediate enhancement, as indicated by a small negative effect size ($d+ = -0.35$). Contrary to prediction, the negative effect size indicates that on average the suppression group actually produced fewer thought intrusions during the initial period than the control group (express or monitor thinking). However, a positive, moderately sized weighted average effect was found ($d+ = 0.30$), indicating a significant rebound effect. The rebound effect size was significantly larger than the initial enhancement effects. The authors concluded that individuals can suppress their thoughts over a short period of time, as indicated by the relative absence of initial enhancement effects. As time progresses, or once people relax their suppression efforts, there is resurgence in the target thought. However, the authors note that even though the rebound effect size was significant, a value of 0.35 is considered quite small. Thus, the postsuppression rebound effect appears to be weaker and more transient than assumed by some reviewers.

Suppression of Neutral Thoughts

A simple review of thought suppression experiments involving *neutral target thoughts* with nonclinical volunteers reveals considerable inconsistency. Some studies found evidence of rebound effects (D. M. Clark, Ball, & Pape, 1991; D. M. Clark, Winton, & Thynn, 1993; Harvey & Bryant, 1999; Kelly & Kahn, 1994, experiment 2; Wegner et al., 1987, experiments 1 and 2; Wegner, Schneider, Knutson, & McMahon, 1991), others found no significant differences (Davies & D. M. Clark, 1998; Gaskell, Wells, & Calam, 2001; McNally & Ricciardi, 1996; Merckelbach, Muris, van den Hout, & de Jong, 1991; Muris, Merckelbach, & de Jong, 1993; Roemer & Borkovec, 1994; Rutledge, Hollenberg, & Hancock, 1993, experiment 1; Smári, Sigurjónsdóttir, & Sáemundsdóttir, 1994; Wegner, Shortt, Blake, & Page, 1990), and a very few researchers reported an initial enhancement effect (Lavy & van den Hout, 1990; Muris, Merckelbach, van den Hout, & de Jong, 1992; Wegner et al., 1987, experiment 1).

In four experiments Rutledge and her colleagues (Rutledge, 1998; Rutledge et al., 1993, experiment 2; Rutledge, Hancock, & Rutledge, 1996, experiments 1 and 2) found that only a minority of individuals exhibit the rebound effect. In three studies involving nonclinical participants and the white bear target thought, between 19–23% of participants met the defining criteria for rebound effect (Rutledge et al., 1993; Rutledge, Hancock, & Rutledge, 1996). Overall, then, the paradoxical effect of thought suppression is clearly a weak and inconsistent phenomenon, at least for nonclinical subjects suppressing neutral thoughts (see Rassin, Mercekelbach, & Muris, 2000, for an opposite conclusion).

Suppression of Personal, Emotional Thoughts

Wegner proposes that active, intentional thought suppression plays a causal role in the etiology of the unwanted thoughts that characterize many clinical disorders (Wegner, 1994a; Wenzlaff & Wegner, 2000). For example, Wegner (1994a, p. 167) states that "an obsession can grow from nothing but the desire to suppress a thought." If we assume that thought suppression is a critical process in the persistence of unwanted negative thoughts like obsessions, then we would predict that the paradoxical effects of suppression might be stronger with personal or emotionally charged target thoughts, or with clinical subjects. At the very least, given doubts that findings from experiments on the suppression of neutral thoughts can be generalized to the types of persistent cognitive activity we see in clinical disorders (Muris et al., 1992; Purdon, 1999), research on the suppression of more clinically relevant cognitive material is necessary.

In one of the first studies on the suppression of emotional thoughts, Wenzlaff, Wegner, and Roper (1988) found that highly dysphoric students who suppressed thoughts about a negative event over a 9-minute interval showed a significant increase in the target thought during the final 3-minute time interval. The low dysphoric group showed a steady decline in the frequency of the target thought. Moreover, the effect was not as pronounced when the dysphoric participants suppressed thoughts of a positive event. Further analysis revealed that the nondysphoric students tended to use positive thoughts to distract themselves from the target, whereas the dysphoric students used other negative thoughts as distracters because they were more accessible. The findings of Wenzlaff et al. (1988), then, suggest that individuals with a clinical disturbance might be less effective in suppressing disorder-relevant thoughts (i.e., more likely to experience resurgence in unwanted thoughts) because they use less effective control strategies (i.e., distracters that are more likely to cue the to-be-suppressed thought).

In the past decade, a number of other researchers have investigated the suppression of personal, negative thoughts. Among nonclinical participants who suppressed either normative or idiosyncratic, personally relevant negative material, initial enhancement or postsuppression rebound was found in some studies (Davies & D. M. Clark, 1998) but not in others (Gaskell et al., 2001; Muris et al., 1992; Rassin, 2001; Roemer & Borkovec, 1994; Rutledge et al., 1993, experiment 1). In fact, Kelly and Kahn (1994) found a rebound effect for suppression of white bear thoughts, but not when individuals suppressed their own intrusive thoughts. They concluded that intentional suppression of an individual's personal thoughts will diminish the subsequent occurrence of these thoughts. Unfortunately, experiments involving analogue samples (high scores on a symptom measure) or clinical patients have not produced clearer results (see Becker, Rinck, Roth, & Margraf, 1998; Conway et al., 1991; Harvey & Bryant, 1998, 1999). Salkovskis and Reynolds (1994) obtained evidence that individuals trying to quit smoking experienced initial enhancement but not a rebound effect when they tried to suppress smoking-related intrusive thoughts.

Together the findings from these studies indicate that the paradoxical effects of suppression are not stronger when nonclinical subjects suppress more personal, or even distressing, thoughts. In fact, suppression of personal unwanted thoughts may be more effective than suppression of a neutral or irrelevant thought like "white bears." For individuals with high negative affect or a clinical disturbance, initial enhancement or postsuppression rebound may not be more apparent, even when individuals attempt to suppress distressing cognitions. However, it may be that individuals with a clinical disturbance are relatively less successful at suppressing their unwanted distressing thoughts than nonclinical subjects. What is less clear is whether this "impaired mental control" actually translates into the paradoxical effects of thought suppression (i.e., enhancement or rebound) predicted by Wegner's model. Purdon (1999) provides a detailed review and critique of the role of thought suppression in psychopathology.

Thought Suppression and OCD

The ironic effects of thought suppression should be evident in the pathogenesis of obsessions. Deliberate suppression of obsessions should have adverse effects, because it terminates exposure to the obsession, thereby preventing natural habituation of obsessive–compulsive anxiety (Purdon, 1999). Moreover, suppression inadvertently reinforces beliefs about the significance of the obsession and the need to prevent the perceived negative consequences linked to the obsession. Together, these adverse consequences of thought suppression should cause an increase in thought frequency and the urge to neutralize.

Nonclinical Intrusive Thought Studies. A number of studies investigated paradoxical suppression effects on unwanted intrusive thoughts in nonclinical samples. In a modified thought suppression experiment, Salkovskis and Campbell (1994) found that students who reported a high frequency of negative intrusive thoughts experienced an enhancement, but no rebound effect, when they suppressed a personally relevant negative thought. The "monitor only" group had significantly fewer intrusive target thoughts than the suppression group. Even outside the laboratory, students instructed to suppress a negative intrusive thought over a 4-day period experienced more target thought intrusions, greater discomfort, and more effort to suppress the thought than the "monitor only" or "think through" controls (Trinder & Salkovskis, 1994). Effort to suppress and discomfort were correlated ($r = .51$), indicating that the harder a person tried to suppress the unwanted intrusion, the more discomfort he or she experienced from the intrusion. However, results from the Maudsley Obsessional Compulsive Inventory (MOCI) and target thought frequency or discomfort were uncorrelated.

Other studies have failed to find strong evidence of paradoxical effects for suppression of negative target thoughts. McNally and Ricciardi (1996) reported only a weak trend for negative thoughts to rebound after initial suppression, whereas Kelly and Kahn (1994) found rebound effects when participants suppressed "white bear" thoughts but not when they suppressed an anxious or worrisome thought. Rutledge (1998) calculated individual enhancement and rebound scores for students who suppressed and then expressed a personally negative intrusive thought. She found that only 4 individuals (4%) exhibited true enhancement (increased thought frequency during suppression) and 17 (16%) showed a rebound effect (increased frequency during the second expression period).

In a thought suppression experiment conducted in our laboratory, students were randomly assigned to initially suppress or monitor a neutral thought (e.g., white bear), a personally relevant pleasant thought, or a personally relevant obsessive intrusive thought. There was no evidence of immediate enhancement or rebound for the suppression versus monitor-only groups (Purdon & Clark, 2001; see also negative results reported by Purdon, 2001). However, there was evidence that suppression might interfere with the natural habituation that occurs with repeated exposure to thought occurrences (Purdon, 2001, reported a similar finding). In addition, less success at suppressing obsessional intrusive thoughts was associated with more negative postexperimental mood (Purdon & Clark, 2001; see also Markowitz & Borton, 2002). Purdon (2001) also found that faulty appraisal of thought recurrences in a suppression experiment predicted a more negative mood state. Overall, these findings indicate that suppression of intrusive thoughts may have a significant negative impact on mood. In addition, dysfunctional appraisals of target thought recurrences will lead to greater efforts to control the thoughts and a subsequent decline in mood state.

A number of studies have examined the relationship between self-report measures of obsessionality and suppression effects. Smári, Birgis-dóttir, and Brynjólfsdóttir (1995) found that students with high MOCI scores had significantly more target thoughts during suppression, felt more distressed by unwanted thoughts, and tried hard to suppress the personally relevant intrusive thought during the suppression period. However, there was no evidence of enhancement or rebound for personally distressing intrusive thoughts. Other studies have not found a relationship between enhancement or rebound effects and heightened obsessionality (Smári et al., 1994; Trinder & Salkovskis, 1994). In fact, Rutledge et al. (1996) reported a *negative* correlation between the MOCI and thought rebound scores. That is, less obsessionality actually predicted more thought rebound in their experiment.

In summary, there is no evidence of greater paradoxical effects resulting from suppressing personally relevant negative thoughts than from suppressing neutral thoughts. In fact, it may be that postsuppression rebound is more likely with neutral thoughts than with personally distressing cognitions. It is possible that individuals are already naturally suppressing their negative thoughts, so that thought suppression instructions have little impact (Tolin, Abramowitz, Przeworski & Foa, 2002). It may also be that the greatest impact of thought suppression is on negative mood and appraisal of the target thought. Finally, the lack of association between thought suppression and measures of obsessive–compulsive symptoms calls into question the relevance of this experimental paradigm for understanding OCD.

Self-Report Measures of Thought Suppression. Retrospective self-report measures of mental control, such as the White Bear Suppression Inventory (WBSI; Wegner & Zanakos, 1994), do correlate moderately with measures of obsessional symptoms. However, it is also clear that these mental control measures are equally correlated with indices of other emotional states like anxiety or depression (Smári & Hólmsteinsson, 2001; Wegner & Zanakos, 1994). Rassin, Diepstraten, et al. (2001) found that pretreatment WBSI scores did not predict symptom improvement in patients with OCD who received cognitive-behavior therapy (CBT).

Rassin, Merckelbach, Muris, and Stapert (1999) found that students with elevated scores on the WBSI also reported a more intense urge to engage in their rituals, more discomfort from the rituals, and more resistance against their ritualistic urges than low scorers. There were no differences in frequency of actual ritualistic behavior or in success in resisting the urge to titualize. Höping and de Jong-Meyer (2003) factor analyzed the White Bear Suppression Inventory and found that the Thought Suppression factor had practically no relationship with self-report symptom measures. Along with the correlations reported in the experimental studies, these findings raise serious doubts on whether thought suppression and its consequences have a specific relationship with obsessive–compulsive symptoms.

Thought Suppression in OCD Samples. Two published clinical studies provide a direct test of the role of thought suppression in OCD. Janeck and Calamari (1999) compared 32 patients with DSM-IV OCD with 33 nonclinical control subjects on their ability to suppress negative intrusive thoughts. The target thought was based on participants' response to the Intrusive Thoughts Questionnaire. The patients with OCD reported more negative intrusive thoughts and more distress associated with the intrusions than the nonclinical control subjects. However, neither the OCD group nor the nonclinical group showed any evidence of immediate enhancement or rebound effects. Based on the criteria of Rutledge et al. (1996) for defining enhancement or rebound, Janeck and Calamari found that only 25% of the patients with OCD assigned to the suppression condition showed rebound effects, and 31% an immediate enhancement effect.

Tolin, Abramowitz, Przeworski, and Foa (2002) utilized a within-subject experimental design in which OCD, anxious, and nonclinical control subjects monitored, suppressed, and then monitored again, a standard neutral thought. A neutral target thought (i.e., white bear) was used to test whether individuals with OCD have a general deficit in thought suppression. Analysis revealed that only those in the OCD group showed a significant immediate enhancement effect, with more white bear thoughts occurring during suppression than during the baseline period. None of the groups evidenced a rebound effect. In a second experiment involving a lexical decision task, those in the OCD group again evidenced immediate enhancement but no rebound effect (Tolin, Abramowitz, Przeworski, & Foa, 2002). Only the participants with OCD evidenced significantly faster response times for suppressed words as compared with nonsuppressed words. These findings indicate that the immediate enhancement effect is not simply an artifact of self-report biases. Furthermore, it appears that the act of suppression may prime target thoughts, thereby making the thoughts more accessible and likely to intrude into consciousness.

The results of these studies are somewhat troubling in regard to the role of thought suppression in OCD. One would expect that individuals with persistent, distressing obsessions would be especially susceptible to the paradoxical effects of thought suppression. Even with the more positive findings of Tolin, Abramowitz, Przeworski, and Foa (2002), the enhancement effect size was only small to moderate, and it correlated with Yale-Brown Obsessive–Compulsive Scale (YBOCS) symptom severity only in the first study. Together these results indicate that the paradoxical effect of thought suppression may not be a robust phenomenon in obsessional states.

A Critical Postscript on Thought Suppression

Current Status

After considerable research, the lack of evidence for the paradoxical effects of thought suppression in clinical disorders like OCD is quite discouraging. The effects of thought suppression have proven weaker and more transient than previously expected. It may be helpful to review what has been learned about the effects of intentional thought suppression on the persistence of negative cognition. Table 6.1 provides a summary of current findings.

All studies found that both clinical and nonclinical individuals are unable to attain complete suppression of a target thought, regardless of its valence or personal relevance. Suppression may be less successful over longer periods of time, but in the short term the most consistent finding is that suppression results in less frequent target intrusions in subsequent time periods (Abramowitz et al., 2001). Nonclinical individuals can sup-

TABLE 6.1. Thought Suppression Effects on Frequency of Unwanted Cognitions

1. Complete suppression of neutral or clinically relevant thoughts is rarely obtained.
2. Individuals are able to suppress unwanted thoughts in the short term.
3. Suppression of unwanted thoughts usually leads to less frequent target thought intrusions even after suppression efforts cease.
4. Only a minority of individuals show immediate enhancement or rebound effects after suppression of unwanted thoughts.
5. Personally relevant and negative unwanted thoughts are not more susceptible to the paradoxical effects of thought suppression than neutral thoughts.
6. Subclinical and clinical individuals are less successful in suppressing unwanted negative thoughts, but this relative failure in suppression does not result in a later resurgence of target thought frequency. Because of less effective suppression, clinical and analogue individuals may be more likely to show immediate enhancement effects.
7. Presence of obsessional symptoms or disorder may not necessarily increase the likelihood of paradoxical thought suppression effects.
8. Suppression of unwanted negative thoughts may interfere with natural habituation associated with thought repetition.

press personally relevant negative target thoughts as well as they can suppress neutral thoughts. Individuals with clinical or subclinical disorders may find negative cognitions more difficult to suppress. Occasionally, this may even result in an initial enhancement effect.

It is clear that the paradoxical effects of thought suppression are evident in only a minority of individuals. Moreover, personally relevant emotional thoughts may be *less* susceptible to the paradoxical effects of suppression than neutral material (see Kelly &Kahn, 1994; Muris et al., 1992). Thus, the relevance of thought suppression for understanding the escalating cycle of obsessional intrusive thoughts remains in doubt. The most plausible explanation for the effects of thought suppression on frequency of intrusions may be that it interferes in the natural decline in target thought occurrence evident after repeated expression of cognition (see Purdon & Clark, 2001; Purdon, 2001; Roemer & Borkovec, 1994). Rassin, Mercekelbach, and Muris (2000) noted that there is little evidence that thought suppression *causes* frequent unwanted intrusive thoughts in clinical disorders. In fact, it may be more likely that thought suppression is a *consequence* and not the cause of frequent distressing cognitions.

Wenzlaff and Wegner (2000) state that the paradoxical effect of thought suppression is strongest when mental control is disrupted during suppression. They cite a number of studies indicating that the imposition of a cognitive load during suppression (e.g., time pressure, concurrent memory task, etc.) results in greater enhancement and rebound effects as compared with no-load conditions (e.g., Wegner & Erber, 1992). In addition, there is evidence that rebound effects may be more pronounced when individuals use multiple distracters during suppression or when the environmental context or mood state during suppression is reinstated (e.g., Wegner et al., 1991). Conway et al. (1991) found that dysphoric students are worse at thought suppression than nondysphoric individuals, which suggests that negative mood interferes with the ability to exercise mental control. This may be due to dysphoric individuals' use of more negative distracters that inadvertently prime the target thought (see Wenzlaff et al., 1988).

Other researchers note that the exclusive focus on thought frequency as the primary dependent variable in thought suppression research may be misguided. Purdon (1999) argued that suppression may have its greatest impact on appraisal and emotional response to an intrusion, as well as on beliefs about thought control and on current mood state. In a number of experiments, thought suppression causes more anxiety or distress in response to recurrences of the unwanted target thought (Kelly & Kahn, 1994; Purdon & Clark, 2001; Roemer & Borkovec, 1994; Trinder & Salkovskis, 1994). However, others have reported no relationship between suppression and negative mood (Davies & D. M. Clark, 1998). Rassin (2001) also reported that suppression of thoughts about accidents did not affect mood state and that thought suppression may actually reduce stress and discomfort caused by TAF bias.

Limitations

The inconsistent findings across thought suppression studies may be due to various methodological problems evident with this experimental paradigm (see reviews by Abramowitz et al., 2001; Purdon, 1999; Purdon & Clark, 2000; Wenzlaff & Wegner, 2000). Table 6.2 provides a summary of the shortcomings evident in the thought suppression research.

A number of methodological problems are inherent in the experimental design of thought suppression research. Because participants are instructed to suppress thoughts, experimental demand characteristics could influence results by decreasing participants' willingness to report target thought occurrences (Abramowitz et al., 2001). Studies differ as to what constitutes a target thought occurrence, a very specific thought statement (e.g., white bear), or any thought related to a target story. Moreover, there is no consensus on the best method for assessing thought frequency. Questions can also be raised about the generalizability or ecological validity of laboratory-based thought suppression. Can it be assumed that brief periods (3–5 minutes) of mental control initiated in response to experi-

---

TABLE 6.2. Issues and Limitations in Thought Suppression Research

Methodological

- Demand characteristics may be present in though suppression research.
- There is no consensus across studies in the definition of what constitutes target thought occurrences (i.e., discrete thoughts like "white bear" vs. thought segments like "any idea involving white bears").
- A variety of methods are used by researchers to assess thought frequency (i.e., stream-of-consciousness verbalization vs. event marking).
- Researchers disagree on which control condition is most appropriate (i.e., express vs. monitor only).
- Participants may differ in their willingness to report unwanted intrusions.
- Individuals may engage in natural or spontaneous suppression in the control condition.
- The findings may not generalize beyond the laboratory.

Conceptual

- Thought suppression experiments simulate a low responsibility condition.
- Individuals may use different mental control strategies.
- Thought suppression experiments confound frequency and duration of target thoughts.
- Thought suppression fails to address motivational aspects of thought control.
- Thought suppression experiments focus mainly on prevention rather than dismissal of unwanted thoughts.

menter instructions in a laboratory setting are comparable to spontaneous mental control efforts sustained over longer time periods in an uncon-
trolled environmental context?

A number of related conceptual problems are apparent in the
thought suppression experiments. Instructing participants to suppress or
not suppress a distressing target thought represents a subtle *responsibility
manipulation.* Individuals with OCD could construe this as a low responsibility condition (e.g., "The experimenter is telling me not to think about
the obsession"). Any occurrence or perceived negative consequence associated with the obsession during the experiment could be attributed to
the experimenter. Under such conditions, the frequency and intensity of
obsessive intrusive thoughts would be diminished. Rassin, Mercekelbach,
and Muris (2000) also noted that thought suppression should not be considered a unitary phenomenon. People may use different strategies to suppress or control intrusive thoughts, and the effects of such control strategies may have different effects on outcome, depending on the type and
content of the unwanted thought.

Another problem for the study of obsessions is that the thought suppression experimental design confounds the frequency and duration of
target thoughts. Under instructions to engage in suppression, a person
may have great difficulty suppressing his or her obsession so that the person would experience a low rate of separate target thought reoccurrence
(i.e., fewer intrusions of long duration). On the basis of frequency rate,
one might assume that the person had good control over the target
thought. In reality, the person may have had a near continuous experience
of the thought throughout the suppression period. Although a number of
researchers attempted to address this issue by examining the percentage
of time devoted to target thoughts, the very fact that many individuals
with severe OCD report that the obsessions never really leave their minds
makes this experimental paradigm ill suited for the study of obsessions.

Whether individuals engage in thought suppression may not be the
most important question in disorders like PTSD or OCD, which are
characterized by persistent, uncontrollable thought intrusions. Rassin,
Mercekelbach, and Muris (2000) argued that thought suppression may
play a relatively minor role in the pathogenesis of obsessions, given evidence that the cognitive factors emphasized in cognitive-behavioral theories of OCD may be more important to the disorder. Thus, the more important question may be, *What motivates individuals to continue to put so
much effort into suppressing these thought intrusions when their efforts are so futile and counterproductive?* (see Purdon, 1999, for further discussion). The
thought suppression literature is less informative on the motives that
drive habitual natural resistance to an intrusion. This is because thought
suppression theory and research focus on the question of "thought prevention." What is the consequence of trying to prevent oneself from think-

ing a target thought? Although this question is relevant to OCD, it is not the most pressing question in a theory of obsessions.

Instead, there are two critical questions that must be addressed in the control of obsessions. First, what is the impact of intentional, effortful attempts to dismiss a thought once it occurs? That is, what happens after the obsession occurs? What is the effect of trying to remove the thought from conscious awareness? And second, why are individuals with OCD so highly motivated, even compelled, to engage in habitual naturally occurring resistance (i.e., suppression) to the obsession despite the counterproductive effects of their efforts? The typical thought suppression paradigm cannot address these questions. Instead, we must turn to the less developed research on thought dismissal.

THOUGHT DISMISSAL

For individuals with OCD, the primary control issue is not the prevention of obsessions through suppression, but rather the quick and efficient removal of an unwanted distressing intrusive thought. A recent study by Purdon, Rowa, and Antony (2002) highlights the importance of distinguishing prevention and removal in OCD. Thirty-seven individuals with OCD kept diaries of attempts to suppress their obsessions over 3 consecutive days. Analysis revealed that significantly more of the thought suppression attempts were reactive (74%; suppression of thought after it occurred) than proactive (26%; suppression designed to keep the thought from occurring). This finding supports my contention that difficulty with thought dismissal is more germane to the problem in OCD than thought suppression or prevention.

An experimental research design called *thought dismissal* may be more helpful for investigating mental control, because it targets "reactive suppression." Figure 6.1 illustrates a typical thought dismissal experiment.

There are two key dependent variables in the thought dismissal experiment: time taken to form the target thought (thought formation latency) and time taken to dismiss the thought (thought dismissal latency). Typically, the experiment begins by identifying a personally relevant target thought that is specific to each participant. After establishing the preexperimental mood state, the experimenter instructs participants to form the target thought. The time interval from the end of thought formation instructions to participants' signal that they have formed the cognition is considered the *thought formation latency*. Individuals hold the target thought for a standard time interval (i.e., 15–30 seconds). At the end of this mentation period, participants are instructed to dismiss the thought. The time between instructions to dismiss and participants' signal

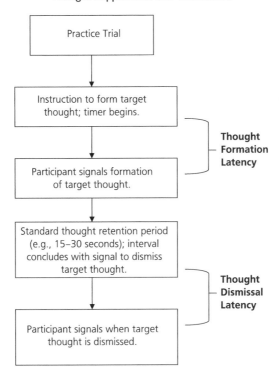

FIGURE 6.1. Typical thought dismissal experimental procedure.

that the thought is removed from conscious awareness is the *thought dismissal latency*. The experiment usually ends with postexperimental mood ratings and, possibly, various appraisal ratings of the target thought. Repeated trials of thought dismissal can be employed to study habituation effects, and the controllability of different thought content can be compared across trials.

Two caveats must be noted before considering the few studies on thought dismissal. First, it is obvious that the thought dismissal signal will cue further occurrence of the target thought. Thus, by signaling that they have dismissed the thought, participants will be instantly reminded of the target cognition. Clearly, thought dismissal latency is not a true measure of a person's ability to remove thoughts from conscious awareness. Instead, it is a measure of subjective judgment that the person has achieved a satisfactory level of control so that the target thought no longer dominates conscious awareness. Second, it is likely that target thought dismissal occurs through the use of thought substitution. That is, a person can signal that a target thought is dismissed because he or she is thinking of another thought. Thought replacement, covert distraction, and similar substitution strategies are the most common forms of mental control reported in clinical and nonclinical samples (see Chapter 2). Thought dismissal latency, then, can be construed as an indication of a person's ability to replace the target thought with a replacement cognition.

Empirical Studies

Thought dismissal has been used in only a few studies to investigate the parameters of mental control in unwanted intrusive or obsessive thoughts. Rachman and de Silva (1978) found that patients with OCD and nonclinical control subjects evidenced increasing difficulty in forming and retaining their obsessions or unwanted intrusive thoughts over repeated thought dismissal trials. This suggests that obsessions are subject to habituation with repeated practice (see also Parkinson & Rachman, 1980). Likierman and Rachman (1982) used thought dismissal to assess the effectiveness of four trials of thought stopping versus habituation training in 12 patients with obsessional ruminations.

The validation of thought dismissal as a measure of mental control has been confirmed in a few nonclinical studies. In a study based on 32 nonclinical individuals, Sutherland et al. (1982) gave all participants six trials of thought formation, retention (5-second duration), and dismissal of an unwanted intrusive and neutral thought under happy and sad mood inductions. Thought dismissal, but not formation latency, proved a sensitive indicator of mental control, with intrusive thoughts under a sad mood induction taking significantly longer to dismiss.

In a psychophysiological experiment involving thought dismissal, I found that students who reported more frequent and distressing intrusive thoughts took significantly longer to dismiss the intrusive thoughts than a control group, with longer dismissal times positively associated with postexperimental negative mood and subjective ratings of control (D. A. Clark, 1984, 1986). Edwards and Dickerson (1987) found that participants in their thought dismissal experiment took significantly longer to replace (i.e., dismiss) intrusive thoughts than neutral cognitions, even when formation time for the neutral thought was held constant. These authors concluded that the slower dismissal times for intrusive thoughts were more likely due to difficulties in disattending to the target thought rather than a problem of accessing replacement thoughts.

Although it is premature to draw any conclusions about the reliability and validity of the thought dismissal experimental paradigm, the initial findings are encouraging. They suggest that time taken to dismiss thoughts within a laboratory setting may be an appropriate experimental analogue for studying mental control. However, much more research is needed to understand the parameters that affect thought dismissal latency and its relation to psychopathology. In particular, little is known about how individuals with OCD respond under thought dismissal instructions. Christine Purdon and I are in the process of exploring a number of questions about mental control, using the thought dismissal paradigm in a 3-year research program funded by a grant from the Social Sciences and Humanities Research Council of Canada.

SUMMARY AND CONCLUSION

Is OCD characterized by a breakdown in mental control? Phenomenological and experimental research on this question has produced few definitive answers. Certainly, individuals with OCD appear to try too hard to control their unwanted intrusive thoughts or obsessions. Moreover, this excessive mental control is not necessarily a pervasive phenomenon but seems focused on specific unwanted intrusive thoughts that are considered particularly significant and threatening to the individual.

When they are placed under laboratory conditions, it is not clear that individuals with OCD are less effective in controlling their obsessions or suffer more adversely the paradoxical effects of intentional thought suppression. Experimental studies on thought suppression have produced few tangible results about the control of unwanted intrusive thoughts or obsessions. Most researchers now conclude that the adverse effects of thought suppression (i.e., immediate enhancement or postsuppression rebound effects) may play, at best, a minor role in the persistence of obsessions. A number of problems with the thought suppression research were raised that limit its relevance to OCD. Although the thought dismissal experimental paradigm may prove a better method for investigating mental control of persistent and repetitive unwanted intrusive thoughts or obsessions, too few studies have been conducted to evaluate its usefulness.

We know from clinical observation that control is an important issue in the persistence of obsession. If the effects or outcome of thought suppression do not play a prominent role in the persistence of obsessions, it may be that other aspects of mental control are more important. For example, it is obvious that perfect suppression or control over our unwanted thoughts is impossible. Could it be that the problem in OCD is a maladaptive or faulty appraisal of one's mental control efforts? This possibility is explored in the next chapter.

CHAPTER 7

Cognitive Control

A New Model of Obsessions

In OCD, dysfunctional mental control is a cardinal feature of the disorder. Individuals with obsessions struggle to exert even a modicum of control in preventing or removing obsessive thoughts from conscious awareness. Haunted by recurring upsetting thoughts of violence, disease, doubt, or the like, individuals with OCD can devote much of their days struggling against obsessions. This apparent breakdown in mental control is not a general dysfunction, but rather occurs with specific types of thought content that are idiosyncratic to the personal concerns and values of the individual. This specific breakdown in control may be due, in part, to greater reliance on dysfunctional mental control strategies (Amir, Cashman, & Foa, 1997; Ladouceur et al., 2000). It may also be blamed on the adverse effects of intentional mental control, although we now believe that this may play a relatively minor role in the persistence of obsessions.

This chapter presents a different perspective on the problem of mental control in OCD. In contrast to viewing poor control over obsessions as a general breakdown in self-control processes or the adverse effects of excessive control efforts, it is proposed that faulty appraisal of control and its consequences is a central cognitive process in the persistence of obsessions. As noted in Chapter 5, current cognitive-behavioral theories of OCD focus exclusively on the faulty appraisals and beliefs associated with the obsession. I propose that individuals with OCD not only misinterpret the obsession, but they also engage in a faulty evaluation of their mental control efforts, as well as the perceived consequences of failure to control the obsession. This secondary appraisal of one's response to the obsession interacts with the primary appraisals of the obsession to ensure continued preoccupation with obsessional content. The cognitive control model described in the following discussion is an elaboration and extension of the cognitive-behavioral theories of OCD presented in Chapter 5.

COGNITIVE CONTROL THEORY OF OBSESSIONS

General Description of the Model

The cognitive control theory of obsessions outlined in Figure 7.1 proposes that a number of cognitive constructs may be involved in the uncontrollability and persistence of obsessions. This expanded and more elaborated formulation focuses on factors that may explain the strong motivation for persistent natural resistance to an obsession and the poor re-

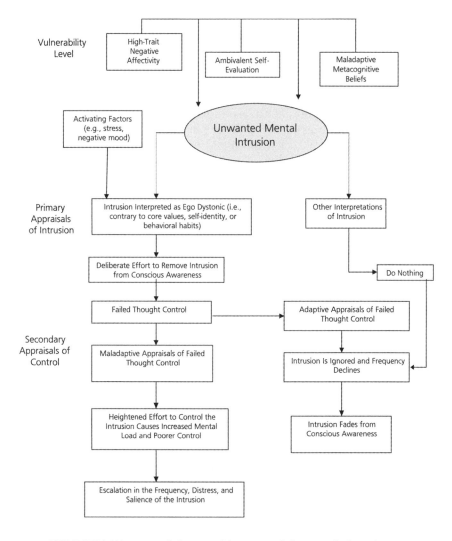

FIGURE 7.1. Diagram of the cognitive control theory of obsessions.

sults associated with active attempts at thought dismissal. The main proposition of this model is that an important contributing factor in the persistence of obsessions is *the presence of faulty misinterpretations of mental control over unwanted intrusive thoughts that arise from the perceived negative consequences associated with failed thought control.*

Clinical observation indicates that individuals with OCD are often worried about anticipated repercussions if they relinquish their attempts at mental control over an obsession. For example, individuals with molestation obsessions worry that if they do not actively try to suppress such thoughts, the frequency and intensity of the obsession will build to the point where they might act on the thoughts. From this perspective, failed mental control may lead to a catastrophic act of violence toward an innocent child. For individuals with obsessions about contamination, avoidance and washing compulsions are the primary control strategies for the obsession. The fear may center on becoming overwhelmed with the frequency and intensity of the obsession if they do not exercise continued control over the thought. For a devoutly religious person, the existence of unwanted sexual obsessions and his or her lack of control over them may be interpreted as proof of a sinful and unspiritual nature, possibly even demon possession in extreme cases. In all of these examples, failure to control a primary obsession is considered a highly threatening, in some cases catastrophic, consequence that the person must continually struggle against. What is interesting in this regard is that most people with OCD realize that they have poor control over the obsession. What they are trying to avert, however, is an even worse perceived state of uncontrollability should they ease up on their current control efforts.

A number of constructs are proposed in Figure 7.1 that may be involved in the persistence of obsessions and continued mental control attempts. These constructs occur at three conceptual levels. At a *vulnerability level* we find the enduring cognitive structures or schemas (i.e., beliefs) that represent the organization and storage of information that guides the processing of information (Ingram & Kendall, 1986). These schemas constitute an underlying vulnerability or predisposition to experience obsessions. In this sense, vulnerability is understood as an enduring, trait-like, endogenous construct that remains latent until it is triggered by a critical experience, thereby causally contributing to the onset of disorder (Ingram & Price, 2001). In the present model, three vulnerability domains are proposed that may predispose individuals to have a higher frequency of unwanted, ego-dystonic intrusive thoughts, images, or impulses.

A variety of cognitive factors related to mental control are activated with the occurrence of an unwanted intrusive thought. These are categorized as *primary appraisals of the intrusion* itself and *secondary appraisals of control.* The notion of an initial primary appraisal of an intrusion is consistent with the theories of Carr (1974) and McFall and Wollersheim (1979) (see Chapter 5 for discussion). Salkovskis and Wahl (2003) also proposed that individuals with OCD try too hard to control their obsessions because of primary appraisals that exaggerate the probability and consequence of perceived threat from the obsession and secondary appraisals in which their ability to cope and be rescued from the perceived threat is underestimated. However, in contrast to the present formulation, Salkovskis and Wahl consider the secondary appraisal of coping and rescue part of the initial appraisal of threat.

In the current context, primary appraisals reflect evaluations of the importance, threat, and inflated responsibility of the obsession, whereas the secondary appraisals focus on the importance and perceived consequences of failed mental control. This formulation is also consistent with the information-processing model of anxiety proposed by Beck and D. A. Clark (1997), in which primary appraisal of the intrusion occurs at the *immediate preparation stage*, involving activation of a threat mode, and secondary appraisal of control occurs at the *secondary elaboration stage*, in which coping resources and their probable effectiveness are evaluated.

Vulnerability to Unwanted Mental Intrusions

There are no published prospective psychological studies on the development of OCD in adulthood (McNally, 2001b). A number of twin and family studies have been conducted, but the findings are not at all clear or consistent. Although there is evidence that genetic factors play a role in OCD, some studies suggest that what is inherited is a general susceptibility to anxiety disorders and not a specific inheritance of OCD (Alsobrook & Pauls, 1998; Tallis, 1995). Hanna (2000) concluded from his review of the literature on childhood OCD that it "is a common, heterogeneous illness of unknown etiology" (p. 97). Clinical researchers have speculated on possible psychological vulnerability factors, based mostly on clinical observation (McNally, 2001b). Salkovskis and colleagues proposed that preexisting beliefs about excessive responsibility resulting from early childhood experiences may result in greater susceptibility to misinterpreting unwanted intrusive thoughts (Salkovskis, 1998; Salkovskis & Wahl, 2003; Salkovskis et al., 1999). Rachman (1993, 1997, 2003) suggested that high premorbid moral standards, preexisting TAF beliefs, depression, and anxiety-proneness may all constitute a vulnerability to making catastrophic misinterpretations of significance for unwanted intrusive thoughts.

Figure 7.1 presents three personality vulnerability constructs that may increase the frequency of unwanted intrusive thoughts and a tendency to generate faulty primary and secondary appraisals. Like those of other OCD researchers, these speculations are based on theoretical and clinical experience rather than empirical research.

Negative Affectivity, Neuroticism, and Anxious Apprehension

Tellegen (1985) and Watson and L. A. Clark (1984) proposed a broad personality/mood disposition termed *negative affectivity* (NA) that may increase susceptibility to a variety of negative emotional states, including anxiety and depression. High-NA individuals tend to worry, to be anxious, tense, distressed, angry, pessimistic, and resentful, to have negative appraisals of self and others, to report somatic complaints, and to have low self-esteem. Given this enduring personality predisposition to experience generalized distress or negative emotions, high-NA individuals are at greater risk for anxious and depressive symptoms and disorders (Watson, L. A. Clark, & Harkness, 1994). Watson, L. A. Clark, and Carey (1988) reported significant correlations between trait NA and number of obsessive–compulsive symptoms, obsessions about dirt and contamination, and checking/repeating compulsions in 150 twins or cotwins with psychiatric diagnoses. High-trait NA maps very closely with Eysenck's earlier concept of neuroticism (Eysenck & Eysenck, 1985). There is evidence from earlier studies that the neurotic–introverted quadrant may characterize obsessional states. Although the necessary longitudinal research has not been done, high-NA or neurotic individuals are likely to experience more unwanted, distressing intrusive thoughts and to find these thoughts more intense and distressing.

More recently Barlow (2002) proposed that three interacting vulnerabilities are involved in the etiology of anxious apprehension and anxiety disorders. The first is a generalized biological vulnerability represented by a genetic predisposition to be nervous, emotional (i.e., have high-NA or neurotic temperament), or to be highly reactive biologically to environmental changes. The second is a generalized psychological vulnerability of diminished sense of control. This is evident as a "chronic inability to cope with unpredictable uncontrollable negative events" (Barlow, 2002, p. 254). Early childhood experiences such as parental insensitivity to a child's expressive, independent behaviors or high protection, intrusiveness, and lack of warmth could possibly foster a sense of personal uncontrollability, which might in turn contribute to the development of anxious apprehension, anxiety, or depression if this occurs within the context of a generalized biological vulnerability. The third factor is a specific psychological vulnerability that predisposes the individual to focus anxious apprehension on a specific object or event. Barlow called this third vulnerability "learning what is dangerous" and suggested that this vulnerability arises from early learning experiences. In OCD the person learns that certain obsessional thoughts, images, or impulses are dangerous.

Fragile, Ambivalent Self-Evaluation

The proposal in the current model, that high-trait NA or neuroticism pre-disposes a person to anxiety disorders like OCD, falls within Barlow's conceptualization of generalized biological and psychological vulnerabilities. However, it is suggested that two further vulnerability constructs are important for understanding a specific predisposition to misinterpret unwanted intrusive thoughts as dangerous (i.e., a predisposition for obsessional complaints). The first is the presence of an *ambivalent, uncertain self-evaluation.* Guidano and Liotti (1983) proposed that obsession-prone individuals have a conflictual, ambivalent, uncertain, and fragile self-image that causes them to seek perfectionism, certainty, and an absolute correct solution for human problems. Unfortunately, this drive for certainty invariably leads to doubts about everything. Obsessions and compulsions reflect a preoccupation with self-worth and a desire to resolve these feelings of ambivalence. Unwanted intrusive thoughts or obsessions are interpreted as threats to a positive view of the self because they defy internalized standards of moral purity and social approval (see Bhar & Kyrios, 2001, for further discussion).

Research on whether an ambivalent and fragile self-concept is relevant to OCD is very limited. Bhar and Kyrios (2001) found that high self-ambivalence in a nonclinical sample was related to self-reported obsessive–compulsive symptoms and dysfunctional beliefs about perfectionism, and to the importance and control of intrusive thoughts. Although empirical research on self-worth issues in OCD is scarce, it is plausible that self-esteem issues are involved as a specific vulnerability for obsessionality. The propensity to misinterpret certain unwanted intrusive thoughts, images, or impulses as a threat to core personal values and ideals must be considered within the context of a fragile view of the self. This notion is discussed further in the consideration of the primary appraisals of intrusive thinking.

Maladaptive Metacognitive Beliefs

A second construct specific to obsessionality and presented in Figure 7.1 at the vulnerability level concerns enduring dysfunctional beliefs or schemas about the nature and function of cognition, especially unwanted intrusive thoughts, images, and impulses. The ability to monitor and regulate the information-processing system is an important human capacity that Flavell (1979) referred to as *metacognition* or "thinking about thinking." In OCD pre-existing beliefs about the function and meaning of unwanted thoughts, images, or impulses (i.e., *metacognitive beliefs*) may constitute a specific vulnerability to misinterpreting the significance of particular unwanted thought intrusions.

In earlier writings I proposed that obsession-prone individuals might hold unrealistic beliefs about the personal importance of particular types of unwanted intrusive thoughts and the need to control such thoughts in order to avoid dire consequences (Clark, 1989; Clark & Purdon, 1993). Specific metacognitive beliefs that certain types of unwanted intrusive thoughts are important and that absolute mental control over these thoughts is both possible and highly desirable are learned rules and assumptions about the mind. They are enduring ideas about the nature and function of mind that can influence whether a person appraises an unwanted intrusive thought in an adaptive or maladaptive fashion.

For example, if you believe that spontaneous violent thoughts (e.g., a thought of stabbing your child with a knife) are indicative of unconscious desires or impulses, or a sign of true inner evil or sinfulness, then you might also believe that such thoughts must be totally eradicated from the mind because of their inherent evilness or potential to lead to real harm. A person who holds such beliefs is much more likely to appraise unwanted intrusive violent thoughts in a maladaptive manner. Of course, we all have metacognitive beliefs about intrusive thoughts. Some people believe that intrusive thoughts can be a sign of creativity and inspiration. Others believe that intrusive thoughts reflect a person's true inner emotional being and so they should be attended to and acted on. Still other people may view certain intrusive thoughts as spiritual insight or instruction. People also differ in their beliefs about the importance, nature, and effectiveness of mental control of intrusions. Clearly, then, the beliefs a person holds about unwanted intrusive thoughts and their control should play an important role in determining the primary and secondary appraisals of these intrusions.

Wells and Mathews (1994) also proposed a metacognitive model of OCD in which the core dysfunction is an excessive monitoring for instances of a particular unwanted intrusive thought and the activation of metacognitive knowledge (i.e., beliefs) about the importance of controlling the unwanted intrusion via various coping strategies such as suppression, avoidance, continued rumination, and the like. Later Wells (1997) noted that three types of metacognitive beliefs may be particularly important in OCD: beliefs about the equivalence of thought and action, beliefs about the positive and negative effects of rumination, and beliefs about the need to neutralize. Wells and Mathews (1994) also proposed that OCD is the result of an impairment in metacognitive skills that manifests itself as a difficulty in distinguishing fantasy from reality.

A predisposition or heightened susceptibility to generate the faulty appraisals of unwanted intrusive thoughts that lead to obsessive and compulsive symptoms is the interactive outcome of general and specific vulnerabilities that are activated by certain contextual factors. Individuals with the generalized biological and psychological vulnerability to reacting with anxious apprehension and who also possess certain metacognitive beliefs about the importance and control of unwanted mental intrusions will have a greater tendency to appraise particular unwanted intrusive thoughts as threatening, especially when under stress or during a negative mood state. For these psychologically vulnerable individuals, the primary and secondary faulty appraisals of intrusions described in the following discussion occur as an effortless, "natural" response to a troubling mental intrusion.

Primary Appraisals of Intrusions

The model outlined in Figure 7.1 readily acknowledges the importance of primary appraisals of threat, significance, and responsibility described by Rachman, Salkovskis, Freeston, and others, as well as the critical role played by neutralization and other efforts to control an unwanted intrusive thought or obsession. However, another feature of the primary misinterpretation of significance and threat that has not been emphasized in cognitive-behavioral theories of obsessions is the role of *ego dystonicity.*

In Chapter 2 ego dystonicity was identified as one of the five defining features of obsessions. As noted by Rachman (1998), the unwanted intrusive thoughts that are most likely to lead to faulty primary appraisals of significance and threat are those that are contrary to or threaten the person's system of values. For example, individuals who value courteous and gentle behavior will be most upset by intrusive aggressive thoughts and impulses. If obsession-prone individuals have a preexisting ambivalent or fragile self-view, then unwanted intrusive thoughts that are completely contrary to core elements of this self-view are more likely to be interpreted as highly significant and threatening. That is, vulnerable persons are more likely to appraise their unwanted intrusive thoughts as alien to their fragile self-identities.

This can be illustrated by a woman with persistent troubling obsessions concerning whether she might be prone to commit violent sexual acts against others. She was distressed by such thoughts because she was, by nature, an introverted, conscientious, and gentle person who valued kind and fair treatment toward all. Unwanted thoughts of sexually violating other people, especially children, were abhorrent to her because they were so contrary to her value system and her self-view. Her misinterpretation that these thoughts were personally significant and threatening stemmed in part from their highly ego-dystonic or alien content. In sum, *the critical primary appraisal that leads to the spiraling escalation of obsessional rumination occurs when vulnerable individuals misinterpret an unwanted intrusive thought as a significant threat to important values or self-attributes (i.e., ego dystonic).* They then conclude that they are responsible for preventing any possibility of harm or dire consequences that might occur as a result of continued preoccupation with the mental intrusion.

Once an unwanted intrusive thought is considered a significant personal threat, deliberate efforts are made to dismiss or remove the intrusion from conscious awareness. As discussed previously, a variety of mental control strategies may be used to divert attention away from the unwanted thought, but with limited success. Unfortunately, the attempt by vulnerable individuals to control or suppress a highly significant, threatening, ego-dystonic intrusive thought is done under the worse possible conditions for successful mental control. As a result, the obsession-prone individual fails to achieve a satisfactory level of control (elimination) of the unwanted thought.

Failure to control a mental intrusion reinforces the faulty primary appraisal that the intrusive thought is a highly significant threat that must be subjected to even greater mental control efforts. This sets the stage for an escalation of the intrusion into a more persistent obsession. At this point, the cognitive control theory of obsessions is highly consistent with the basic cognitive-behavioral appraisal theory presented in Figure 5.1. The major theoretical difference, however, comes after the primary appraisals and failure to suppress an unwanted intrusive thought. Unlike other cognitive behavioral theories, the model presented in Figure 7.1 proposes that additional cognitive processes occur at a secondary appraisal level as individuals evaluate and respond to their failed attempts to achieve a desired state of mental control.

Secondary Appraisals of Control

It is proposed that the misinterpretation of failed thought control plays a more important role in the etiology and persistence of obsessions than previously acknowledged. With perceived failure to achieve satisfactory control over a significant, threatening unwanted intrusive thought, individuals will then engage in a secondary appraisal of their apparent inability to cope successfully with the unwanted mental intrusion. This *secondary appraisal involves an evaluation of the outcome of one's efforts to prevent, suppress, and remove specific unwanted thoughts, images, or impulses from conscious awareness.* The unsuccessful control of unwanted intrusive thoughts can be appraised in an adaptive or maladaptive manner. Several features of the misinterpretation of failed thought control can be identified that will result in further attempts to control the intrusive thought and ultimately result in a paradoxical escalation in the frequency, distress, and salience of the intrusion.

Misinterpretations of Significance

One of the main features of faulty secondary appraisal involves the undue significance or importance of failed control of the intrusion. As discussed in Chapter 6, complete suppression of unwanted thoughts is not possible. Thus, intentional suppression of an unwanted thought will be associated with target thought recurrences. It may be that the central difficulty at this secondary appraisal level is that any instance of thought recurrence is misinterpreted as failed mental control. Furthermore, the perceived inability to achieve complete control over the unwanted intrusive thought is interpreted as a highly significant failure that could portend dire consequences. For example, the vulnerable person may conclude from these recurrences of the unwanted thought, "I am not in control," "This unwanted thought must be important because it keeps returning despite deliberate thought control efforts," "Achieving complete control over this intrusive thought is the only way to get better," or "My inability to control this thought means that I am mentally weak and inadequate." It is this misinterpretation of the significance of failure to achieve complete elimination of the unwanted intrusive thought that leads to even greater efforts at controlling its occurrence. Thus, failed thought control that is interpreted as *highly significant* to one's personal concerns will result in greater effort to control the unwanted intrusive thought.

Appraisals of Threat

The faulty appraisals of failed thought control are considered personally significant because of the perceived threat associated with the obsession. The unwanted, distressing intrusive thought signifies the possibility of future harm or danger. If the mental intrusion can be removed from conscious awareness, then the possibility of an anticipated future catastrophe is averted. Failure to remove the unwanted intrusion may be viewed as threatening because it increases the probability of a highly undesirable, negative consequence. Clinical examples of this type of secondary appraisal include "I must reduce this preoccupation with contamination or I will slip into a clinical depression," "My inability to control the obsession as to whether I am sexually violent will continue to cause me great personal distress and eventually ruin my life," "If I don't control the obsessions and associated anxiety, it will drive me crazy," or "I need to control the obsessions because if I don't I will relapse and get worse again." When failed thought control is interpreted as increasing the probability of future harm or danger to self or others, the result is greater thought control efforts.

Appraisals of Possibility

Implicit in the faulty secondary appraisals of failed thought control is the belief that it is possible and highly desirable to achieve control over a particular unwanted intrusive thought, image, or impulse. No doubt, most individuals believe that they are able to maintain some control over their mental intrusions, but the obsession-prone individual is likely to have a particularly strong belief in the power of thought control. In OCD the person believes that it is possible to intentionally and deliberately rid the mind of offending thoughts and images, as illustrated in the following examples: "I must control all unwanted, upsetting, abhorrent intrusive thoughts that enter my mind," "I must control the obsession or the obsession will control me," "I can control the obsession by washing my hands," or "I must try to shut off my mind, control my thoughts so that God can spontaneously speak through His word or hymns." In each of these examples individuals with OCD believe that mental control can be achieved through a variety of strategies, including neutralization and overt compulsions.

Unrealistic Expectations of Control

Because failure to remove an unwanted distressing intrusive thought from consciousness is considered highly significant and threatening, any recurrence of the obsession is perceived as intolerable. The goal for the obsessional person is not reduction in the frequency of the obsession or improved mental control, but rather the complete elimination of the obsessional intrusive thought. The drive for perfect control over unwanted thoughts is, of course, entirely unrealistic and the goal unattainable. However, such an expectation ensures that the obsession-prone individual will continue to expend considerable effort to control every occurrence of the obsession. This unrealistic expectation of complete or perfect control over obsessions will result in greater effort to suppress every occurrence of the unwanted obsessive intrusive thought.

Inflated Responsibility

Salkovskis (1998) noted that an inflated sense of responsibility can arise from a failure to control thoughts. Once individuals perceive that they are responsible to prevent the harm implied by the occurrence or content of unwanted intrusive thoughts, they will engage in various mental control and other neutralizing strategies to curtail the occurrence of the intrusion and thus lower their inflated sense of personal responsibility. In the current theory of OCD, it is suggested that appraisals of responsibility will contribute to an increased effort to control an unwanted, distressing intrusive thought. In turn, the perceived failure to effectively control the occurrence and consequences of the intrusion will raise the level of perceived responsibility. Thus, the present formulation considers inflated responsibility an important variable in contributing to the vicious cycle of perceived uncontrollability of the obsession. Furthermore, as the obsessional state worsens, the appraisals of inflated responsibility shift from an emphasis on the prevention of anticipated harm to self or others, to a focus on one's responsibility to control every occurrence of the obsession. Thus, inflated responsibility in the current formulation is firmly linked to the perceived control of obsessions. Increased responsibility appraisals for the suppression or removal of unwanted intrusive thoughts will contribute to an increased effort to control the unwanted mental event.

Faulty Inferences of Uncontrollability

A final characteristic important in the secondary appraisal process involves the inferences or conclusions that the obsession-prone individual draws from occurrences of failed thought control. Vulnerable individuals will reach certain conclusions about their unsuccessful efforts at controlling the intrusion that will result in even greater thought control efforts. These faulty inferences about uncontrollability bear a close resemblance to Rachman's (1993) TAF bias. Moreover, the inferences often emerge as conditional statements, or "if–then" clauses, in which success or failure to dismiss an unwanted thought is interpreted as an important sign or test. Examples of faulty inferences of control include "If I can't control unwanted sexual intrusions, then I might lose control over my sexual behavior," If I can't control these unwanted thoughts, then I must be a weak and vulnerable person who is capable of losing control," and "If I successfully remove all sinful thoughts from my mind, then God will be pleased with me and I will feel at peace." Thus, the vulnerable person is highly motivated to engage in mental control because successful removal of the thought is interpreted as having positive effects, whereas failed control is associated with a number of anticipated negative consequences.

Misinterpretations of unsuccessful thought control make an important contribution to the pathogenesis of obsessions because they lead to even greater efforts to control the unwanted intrusive thought. Salkovskis and Forrester (2002) discussed this problem of "trying too hard" in OCD. They noted that obsessional patients often have difficulty in deciding when to stop even routine activities that might be the focus of their obsessional problems (e.g., when to stop washing, checking, recalling what was said in a conversation). Individuals with OCD often adopt two main strategies to decide when to terminate an action: (1) the activity is repeated until it feels right to stop or (2) it is conducted in a way that will ensure a feeling of completeness. Unfortunately, these criteria for deciding when to stop are fairly vague and difficult to remember, often resulting in many repetitions before "closure" is achieved.

Salkovskis and Forrester's (2002) analysis can also be applied to issues of mental control over the obsession. Thus, obsession-prone individuals may also have difficulty deciding when they have successfully removed an unwanted obsessive intrusive thought from conscious awareness. This, combined with their faulty misinterpretations of thought uncontrollability, will result in the intense and persistent preoccupation with resisting the obsession that has become the hallmark of OCD. Together, these cognitive processes ensure that successful and enduring mental control of the obsession will continue to remain beyond the grasp of the individual with OCD. Greater attentional resources devoted to the control of the obsession will result in more cognitive load and poorer perceived control over the obsession. The end result is a spiraling escalation in the frequency, intensity, and distress associated with the obsession.

Adaptive Appraisals of Control

As indicated in Figure 7.1, there are two pathways that can lead to a healthy or adaptive appraisal of unwanted intrusive thoughts, images, or impulses. First, at the initial occurrence of an intrusion, individuals might view the thought as irrelevant, stupid, or a "quirk" of the current context or mood state. In this case they are likely to do nothing and so ignore the thought. In other instances, they may generate an initial primary appraisal that the thought might be significant and so attempt to exert some degree of mental control (e.g., try to distract themselves from the thought). On the basis of thought suppression research, we know that even under optimal conditions their control efforts will be less than completely effective. However, if this partial failure in mental control is associated with an adaptive interpretation (e.g., "This thought will eventually go away if I just leave it alone"), then once again the person will avoid preoccupation with the intrusion. On the basis of this model, cognitive-behavioral treatment of obsessions should focus not only on the reduction of maladaptive primary and secondary appraisals, but also on fostering more adaptive approaches to the control of obsessions.

EMPIRICAL STATUS OF COGNITIVE CONTROL THEORY

The proposed cognitive control perspective on obsessions is a recent formulation. Direct empirical research on faulty appraisals of mental control in OCD has not yet been conducted. However, there are a few studies that provide indirect support for some aspects of the model.

There is evidence that beliefs and appraisals of thought control are critically involved in the heightened frequency and persistence of unwanted mental intrusions in clinical and nonclinical subjects (see review of Purdon & Clark, 2002). Individuals with subclinical or clinical obsessive–compulsive symptoms report more attempts to control their unwanted intrusive thoughts with less perceived success than nonclinical control subjects (Freeston & Ladouceur, 1997b; Ladouceur et al., 2000). Purdon et al. (2002) reported wide variability in the number of daily thought suppression attempts recorded by the 37 patients with OCD who participated in their 3-day diary study. The number of suppression attempts correlated with the YBOCS item assessing time spent having obsessions and interference due to obsessions. Furthermore, the number of daily suppression attempts also correlated with the appraisals of importance attached to unwanted obsessive intrusive thoughts. Even though patients rated their suppression attempts as completely successful only 14% of the time, the unwanted thoughts eventually disappeared with continued effort 59% of the time. Generally, participants viewed the act of thought suppression as having only a slight negative impact on daily functioning. Together these findings indicate that individuals with OCD may too readily react to their primary unwanted obsessive intrusive thoughts with mental control efforts that are relatively unsuccessful. Yet it may be that they perceive just enough success to reinforce their thought control attempts.

Appraisals of failed mental control also predicted self-rated efforts to suppress unwanted cognitions in a thought suppression experiment (Purdon, 2001). Furthermore, dysfunctional beliefs about mental control may interact with actual efforts to control unwanted intrusions to predict the subsequent success of individuals' suppression efforts (Purdon, 1997). Together these findings suggest that maladaptive beliefs and appraisals about thought control may influence individuals' motivation to suppress their thoughts. In turn, heightened effort to suppress unwanted thoughts may have a negative impact on the success of actual thought control efforts.

Tolin, Abramowitz, Hamlin, and Synodi (2002) conducted the most direct test to date on reactions to thought control failure in OCD. They selected participants from the Tolin, Abramowitz, Przeworski, and Foa (2000) experiment who demonstrated failure to suppress the target thought. This yielded 17 participants from the OCD group, 11 anxious participants (controls) and 8 nonclinical participants. Analysis revealed that the participants with OCD reported stronger internal attributions for thought control failure than the anxious or nonclinical groups (e.g., failed to control thoughts because of personal weakness), and this difference was not an artifact of paradoxical suppression effects or depression. The groups did not differ on external attributions for thought control failure, nor did thought suppression failure have a significant differential emotional impact on the three experimental groups. The authors concluded that individuals with OCD may attach internal negative meanings to their thought suppression failure, which then leads to greater distress and increased motivation to engage in future suppression.

SUMMARY AND CONCLUSION

A new cognitive-behavioral model of obsessions was presented that emphasizes the role of faulty appraisals of thought control as a critical cognitive process involved in the escalation of obsessions (see Figure 7.1). Like the cognitive-behavioral models discussed in Chapter 5, the present formulation proposes a number of vulnerability factors for OCD. However, the model differs in proposing two conceptual levels of appraisal in the pathogenesis of obsessions. At the primary appraisal level, unwanted intrusive thoughts will persist if considered personally significant, contrary to one's values or ideals (i.e., ego dystonic), and/or threatening because of anticipated negative consequences to self or others. This faulty appraisal, along with a heightened sense of responsibility, will lead to greater thought control efforts, including compulsions and neutralization.

At a secondary appraisal level, evaluations of failed thought control will also be a major contributor to an increase in the frequency, salience, and distress associated with the obsession. In the end, the person with OCD not only "tries too hard" to control the obsession, but "cares too much" about the consequences of incomplete thought control. If this analysis is correct, then cognitive assessment and intervention directed at the modification of dysfunctional thought control beliefs and appraisals will be a critical element in the treatment of obsessions. Part III, which follows, presents a comprehensive cognitive-behavioral perspective on assessment, case conceptualization, and treatment of OCD that is derived from the model illustrated in Figure 7.1.

Cognitive-Behavioral Therapy

CHAPTER 8

Cognitive-Behavioral Assessment of OCD

The implementation of effective treatment depends on a thorough understanding of a disorder and its presentation in each individual. Treatment planning should be based on a theoretically derived and empirically based assessment strategy that combines both nomothetic standardized measurement and idiographic approaches so that a case formulation is developed for each treatment seeker (J. S. Beck, 1995; Persons, 1989; Persons & Davidson, 2001). Moreover, reliable diagnostic instruments and psychometrically sound measures of obsessive–compulsive symptoms are critical for the evaluation of theories and the treatment of OCD (Taylor, 1998). Given the complex and heterogeneous nature of obsessive–compulsive states, a comprehensive, detailed, and individualized assessment strategy is necessary.

This chapter provides a detailed discussion of a cognitive-behavioral perspective on assessment of obsessions and compulsions derived from the cognitive-behavioral theories and research presented in the previous chapters. Figure 8.1 illustrates the major components of this theory-derived cognitive-behavioral assessment for OCD. Each of the assessment components in Figure 8.1 is discussed in a separate section of the chapter, and relevant assessment tools can be found in Appendices 8.1–8.6. Before discussing specific assessment measures and strategies, the chapter begins by considering the special challenges inherent in the assessment of OCD.

SPECIAL PROBLEMS IN THE ASSESSMENT OF OCD

Obsessional features such as intolerance of uncertainty, exactness, concern about making mistakes, pathological doubt, and indecision are prominent clinical features of OCD that can interfere with assessment. For ex-

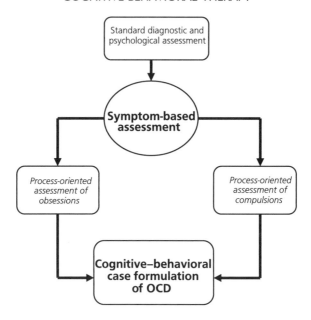

FIGURE 8.1. A diagrammatic outline of a diagnostic and assessment strategy for OCD based on a cognitive-behavioral perspective.

ample, individuals with obsessional checking may show such extreme doubt and concern about making mistakes that they are practically paralyzed when given a questionnaire with numerous items and multiple response options. In this case completing a questionnaire, or even answering questions in a clinical interview, can be extremely anxiety provoking. Under these circumstances, the client may exhibit the very pathology that defines the disorder (i.e., repeated checking of answers) or engage in avoidance behavior. Naturally, avoidance is evident as noncompliance or outright refusal to participate in the assessment.

Summerfeldt (2001) discusses a number of specific issues that arise in the assessment of obsessive and compulsive symptoms. Taylor, Thordarson, and Söchting (2002) also highlight various difficulties in the assessment of OCD, such as the patient's reluctance to describe symptoms, presence of contamination fears, minimization of symptoms, and slowness. In addition, the clinician may have difficulty distinguishing obsessions and compulsions from related clinical phenomena. Table 8.1 provides a summary of pertinent issues in the assessment of OCD, which are categorized as problems intrinsic to the clinical disorder, and difficulties arising from the response style or test-taking behavior of individuals with OCD.

TABLE 8.1. Summary of Possible Difficulties Encountered in the Assessment of OCD

Problems relating to disorder characteristics

- Common features with other symptomatology
- Heterogeneity of symptom content and expression
- Concealment of symptoms
- High comorbidity rate
- Symptom instability and shift
- Symptom multiplicity

Problems involving obsessional response style

- High anxiety resulting from the assessment
- Excessive concern with exactness, correctness, and intolerance of uncertainty
- Pathological doubt and indecision
- Extremely slow response rate
- Elicitation of compulsions like repeating, checking, redoing
- Chronic avoidance of anxiety cues
- Lack of insight; high fixity of belief
- Activation of faulty appraisals of threat, responsibility, or personal significance

Disorder-Related Problems

Because of shared phenomenology, obsessions can be difficult to distinguish from other negative cognitions like depressive and anxious rumination, worry, intrusive thoughts associated with a traumatic experience, jealous ideation, or sexual fantasy (Taylor, Thordarson, & Söchting, 2002). The five core features of obsessions (see Table 2.2) can be helpful in differentiating obsessional ideation from other types of wanted or unwanted mental intrusions. Compulsions and other types of overt or covert neutralization can at times be difficult to distinguish from certain pathological behaviors like tics, impulse control disorders, sexual compulsions, or intentional thought suppression strategies (Summerfeldt, 2001). The distinctive features of compulsive rituals and neutralization discussed in Chapter 2 can be used to make a differential assessment.

Summerfeldt (2001) also notes that there is considerable heterogeneity of symptom content in OCD. The idiosyncratic expression and diverse content of obsessions, in particular, means that each individual can evidence a very specific, highly personalized symptom content. A flexible and comprehensive assessment approach is needed that can accommodate to the variety of symptom manifestations seen in OCD. Individuals with OCD may also deny or minimize their symptoms in an effort to conceal highly upsetting, embarrassing, or immoral obsessions. Newth and Rachman (2001) noted that individuals with repugnant harming and sex obsessions, such as child molestation thoughts, may conceal these intrusions from others. Admitting to such thoughts can be a highly anxious experience, bordering on a panic-like reaction for some individuals. In addition, the high comorbidity rate for disorders like depression, social phobia, and generalized anxiety disorder will increase the multiplicity of symptoms and make it more difficult to determine the disorder specificity of particular clinical phenomena.

Obsessive–compulsive symptoms shift over time, as few individuals maintain the same constellation of symptoms throughout the course of the illness (Summerfeldt, 2001). It is also common for obsessional content to change, so that patients will report a new obsession after weeks or months of preoccupation with a previous theme. Although some individuals with OCD report a single obsession, others can report multiple obsessions. Together these factors can threaten the discriminant validity of assessment measures. At the very least, the clinician's measurement instruments should be more sensitive to OCD symptoms than to the symptoms of other disorders.

Response Style Problems

There are a number of ways in which OCD can also affect an individual's response orientation to the assessment process. For many individuals with OCD, completing questionnaire items or providing answers to structured interview questions is more anxiety provoking and aversive than it is for patients with other clinical disorders. This is because the assessment elicits the very pathology for which they seek treatment. Measurement items may trigger unwanted obsessions and repetitive neutralization responses that are very distressing for the patient. Obsessional persons' excessive concern for exactness, correctness, and intolerance of uncertainty means that they may strive to provide the perfectly correct answer to each question. Because most of our assessment items rely on subjective, personal opinion and evaluation, this increases the ambiguity and vagueness for the person with OCD who is earnestly trying to give the best possible answer. As a result, the assessment triggers continual doubt in the person concerning whether his or her answer really is the most accurate, and so the person can be paralyzed with indecision and uncertainty.

Individuals with OCD may take an inordinate amount of time to complete questionnaires, and the whole process may elicit compulsive rituals like checking and rechecking their answers, repeating statements just made in an interview, or other forms of redoing. Responses to questionnaire items may be accompanied by a detailed explanation of each option that is circled. Moreover, individuals who lack insight into their obsessions may believe that their fears about the assessment process are reasonable.

Particular faulty appraisals and beliefs about the assessment may emerge. For example, some individuals have expressed concern that if they give a wrong answer, this will give the therapist incorrect information about their disorders. As a result, the therapist will arrive at a faulty formulation and their treatment will be ineffective. One can see in this statement an overestimation of threat ("Treatment will be thwarted by my incorrect answers"), inflated personal responsibility ("It is my responsibility to ensure the effectiveness of treatment by providing the most accurate answers possible"), and personal significance ("My answer to this one questionnaire item is absolutely critical for effective treatment"). Given this approach to assessment, it is little wonder that individuals with severe OCD often resort to avoidance. Thus, they may begin assessment but then refuse to continue, or they may refuse even to try, or they may terminate treatment altogether if it depends on completing an assessment protocol.

Strategies for Dealing with Resistance to Assessment

There are a number of strategies the clinician can adopt to improve compliance with assessment in OCD (see also Clark & Beck, 2002; Taylor et al., 2002). These intervention strategies are summarized in Table 8.2.

It is important that the therapist acknowledge, that is, validate, the respondent's anxiety with the assessment process. (See Leahy, 2001, for extensive discussion of validation in response to resistance in cognitive therapy.) The clinician should adopt an empathic, supportive, and collaborative style, similar to the orientation assumed during treatment. The therapist should explain that many people with OCD find answering questions during assessment quite anxiety provoking. It should be noted that this is part of the problem with OCD; that is, assessment is difficult because of the OCD. Validation of the patient's feelings should occur as the

---

TABLE 8.2. Intervention Strategies to Improve Compliance with Assessment in OCD

1. Validate the respondent's anxiety concerning the assessment process.
2. Provide a thorough explanation of the role of assessment in the treatment process.
3. Explain the therapeutic value of assessment for some types of OCD.
4. Be selective and include only the most essential measures.
5. Allow additional time for assessment. It may be necessary to extend formal assessment into the early phases of active treatment.
6. Identify faulty appraisals and beliefs that may interfere in assessment. Use cognitive restructuring to deactivate these beliefs.
7. If necessary, selectively and judiciously offer reassurance during the assessment process and assume some responsibility for the assessment outcome.
8. Explain that assessment is a continuous process, so that the results of assessment are frequently refined, corrected, and elaborated throughout treatment.

person first begins to experience distress with the assessment. Steps should be taken to minimize this distress as much as possible without jeopardizing the validity of the assessment itself. Validation involves acknowledging patients' feelings about the assessment, discussing their fears and anxieties, and allowing sufficient time for expression of these anxieties and reservations. Together the therapist and patient can work out an approach to assessment that may lessen personal anxiety. For example, individuals can review each questionnaire with the therapist beforehand to ensure that they understand each question. The main point that therapists want to convey to a patient is they understand that assessment is very difficult and anxiety provoking, but that a flexible, caring approach will be used to minimize anxiety as much as possible.

It is also important that a thorough and complete explanation about the nature and purpose of the assessment is provided to the patient during the introductory phase. The clinician should explain that the use of questionnaires, interviews, and rating scales is important for providing a detailed understanding of the nature of the patient's disorder, for formulating a treatment plan, and for evaluating the effectiveness of treatment. In addition, the therapist can point out that the very act of participating in the assessment can have a beneficial, therapeutic impact on certain obsessive–compulsive symptoms. For obsessive–compulsive checking, doubting, and indecision, completion of questionnaires and diary rating scales are exercises that exposure individuals to their fears (making decisions) and encourage the prevention of a neutralizing response (rechecking answers). For these individuals, participation in the assessment may have some early therapeutic benefits.

The provision of a full rationale for assessment is intended to lessen the person's anxiety and improve motivation to comply with the assessment process. However, at times anxiety may be so high that a more drastic intervention is necessary. Although it is normally not advisable to offer reassurance (see Chapter 9 for explanation), in order to get the assessment completed it may be necessary to reassure individuals in the early phase of contact and even to assume some degree of responsibility for their responses during assessment. Rachman (1993) indicated that obsessive–compulsive patients will sometimes agree to a temporary *transfer of responsibility* to the therapist for a very specific, well-defined purpose. In the manual for the Clark–Beck Obsessive–Compulsive Inventory (Clark & Beck, 2002), we suggested the following intervention for the person reluctant to complete a questionnaire.

> I understand that it is very difficult for you to answer these questionnaire items. [*validation statement*] Why don't you complete the questionnaire on your own based on your first impression? [*instructions to counter OC symptoms*] I will then look over your questionnaire responses and if I

think that any of your answers seem different or inaccurate given what you have already told me about your psychological problems, I will discuss them with you and we can make the appropriate changes. [*reassurance and transfer of responsibility*] In this way I can take ultimate responsibility for insuring that the questionnaire is completed accurately. (p. 12)

There are two very practical considerations that can improve compliance and the quality of the assessment data: Be highly selective in the instruments chosen for the assessment process, and provide extra time to complete each measure. Because of the difficulty many patients with OCD experience with assessment, the entire process should be kept as brief as possible. Select measures that directly target the individual's core symptomatology and critical disorder-specific cognitive and behavioral constructs. It may be that a certain level of comprehensiveness will be sacrificed, but this is better than outright noncompliance with assessment. The instruments recommended in the following sections were selected with these criteria in mind.

The therapist can also expect most individuals with OCD to take much longer than usual to complete measurement instruments. Therefore, to be flexible and allow extra time. Try to encourage the obsessional person to go with his or her first impression or response, noting that this is often most useful for assessment purposes. Although most therapists prefer to complete an assessment within the first two or three sessions before starting treatment, this sharp distinction between assessment and treatment may not be possible in OCD. Instead, the therapist may have to be content with some initial assessment data at pretreatment and then continue to collect additional, possibly process-related, data during the initial treatment sessions. In this way the full assessment may have to extend over many more sessions than is usual in cognitive therapy for other disorders.

The assessment process will not only elicit obsessive–compulsive symptomatology, it will also activate the very core faulty beliefs and appraisals that characterize the disorder. It is essential that the therapist identifies these faulty appraisals and beliefs and then tests the validity of each using cognitive restructuring (see Chapter 10). For example, assume that a person is extremely slow and hesitant about completing a particular questionnaire. The therapist discovers that the person is thinking that there are so many items in the questionnaire, it will take a very long time to complete, and by that time the anxiety will be intolerable. The therapist could inquire about the evidence for this belief. "Were there other times when this happened to you?" "Were there any times when you did complete a form and your anxiety was less than you expected?" "Are there things that increase or decrease the anxiety?" "What might be done in the current situation to lessen your anxiety?" The therapist could then assign a behavioral task to test the patient's level of anxiety. The individual could be asked to complete just 10 questions at a time and hand in these questions to the therapist. The patient could then complete a second set of 10 questions from the questionnaire, and so on until the instrument is complete. Not only would this strategy result in the eventual collection of complete questionnaire data, but it would be a direct behavioral test of the patient's belief that "I will be overwhelmed with anxiety if I try to fill in this questionnaire."

Finally, many individuals with OCD are concerned that they will provide information that will lead the therapist hopelessly astray in their treatment. The therapist should explain that assessment is an ongoing process that continues as long as the person is in therapy. Consequently, new information is constantly being collected, and the therapist's case formulation and treatment strategy is under continual review for refinement, elaboration, and correction. Thus, there is no patient information that cannot be changed, modified, or corrected later in therapy. It is important that the therapist challenge any misunderstandings patients may have that their answers are static, immutable, and irreconcilable facts about their experiences. In the end, the therapist would like the patient to view assessment as a flexible, dynamic, exploratory, and collaborative process of discovery.

DIAGNOSTIC ASSESSMENT AND SCREENING

A number of reviews have been published on assessment in OCD (Antony, 2001; Feske & Chambless, 2000; Taylor, 1995, 1998; Taylor et al., 2002). Because these reviews provide a comprehensive and critical evaluation of the reliability and validity of a variety of measures used to assess obsessions and compulsions, the present discussion offers a more condensed overview of a select number of instruments that are particularly relevant for the assessment strategy advocated in this chapter.

Diagnostic Interviews

It is important that any assessment of OCD begin with diagnostic instruments that allow for the screening of OCD (Summerfeldt, 2001). Standardized diagnostic interviews like the Structured Clinical Interview for DSM-IV (SCID-IV; First, Spitzer, Gibbon, & Williams, 1996) and the Anxiety Disorders Interview Schedule for DSM-IV (ADIS-IV; Brown, Di Nardo, & Barlow, 1994; Brown, Campbell, et al., 2001) are used most frequently to establish a diagnosis of OCD. The SCID is a semistructured interview developed for the diagnosis of the most frequent Axis I disorders. Interrater reliability for OCD with older versions of the instrument range from low (.59) to very high (1.00) kappa values (Steketee, Frost, & Bogart, 1996; Williams et al., 1992).

The ADIS, however, was developed specifically for anxiety disorders and their associated conditions like depression, substance abuse, and somatoform disorders. In addition to determining whether diagnostic criteria are met, the ADIS provides information on obsessive–compulsive symptom severity, insight into obsessional symptomatology, resistance, and avoidance. The ADIS-IV Lifetime version has high interrater agreement for OCD (kappa = .85) as the principal diagnosis (Brown, Campbell, et al., 2001). Taylor (1998) noted that the SCID-IV and ADIS-IV require that interviewers be well trained in the use of these instruments, although even BA- or MA-level training in psychology is sufficient to achieve good reliability as long as the interviewers are well trained and closely supervised by doctoral-level psychologists. Both Feske and Chambless (2000) and Taylor (1998) concluded that the ADIS-IV might be slightly more reliable in the diagnosis of OCD than the SCID-IV. It also yields more information, but can take 2–4 hours to complete in clinical samples (Summerfeldt & Antony, 2002). The SCID-IV Clinical Version can be obtained from the American Psychiatric Association Press and the ADIS-IV can be purchased from Graywind Publications.

Clark–Beck Obsessive–Compulsive Inventory (CBOCI)

The 25-item CBOCI (Clark & Beck, 2002; Clark, Antony, et al., 2003) is a self-report questionnaire recently developed as a screener for OCD. It adopts a structure and response format that is identical to those of the Beck Depression Inventory–II (BDI-II; Beck, Steer, & Brown, 1996) and so is designed to be used as part of an assessment battery with the BDI-II and the Beck Anxiety Inventory (BAI; Beck & Steer, 1993). The CBOCI items are scored from 0 to 3, with each item consisting of four response option statements. Fourteen items assess core diagnostic features and content areas of obsessions, and 11 items assess the common symptom characteristics of compulsions. The measure was designed to cover the DSM-IV diagnostic criteria for OCD as well as a number of additional symptom features that figure prominently in current cognitive-behavioral theories of OCD. The 14 obsession items assess frequency of dirt/contamination, aggression/harm, and religious/moral/sexual obsessions, as well as uncontrollability, salience, inflated responsibility, doubt, resistance, perfectionism, indecision, daily interference, insight, and cognitive avoidance. The 11 compulsion items assess frequency of cleaning, checking, repeating, and precision/symmetry, as well as mental neutralizing, slowness, distress from prevention of compulsion, daily interference, avoidance, uncontrollability of compulsion, and distress. An Obsessions subscale, Compulsions subscale, and Total Score are derived from the questionnaire.

A psychometric validation study was recently completed involving 83 outpatients with DSM-IV OCD, 43 nonobsessional anxious patients, 32 depressed outpatients, 26 nonclinical adults drawn from the community, and 308 students (Clark, Antony, et al., 2003). On the basis of the OCD sample, internal consistency was high for CBOCI Obsessions (alpha = .90), Compulsions (alpha = .87), and Total Score (alpha = .93), and the scales had acceptable 3-month test–retest stability when administered to a subgroup of the student sample (Obsessions = .69, Compulsions = .79, Total Score = .77). Patients in the OCD sample scored significantly higher on all CBOCI scales than the anxious, depressed, or nonclinical control groups, and the measure was highly correlated with other OCD symptom measures like the Padua Inventory Revised and self-report YBOCS. However, like other obsessive–compulsive symptom measures, the CBOCI was moderately correlated with more general measures of depression, anxiety, and worry, even when controlling for obsessionality.

The diagnostic utility of the CBOCI was assessed in terms of how well the instrument distinguishes individuals with OCD from nonobsessional clinical and nonclinical control subjects. Receiver operating characteristic curves were calculated to determine the optimal cutoff scores for distinguishing groups. Analysis revealed that the cutoff score of 22 on the CBOCI Total Score yielded high sensitivity (90%) and specificity (78%) for distinguishing individuals with OCD from student control subjects. The clinical effectiveness of the scale was 81%. A Schmid–Leiman analysis based on the clinical sample revealed that the CBOCI consists of a high-order General Distress factor (68% of variance) and two lower-order factors of Obsessions (17%) and Compulsions (15%). It was concluded from this that the CBOCI does assess specific symptom features of OCD and so can be useful in identifying this disorder. (For further details, see Clark et al., 2003).

A recommended strategy for establishing a diagnosis of OCD is that clinicians begin by administering one or two self-report symptom screeners such as the CBOCI and the BDI-II. This must be followed by a diagnostic clinical interview, preferably a semistructured interview like the SCID-IV or the ADIS-IV, in order to determine whether OCD diagnostic criteria are met. Once it is clear that the patient meets the diagnostic criteria for OCD, the clinician is ready to progress to the next stage of assessment, a more detailed measurement of obsessive and compulsive symptomatology. The CBOCI and manual are available from The Psychological Corporation.

SYMPTOM-ORIENTED ASSESSMENT

A number of self-report and clinician-administered instruments are available to provide a more detailed measurement of the frequency, severity, and diversity of obsessive–compulsive symptoms. These measures are most useful for quantifying the severity or intensity of OCD and are therefore particularly valuable in evaluating treatment effectiveness. Moreover, most of these measures assess a range of obsessional content, which can be useful in determining OCD subtypes and planning treatment.

Clinician-Administered Symptom Measures

Compulsive Activity Checklist

The Compulsive Activity Checklist (CAC) was originally developed as a 62-item clinician-administered schedule to assess the degree to which obsessive–compulsive symptoms interfere in everyday activities, primarily involving washing and checking compulsions (e.g., retracing steps, washing hands and face, using the toilet, reading, writing, etc.). Items are rated from 0 ("performance of the activity within normal limits") to 3 ("completely unable to perform task or totally avoids due to obsessive fear"). It was first developed by Richard Hallam and reported by Philpott (1975). Since then different researchers have proposed various modifications and reductions so that there are now multiple self-report and interviewer-based versions of the CAC. Marks, Hallam, Connolly, and Philpott (1977) proposed a 39-item interview or self-report CAC; Freund, Steketee, and Foa (1987) published a 38-item interview format that factored into washer and checker dimensions; Cottraux, Bouvard, Defayolle, and Messy (1988) have a 37-item and an 18-item self-report CAC, and Steketee and Freund (1993) proposed a shortened 28-item version based on the CAC of Freund et al.

The self-report versions of the CAC have good internal consistency, and the interview-based CAC has moderate to high observer-rated reliability. Test–retest stability is moderate, and both observer and self-report versions show sensitivity to treatment effects (Cottraux et al., 1988; Freund et al., 1987; Marks, Stern, Mawson, Cobb, & McDonald, 1980). The self-report and observer-rated CACs are highly correlated (.83 to .94), and patients with OCD score significantly higher on the measure than nonobsessional anxious patients and nonclinical control subjects. In addition, the CAC correlates with other obsessive–compulsive symptom measures such as the Maudsley Obsessional Compulsive Inventory (MOCI), the Padua Inventory, and Likert ratings of symptom severity. However, discriminant validity is weak, as indicated by correlations with non-obsessive–compulsive symptom measures that are as high as the correlations with obsessive–compulsive symptom measures (Taylor, 1995).

Taylor (1995) noted that the 38-item version is the most popular form of the CAC. Freund et al. (1987) found differences between assessors in their consistency in CAC ratings. They suggested that observers should be trained in the use of the CAC to ensure observed-based reliability. Because the observer and self-report versions are highly correlated, it may be advisable to use the self-report CAC unless assessors are trained in the use of the instrument. However, the instrument does have weak discriminant validity, and its correlation with other obsessive–compulsive symptom measures, such as the MOCI, is often not as high as one would expect (Antony, 2001). Taylor (1995, 1998) also commented that the CAC provides only an indirect measure of obsessive–compulsive symptoms because it assesses the degree of interference in daily activities rather than the frequency or severity of obsessions or compulsions. Feske and Chambless (2000) concluded that the CAC has little to recommend it over the MOCI other than its use of a 4-point rating scale and assessment of highly specific compulsion-relevant activities (see also Sternberger & Burns, 1990a, for supportive evidence). I suggest that the 38-item self-report CAC may be useful for gauging the extent of interference resulting from OCD and for assisting in the development of a fear hierarchy for exposure-based treatment. However, its contribution to the assessment of OCD is quite limited and will be overshadowed by more comprehensive and accurate obsessive–compulsive symptom measures. The 38-item CAC is reproduced in an appendix in the Freund et al. (1987) article, whereas the 28-item CAC can be found in Steketee and Freund (1993).

Yale–Brown Obsessive–Compulsive Scale

The Yale–Brown Obsessive–Compulsive Scale (YBOCS) is a 10-item clinician-rated scale that assesses the severity of obsessions and compulsions independent of the type (content) or number of symptoms (Goodman et al., 1989a, 1989b). It is widely used to assess the effectiveness of pharmacological and behavioral treatments for OCD and, in fact, has become the "gold standard" for assessment of obsessive–compulsive symptom severity in outcome studies (Steketee, 1994). The YBOCS consists of three sections. First, the interviewer provides the respondent with a definition and examples of obsessions and compulsions. Second, the interviewer uses a checklist of 64 common types of obsessions and compulsions to identify a respondent's pattern of current, as well as past, obsessions and compulsions. Because many patients with OCD will indicate a number of symptoms, the interviewer is instructed to mark the principal current obsessions and compulsions that will be the focus of treatment on a Target Symptom List under the categories Obsessions, Compulsions, and Avoidance.

The third section of the YBOCS consists of 10 core items, a 6-item investigational component, and 3 global ratings. The 10 core and 6 investigational items are each rated on a 5-point scale ranging from 0 (none) to 4 (extreme or severe). A descriptive statement is associated with each of the response options. Only the 10 core items are included in the total and subscale scores, and all of the psychometric data on the YBOCS refer to these first 10 items. Obsessions (items 1–5) and Compulsions (items 6–10) severity scores assess five symptom features: (1) duration/frequency, (2) interference in social or work functioning, (3) associated distress, (4) degree of resistance, and (5) perceived uncontrollability of the obsession or compulsion. The total severity score is most commonly reported by summing the 10 core items. Two additional items, (1b) and (6b) inquire about the longest time period individuals are free of the obsessions or compulsions on a typical day, but these are not included in the total score. The 6 investigational items assess lack of insight, avoidance, indecisiveness, inflated responsibility, slowness, and pathological doubting.

Interrater agreement on the 10 items is excellent, ranging from .76 to .97 across three studies (Goodman et al., 1989a; Nakagawa, Marks, Takei, De Araujo, & Ito, 1996; Woody, Steketee, & Chambless, 1995). Internal consistency for the two subscales and total score was in the acceptable range in three studies (Amir, Foa, & Coles, 1997; Goodman et al., 1989a; Richter, Cox, & Direnfeld, 1994), but unacceptably low in studies by Woody et al. (1995; Obsession = .77, Compulsion = .51, Total = .69) and Steketee, Frost, and Bogart (1996; Obsession = .56, Compulsion = .61, Total = .74). The temporal stability of the YBOCS is excellent over a 1- or 2-week interval (see Taylor, 1995). However, the inconsistent results from different factor analyses suggests that the 10 core YBOCS items may not separate cleanly into Obsessions and Compulsions dimensions (Amir, Foa, & Coles, 1997; McKay, Danyko, Neziroglu, & Yaryura-Tobias, 1995).

The YBOCS subscale and total scores show good convergent validity, with strong correlations with other self-report measures of obsessive–compulsive symptoms. In addition, the YBOCS is sensitive to treatment change and patients with OCD do score significantly higher than nonobsessional patients and normal control subjects (see reviews by Antony, 2001; Feske & Chambless, 2000; Taylor, 1995, 1998). The measure is also sensitive to obsessive–compulsive symptoms in nonclinical subject samples, although one can find considerable variability in YBOCS scores (Frost, Steketee, Krause, & Trepanier, 1995).

A few validation problems have been reported with the YBOCS. On occasion the instrument has not correlated with other measures of obsessive–compulsive symptoms. For example, Goodman et al. (1989b) found that it did not consistently correlate with the MOCI (see also Woody et al., 1995). In studies by the Obsessive Compulsive Cognitions Working Group, the self-report version of the YBOCS had weak correlations with specialized measures of obsessive–compulsive beliefs and appraisals, and low to moderate correlations with the Padua Inventory subscales (OCCWG, 2001, 2003a). Woody et al. (1995) reported low correlations with the behavioral avoidance test and ratings of target symptoms. Like other OCD measures, the YBOCS has weaker discriminant validity, as evidenced by moderate correlations with depression and anxiety measures (e.g., Goodman et al., 1989b; Ritcher et al., 1994; Woody et al., 1995).

Pencil-and-paper or computer-administered self-report versions of the measure are highly correlated with the clinician-administered YBOCS (Baer, Brown-Beasley, Sorce, & Henriques, 1993; Nakagawa et al., 1996; Rosenfeld, Dar, Anderson, Kobak, & Greist, 1992; Steketee, Frost, & Bogart, 1996). The YBOCS is currently under revision to address shortcomings in how resistance and avoidance are assessed (see Antony, 2001). Leckman and colleagues are also working on a dimensional symptom version of the YBOCS (see description by Taylor et al., 2002).

The YBOCS is an essential instrument to include in an assessment of OCD because it gives the clinician a measure of symptom severity independent of content, it is sensitive to treatment effects, and it has such widespread use that considerable normative data are now available. However, the measure also has its limitations, including (1) an inadequate assessment of resistance and failure to include avoidance as a core item, (2) has mixed evidence of subscale internal consistency, (3) has poor factorial support for obsessions and compulsions dimensions, (4) has weak discriminant validity, and (5) produces inconsistent relations with other obsessive–compulsive measures. Given the time-consuming nature of the clinician-administered YBOCS, the self-report version may be given as an alternative, although less psychometric evidence is available for this version of the measure. A copy of the YBOCS is reprinted in Anthony (2001) and the self-report YBOCS can be found in Baer (2000).

Self-Report Symptom Measures

Maudsley Obsessional Compulsive Inventory

The Maudsley Obsessional Compulsive Inventory (MOCI) is a 30-item true–false self-report questionnaire developed by Hodgson and Rachman (1977) to assess the presence of different types of obsessive and compulsive complaints. It consists of a total score and four factorially derived subscales: (1) checking (9 items), (2) washing (11 items), (3) slowness/repetition (7 items), and (4) doubting/conscientiousness (7 items). Taylor (1998) noted that the MOCI is actually a symptom checklist with scores reflecting the amount of time consumed by obsessions and compulsions.

A number of studies have evaluated the psychometric status of the MOCI (for reviews see Antony, 2001; Feske & Chambless, 2000; Steketee, 1994; Taylor, 1995, 1998). Internal consistency is adequate for the total score and the checking, washing, and doubting subscales, but not the slowness subscale. The instrument has moderate test–retest reliability and is sensitive to treatment effects. Patients with OCD do score significantly higher on the measure than nonobsessional anxious and nonclinical control subjects. The MOCI also has substantial correlations with other measures of obsessive–compulsive symptoms, and its significant correlations with measures of other psychopathological states tend to be lower than its association with OCD measures. Thus, there is strong support for the MOCI's convergent validity and, to a lesser extent, discriminant validity. Emmelkamp, Kraaijkamp, and van den Hout (1999) replicated the reliability and factorial validity of the MOCI in a sample of patients with OCD, nonobsessional patients, and nonclinical control subjects, although questions were raised about the sensitivity of the measure to treatment effects and its ability to discriminate OCD from depression.

The MOCI has a number of serious limitations. Some of its items do not deal directly with obsessive–compulsive symptoms, and it does not provide an adequate assessment of obsessional rumination (Taylor, 1995). Even though it primarily assesses compulsive rituals, it overemphasizes washing and checking to the exclusion of other types of neutralizing activities. It also fails to assess important aspects of obsessive–compulsive symptomatology such as interference and resistance. The reliance on a dichotomous (true–false) scaling format limits the measure's ability to quantify the severity of obsessive–compulsive symptoms. Finally, because the MOCI does not provide a broad, balanced representation of obsessive–compulsive symptoms, patients with washing or checking compulsions may score higher than expected for the severity of their illnesses, whereas others with obsessional rumination can score unusually low because so few items assess their primary obsessive–compulsive symptoms (Steketee, 1994; Taylor, 1995). Currently, the MOCI is under revision to address many of these shortcomings (Rachman, Thordarson, & Radomsky, 1995). The original version of the MOCI should be used in conjunction with other obsessive–compulsive measures and is most relevant for individuals with prominent washing or checking compulsions. A copy of the MOCI and scoring key can be found in Rachman and Hodgson (1980) and Antony (2001).

Padua Inventory

The Padua Inventory (PI) is a 60-item questionnaire developed by Sanavio (1988) with an Italian sample to assess the degree of disturbance (distress) associated with a range of obsessive and compulsive phenomena. Each item is assessed on a 5-point scale ranging from 0 (not al all) to 4 (very much). The PI was intended to be an improvement over existing obsessive–compulsive symptom measures by including cognitive as well as behavioral items that assessed both obsessions and compulsions.

Factor analysis on a nonclinical sample of Italian patients ($n = 967$) revealed four distinct dimensions: (1) impaired control over mental activities (17 items), (2) contamination (11 items), (3) checking (8 items), and

(4) urges and worries about losing control of motor behavior (7 items). The PI Total Score had adequate internal consistency and test–retest reliability, and patients with OCD scored significantly higher than an outpatient group with other neurotic disorders. Some studies have replicated the original PI factor structure (Sternberger & Burns, 1990b; van Oppen, 1992), whereas others have not reported the same factor solution (Kyrios, Bhar & Wade, 1996; van Oppen, Hoekstra, & Emmelkamp, 1995).

Two problems with the PI have become apparent. A number of PI questionnaire items are highly correlated with worry, so that the instrument has difficulty differentiating obsessions from worry (Freeston et al., 1994). Moreover, factor analysis of an OCD sample ($n = 206$) revealed that only 42 PI items had high loadings on a five-component structure, but even that was not similar to Sanavio's (1988) original factor solution (van Oppen, Hoekstra, & Emmelkamp, 1995). This discovery led to two revisions of the PI. Van Oppen, Hoekstra, and Emmelkamp (1995) proposed a 41-item PI based on their findings. Burns, Keortge, Formea, and Sternberger (1996) constructed a 39-item PI, referred to as the Padua Inventory–Washington State University Revision (PI-WSUR), that excluded items judged to confound worry and obsessions. The PI-WSUR has five content categories (1) obsessional thoughts of harm to self/others (7 items), (2) obsessional impulses to harm self/others (9 items), (3) contamination obsessions and washing compulsions (10 items), (4) checking compulsions (10 items), and (5) dressing/grooming compulsions (3 items). The PI-WSUR appears to have improved psychometric properties over the original PI, and so it has gained in popularity with OCD researchers (Antony, 2001).

The PI and PI-WSUR have good internal consistency and test–retest reliability. The inventory correlates with other measures of obsessive–compulsive symptoms, and individuals with OCD score higher on the measure than patients with other anxiety disorders. Furthermore, the revised versions of the PI do appear to provide a better discrimination of obsessions from worry, and the measure is sensitive to treatment effects. However, the PI and PI-WSUR also show substantial correlations with measures of anxiety, depression, and other forms of psychopathology (for reviews see Antony, 2001; Feske & Chambless, 2000).

Currently, the PI, especially the PI-WSUR, has much to recommend it as a general self-report measure of obsessive–compulsive symptoms. However, even the revised versions contain items that are somewhat ambiguous, lack specificity, and are possibly less relevant to the primary features of OCD (e.g., "Seeing weapons excites me and makes me think violent thoughts," "I sometimes worry at length for no reason that I have hurt myself or have some disease"). Other characteristics of obsessive–compulsive symptoms such as duration, interference, resistance, and uncontrollability are not assessed, and items reflecting mental rituals and sexual intrusive thoughts are missing (Feske & Chambless, 2000). The PI and PI-WSUR also have lower discriminant validity. A copy of the original PI can be found in Sanavio (1988), and the PI-WSUR has been reproduced in Antony (2001).

Obsessive–Compulsive Inventory

The Obsessive–Compulsive Inventory (OCI) is a 42-item self-report questionnaire designed to (1) assess a broader range of obsessive and compulsive symptom content, (2) provide a greater symptom severity range, and (3) have widespread applicability to clinical and nonclinical subjects (Foa, Kozak, Salkovskis, Coles, & Amir, 1998). Each item is rated on a five-point Likert scale for frequency and distress. This yields frequency and distress total scores, as well as separate frequency and distress scores for seven rationally determined subscales: (1) washing (8 items), (2) checking (9 items), (3) doubting (3 items), (4) ordering (5 items), (5) obsessing (8 items), (6) hoarding (3 items), and (7) mental neutralizing (6 items).

The initial psychometric data on the OCI appeared most promising. Foa, Kozak, et al. (1998) based their analyses on 114 individuals with OCD, 58 with generalized social phobia, 44 with posttraumatic stress disorder, and 194 nonclinical subjects who were primarily students. Internal consistency of the Frequency and Distress total scores and most of the seven subscales (with the exception of mental neutralizing) were within an acceptable range (greater than .70). Two-week test–retest ranged from .68 to .97. Although the OCD group had similar Frequency and Distress scores, the remaining groups scored significantly higher on the Frequency scale than on the Distress scale. The OCD group scored significantly higher than those with other anxiety disorders and nonclinical control subjects on all OCI scales except Hoarding. In the sample of patients with OCD, the OCI Frequency and Distress Total Scores had strong correlations with the MOCI and CAC total scores, but correlations with the interview YBOCS were low. However, the OCI Frequency and Distress total scores also had substantial correlations with trait anxiety and with self-reported anxious and depressive symptoms. A subsequent nonclinical study supported the internal consistency and temporal stability of the OCI subscales (Simonds, Thorpe, & Elliott, 2000). Strong correlations were also obtained between the OCI and MOCI Total Scores and subscales.

An 18-item short form of the OCI (OCI-R) was developed by Foa, Huppert, et al. (2002). The instrument was factored into six dimensions (Washing, Checking, Ordering, Obsessing, Hoarding, and Neutralizing), and subscales based on this factor structure showed acceptable internal consistency and good test–retest reliability. Although the OCI-R correlates moderately with the YBOCS (r = .53) and very highly with the MOCI (r = .85), it also has substantial correlations with depression measures (BDI, r = .70). Patients with OCD scored significantly higher than those with generalized social phobia and posttraumatic stress disorder on all subscales except Hoarding. However, analysis of the optimal OCI-R cutoff score revealed that only 66% of the sample of patients with OCD was correctly distinguished from nonanxious students (64% of students were correctly classified). The OCI-R Obsessing subscale did yield better classification rates. Clearly, more research is needed on the diagnostic utility and discriminant validity of the OCI-R before it can be accepted as a standard measure of obsessive–compulsive symptoms. One of the significant limitations of the measure is that only three items assess obsessions. Because it is primarily a measure of compulsions, the OCI-R is subject to some of the same criticisms as the MOCI. A copy of the original OCI is reproduced in Antony (2001), and the short form OCI-R appears as an appendix to the Foa, Huppert, et al. (2002) article.

PROCESS-ORIENTED ASSESSMENT OF OBSESSIONS

A complete assessment of OCD for the purpose of case formulation and treatment planning can not rely solely on clinician-based or self-report global measures of symptom frequency or severity. Rather, idiographic measures are needed that target specific obsessive–compulsive symptoms and parameters (Taylor, 1995). This section discusses a specific assessment strategy for obtaining individualized data on cognitive, behavioral, and situational features of obsessions that will be invaluable in formulating a treatment intervention. The emphasis here is on obtaining *in vivo*, online data on the variables responsible for the maintenance of obsessive and compulsive symptoms. This can be obtained within the therapy session through the creation of "simulations" that induce obsessive–compulsive symptoms (e.g., Purdon, 2001).

For example, a therapist might expose a client with dirt and contamination obsessions to a series of provoking stimuli (e.g., touch a doorknob, handle money, wipe hands on floor, etc.) in order to record the person's level of distress, latency to formation of the obsession, urge to neutralize, and the like. Alternatively, the therapist can provide the client with rating scales and recording sheets to self-monitor his or her experience of obsessions and compulsions between therapy sessions. In fact, the use of between-session self-monitoring exercises will be necessary in order to assess the individual's experience of obsessions and compulsions in a naturalistic setting. Moreover, a specialized semistructured interview designed to obtain general and specific information on obsessions and compulsions can be helpful (see examples provided by Rachman, 2003; Steketee, 1999).

Situational Analysis

As part of the assessment process, it is important to gather specific information on the situations or stimuli that trigger the patient's primary obsessions. These data will be invaluable for constructing the graded fear hierarchy that is important for developing a cognitive-behavioral treatment plan that includes exposure and response prevention. Appendix 8.1 presents a recording form that can be used to identify situations that most often trigger a primary obsession. In addition to providing a description of each situation, the patient is asked to rate the level of distress experienced when exposed to the situation, the likelihood that the primary obsession will be triggered when in the situation, and the likelihood that the person will try to avoid the situation. Information on distress, probability of provocation, and extent of avoidance will be important in ordering situations from least difficult to most difficult when planning exposure exercises. For patients with multiple primary obsessions, a separate situational analysis should be conducted for each obsession. Foa and Kozak (1997) provide additional clinically useful information on situational assessment of obsessions and compulsions in their *Mastery of Obsessive–Compulsive Disorder: Client Workbook.*

Self-Monitoring Diaries

It is, of course, essential to obtain specific information on the daily frequency and distress of the patient's primary obsessions. These data are not only important for assessing the severity of OCD, but will be necessary information for building a treatment program and for judging the effectiveness of an intervention. The primary indicator of treatment success will be reductions in the patient's daily experience of obsessions. Thus, it is critical to obtain a pretreatment baseline assessment of the frequency and intensity of target obsessions over at least a 2-week period. Additional discussion of guidelines and use of self-monitoring forms and diaries in the ongoing assessment of obsessions and compulsions can be found elsewhere (Foa & Kozak, 1997; Freeston & Ladouceur, 1997a; Salkovskis & Kirk, 1989; Steketee, 1999).

Appendix 8.2 presents a daily self-monitoring or diary form that can be used to collect pretreatment baseline data on primary obsessions. On the basis of the prior diagnostic and symptom assessment, the therapist identifies, in collaboration with the patient, the primary obsession(s) that will be targeted for treatment. The individual is then asked to complete a 2-week *in vivo* record of the daily frequency and emotional distress of the obsession, using the form in Appendix 8.2. In addition, patients are asked to make a daily record of their effort to control the obsession and the intensity of their urge to initiate a compulsive or neutralization response.

Cognitive Appraisals and Beliefs

In order to provide cognitive-behavioral therapy (CBT) for obsessions, it is important to obtain information on the cognitive appraisals and beliefs that are considered critical in the pathogenesis of obsessions. The therapist can use standardized self-report measures that have been developed to assess the specific cognitive features of obsessions. Moreover, the therapist should collect more idiographic, *in vivo* ratings of obsessional appraisals in order to tailor the treatment plan to each patient's pathology (for helpful discussion and case illustration on eliciting appraisals in OCD, see McLean & Woody, 2001).

It is beyond the scope of this discussion to provide a comprehensive and detailed review of the numerous measures that have been developed to assess appraisals and beliefs implicated in OCD. Antony (2001), Tallis (1995), and Taylor (1995) offer a brief overview or commentary on a select number of these measures. Most of them have been used only for research purposes and have not achieved a level of psychometric support that would justify their widespread clinical adoption. The following paragraphs do, however, highlight a few measures that the cognitive-behavioral therapist might utilize to provide supplementary information on key cognitive factors of obsessions.

The Thought–Action Fusion Scale (TAF Scale) is a 19-item self-report questionnaire developed by Shafran, Thordarson, and Rachman (1996) to assess the three aspects of TAF: Moral (12 items), Likelihood Others (4 items), and Likelihood Self (3 items). Individuals with OCD tend to score higher on the TAF Scale than nonclinical subjects (although to a lesser extent for TAF Moral), and TAF does correlate with measures of obsessive–compulsive symptoms and other obsession-related cognitive constructs. However, findings are mixed on whether TAF is specific to OCD or has more general relevance, and whether the construct fluctuates over time and situations (Amir et al., 2001; Coles et al., 2001; Rassin, Muris, et al., 2000; Rassin, Merckelbach, et al., 2001; Shafran, Thordarson, & Rachman, 1996; Smari & Hólmsteinsson, 2001). Still, at this time there is some evidence that the TAF Scale may assess an appraisal and belief construct that is a salient feature of obsessional thinking.

Salkovskis and colleagues developed the 26-item Responsibility Attitude Scale (RAS) to assess general attitudes and beliefs about responsibility, and the 22-item Responsibility Interpretations Questionnaire (RIQ) to measure the frequency of, and strength of belief in appraisals of responsibility associated with, intrusive thoughts (Salkovskis et al., 2000). In the validation study (Salkovskis et al., 2000), patients with OCD scored significantly higher on the RAS and RIQ Frequency and Belief scales than anxious and nonclinical control subjects, and the measures showed strong correlations with self-reported obsessive–compulsive symptoms, although

the specificity of the RAS and the RIQ has not been adequately investigated. An earlier measure, the Inventory of Beliefs Related to Obsessions
(IBRO), predates much of the more recent theoretical work on the cognitive basis of OCD and so is not as useful in measuring current cognitive
constructs of OCD (Freeston et al., 1993).

Two measures recently developed by the OCCWG provide the most
promising approach to the self-report assessment of obsessional appraisals and beliefs. The 31-item Interpretation of Intrusions Inventory (III)
was designed to assess appraisals of responsibility, overimportance of
thought intrusions, and control of intrusions. The 87-item Obsessive Beliefs Questionnaire (OBQ) was developed to assess more enduring beliefs
that constitute vulnerability to OCD. The III and OBQ have now been investigated in two large studies involving more than 300 individuals with
OCD, nonobsessional anxious control subjects, and nonclinical samples
of subjects across multiple sites (OCCWG, 2001, 2003a). Overall, both
measures have high internal consistency and moderate test–retest reliability. Patients with OCD scored significantly higher than anxious patients
on OBQ Control of Thoughts, Importance of Thoughts and Responsibility, and on III Control of Thoughts, and Responsibility (OCCWG, 2003a).
Both measures had strong correlations with obsessive–compulsive symptom measures but lower discriminant validity. Factor analysis of the two
measures reveals that the III is a single-dimension instrument and thus
only the Total Score should be used. Factor analysis of the OBQ indicated
that a 44-item version proved as psychometrically strong as the OBQ-87.
The OBQ-44 consists of three subscales, Responsibility/Threat Estimation, Perfectionism/Certainty, and Importance/Control of Thoughts
(OCCWG, 2003b). Despite certain limitations, the OBQ and III are the
best normative self-report instruments currently available for assessing
the contemporary core cognitive constructs of obsessions.

Even when standardized self-report cognition measures are utilized,
it is important to include more individualized, therapy-oriented record
forms and rating scales to obtain a fine-grained assessment of individuals'
core appraisals and beliefs of their obsessions. Appendix 8.3 presents a
form that can be used to identify the perceived negative or harmful outcomes associated with an obsession. It is important that the therapist understand all of the anticipated consequences that individuals imagine are
connected with their obsessions. These can include outcomes such as "I
will become seriously ill or contaminated," "My anxiety will continue to
escalate until I can't stand it," "I will eventual go crazy," "I will lose control
and do something awful," "Someone will get seriously hurt," and the like.
In order to develop an effective cognitive intervention, it is important to
obtain a comprehensive and detailed assessment of all the anticipated
dreaded consequences that could result from a failure to terminate the
obsession. In addition to identifying the consequences, the form also pro-

vides for rating the expected level of distress if an outcome were to occur, the perceived probability that the outcome could occur, and the importance to the patient of preventing this outcome.

A final set of ratings that can prove useful in the assessment of core appraisals of obsessions is a series of rating scales adapted from the Revised Obsessional Intrusions Inventory (Purdon & Clark, 1994b). As presented in Appendix 8.4, individuals are asked to rate their appraisal and experience of a designated primary obsession. The parameters selected in Appendix 8.4 are the key emotion and appraisal variables that characterize obsessions. In addition, Rachman (2003) developed rating scales for assessing appraisals of personal significance, responsibility, and obsessional activity.

PROCESS-ORIENTED ASSESSMENT OF COMPULSIONS

Specific, idiographic data on an individual's experience of compulsions and other neutralizing strategies used to control primary obsessions are also needed in treatment planning. Behavior therapists employing exposure and response prevention have long recognized the need for accurate information on the frequency, intensity, and level of success associated with compulsive rituals. The following discussion gives only a short overview of the behavioral assessment of compulsions and refers the reader to a number of excellent descriptions provided in the behavioral literature (e.g., Foa & Kozak, 1997; Steketee 1993, 1994, 1999; Steketee & Barlow, 2002; Taylor, 1995). In addition, the cognitive-behavioral therapist must assess more broadly for any behavioral or cognitive response strategy that may be used to neutralize or control unwanted obsessions.

Behavioral Avoidance Tests (BATs)

The BAT was originally developed to measure *in vivo* fear and avoidance in specific phobias (Lang & Lazovik, 1963). Rachman and colleagues adapted the procedure for use in OCD (Hodgson, Rachman, & Marks, 1972; Rachman et al., 1979; Rachman et al., 1971). Patients were asked to perform a variety of activities (e.g., five tasks) that provoked their compulsive ritual. An assessor rated whether each activity was executed (score of 1) or avoided (score of 0), and a discomfort rating (0–8) was obtained for each task. A BAT score was calculated in terms of the number of tasks completed and the summed discomfort rating across all tasks.

Although the BAT is a clinically useful instrument for obtaining *in vivo* data on the extent and severity of avoidance and compulsive rituals, it is best suited for assessing fear of dirt/contamination and washing compulsions. Refinements have been made to the BAT (Steketee, Chambless,

Tran, Worden, & Gillis, 1996), and it is correlated with other obsessive–compulsive symptom measures. It is also sensitive to treatment effects, and there is evidence of divergent validity. However, psychometric data on the use of BATs for OCD is limited, it may be difficult to construct the tests for many types of compulsions, there is no standardized protocol for administration, and the tests are time-consuming (Taylor, 1995; Taylor et al., 2002). Nevertheless, a BAT can provide valuable *in vivo* pretreatment information in constructing an exposure/response prevention intervention, especially when there is evidence of extensive avoidance of situations and overt behavioral compulsions. Steketee, Chambless, et al. (1996) and Steketee and Barlow (2002) provide case illustrations of the multiple-step/multiple-task version of the BAT.

Self-Monitoring Forms

It is also useful to have patients self-monitor their rituals between sessions in order to track the frequency of ritualistic behavior, the situations that provoke the compulsions, the amount of time taken up in ritualizing, and the associated discomfort level. Foa and Kozak (1997) provide a self-monitoring form that can be used by patients to monitor their rituals (see also Steketee, 1999). Foa and Kozak (1997) note that self-monitoring one's rituals can have a therapeutic benefit because it can help the patient to become aware of compulsive actions that may be performed quite automatically. In this way the self-monitoring process, though somewhat onerous, is an important first step toward gaining control over a compulsion.

Assessing Covert Neutralization and Mental Control

In addition to obtaining accurate information on the type of control strategies utilized in response to obsessions, it is important that therapists obtain data on the appraisal variables associated with the strategy (see Chapter 7). This information will be especially important in formulating a comprehensive cognitive-behavioral treatment program.

Appendix 8.5 presents a record form for identifying the types of control strategies that patients may use to control their obsessions. The 12 strategies are based on the research of Freeston and Ladouceur (Freeston & Ladouceur, 1997b; Ladouceur et al., 2000; Wells & Davies, 1994; Purdon & Clark, 1994b). Each strategy is rated for its frequency, perceived effectiveness in dealing with the obsession, and perceived effectiveness in reducing distress. When used at pretreatment, this measure will provide the clinician with critical information on the compulsive rituals, neutralization, and intentional mental control strategies that should be targeted in the treatment program. Even more important, the clinician can determine the individual's appraisals of control associated with each strategy.

This information will be critical in constructing cognitive interventions for countering the dysfunctional appraisals that maintain individuals' futile efforts to control their obsessions. Rachman (2003) also presents a work sheet that provides an idiographic assessment of responses to unwanted intrusive thoughts.

COGNITIVE-BEHAVIORAL CASE FORMULATION

As noted in Figure 8.1, the various components of the cognitive-behavioral assessment of OCD converge in the development of a case formulation that will assist the therapist in the provision of effective treatment. Persons and Davidson (2001) define cognitive-behavioral case formulation as "an idiographic (individualized) theory that is based on a nomothetic (general) cognitive-behavioral theory" (p. 86). The case formulation in the present context is based on the cognitive-behavioral theories of OCD described in Chapters 5 and 7. It focuses on formulation at the *problem level* by enumerating the various processes involved in the etiology and persistence of an individual's obsessions and compulsions. In this sense the cognitive-behavioral case formulation for OCD presented in Appendix 8.6 is more similar to the cognitive conceptualization offered by J. S. Beck (1995) than the broader case formulation described by Persons and colleagues (Persons, 1989; Persons & Davidson, 2001). Whether at the level of the case, the syndrome, or the situation, all formulations are considered hypotheses that the therapist continually revises throughout treatment (Persons & Davidson, 2001).

The problem-focused case formulation presented in Appendix 8.6 is designed to facilitate the development of a "working hypothesis," which Persons and Davidson (2001) describe as the "heart of the formulation" (p. 94). According to these authors, the working hypothesis describes the relationships between problems and the various processes thought to maintain these problems, based on a particular theory of the syndrome or disorder. Persons and Davidson (2001) provide an excellent explanation of cognitive-behavioral case formulation and the working hypothesis, in particular, with case illustration and discussion of their integration with treatment planning and implementation.

Taylor et al. (2002) offer an alternative case formulation for OCD that comprises a problem list, problem context, dysfunctional beliefs, working hypothesis, treatment plan, and treatment obstacles. Their approach does not provide the fine-grained analysis of the cognitive basis of obsessions and compulsions represented in Appendix 8.6. Rather, it includes much broader aspects of clinical disorder, such as diagnosis and current symptomatology, personal and family history, predisposing and protective factors. In this way it is more streamlined than the present cognitive-behavioral case formulation. However, both types of case formulation should lead to a working hypothesis, treatment plan, and evaluation.

Distal and Proximal Contributors

The cognitive-behavioral case formulation in Appendix 8.6 is essential for offering the type of therapy for obsessions and compulsions described in the following chapters. The therapist first lists all the current events and experiences that have contributed or even provoked the occurrence of obsessions and compulsions. This information can be obtained from the diagnostic and psychological assessment conducted with the patient. It may include the following types of information:

- Major or even minor life events,
- Critical learning experiences involving unlucky or improbable events that crystallize the person's doubts and irrational assumptions (Rhéaume et al., 1998),
- A comorbid condition like depression or another anxiety disorder,
- Particular personality vulnerabilities such as introversion, low self-esteem, or excessive conscientiousness, and/or
- Other clinical phenomena such as worry or overvalued ideas.

The therapist should also note any distal factors arising from the patient's childhood or family experiences that may have contributed to the development of OCD, as well as any current family or marital factors that may be involved in the persistence of the obsessional state. Together, the contributing factors and determinants noted in the case formulation provide some general indications of distal and, even more so, proximal factors that may be involved in the etiology of the person's OCD.

Core Symptom Features

At the heart of the case formulation is the specification of the primary obsessions and compulsions that will be targeted for treatment. This information is obtained from the diagnostic interview, symptom-based obsessive–compulsive measures, and self-monitoring records administered during the assessment. In many cases multiple obsessions and compulsive rituals may be present. All significant obsessions and compulsions should be noted, but some effort should be made to prioritize which symptoms are primary and which are secondary. Normally, the therapist begins treatment with the primary obsessions and compulsions. At this level, additional information should be noted about the obsessive–compulsive symptoms, such as their frequency, duration (amount of time), level of interference in daily activities, and situational triggers (context). It should also be noted whether there are any additional factors that worsen the symptoms or that enable some reprieve from the obsessions. The clinician should also highlight any factors that may be especially important to the success or failure of treatment, such as the patient's level of motivation, expectation for success, compliance with the assessment, treatment history, or any indications of resistance to therapy.

Cognitive Profile of Obsessions

An important component of the case formulation is the cognitive profile of obsessions, which represents what is most unique about the cognitive-behavioral approach. Here the therapist focuses on specific cognitive content, processes, and structures, which are considered critical in the persistence of obsessions and compulsions and are therefore important targets of intervention. One begins by specifying the affective experience associated with the obsession. Does the obsession primarily elicit anxiety or fear, or are there elements of guilt, anger, or even sadness? What makes the obsession so salient for most individuals with OCD is that it is associated with such intense negative affect. Thus, it is important to understand the nature and intensity of the emotional state associated with the obsession.

The therapist then identifies the core appraisals of the obsession. The process focuses on such constructs as responsibility, threat estimation, intolerance of uncertainty, overimportance of thought, control of thoughts, and the like. This information can be obtained from specific cognitive measures and the idiographic self-monitoring and rating scales previously described. From the types of appraisals associated with the obsession, the therapist will be able to infer the core obsessional beliefs that are maintaining the individual's obsessional symptoms. This part of the case formulation is vital to developing the working hypothesis that guides the cognitive interventions to be used in the cognitive-behavioral treatment that follows.

Cognitive Profile of Compulsions

Another important component of the case formulation is the specification of the cognitive and behavioral factors involved in the person's attempts to control the obsession and its associated distress. In addition to noting the frequency and intensity of compulsive rituals, the therapist includes any other overt or covert neutralization activities or intentional mental control strategies used to deal with the obsession. Information on the frequency and context of these responses to the obsession should be noted. The extent of cognitive or behavioral avoidance should also be recorded. The therapist should then note the main appraisals of control associated with the primary control strategies. How intense is the person's urge to perform the compulsion or other control strategy? Does he or she perceive that the strategy is effective in terminating the obsession or reducing distress? What consequences are expected if the compulsion or other control activities are not performed? From these appraisals of the compulsion, the therapist can identify core beliefs about control that are important in the persistence of the compulsion.

Working Hypothesis

The final phase of the cognitive behavioral case formulation is the development of a *summary statement of the working hypothesis* (Persons & Davidson, 2001). This involves an overall statement of the key variables involved in the etiology and persistence of the individual's obsessions and compulsions. The hypothesis specifies how these key variables interrelate to perpetuate obsessive–compulsive symptomatology. In this way the working hypothesis feeds into the treatment goals and provides guidance for the implementation of the cognitive-behavioral intervention.

SUMMARY AND CONCLUSION

A problem-oriented assessment strategy for OCD is proposed that is derived from cognitive-behavioral theory and research on obsessions and compulsions. This cognitive-behavioral assessment for OCD includes diagnostic and psychological interviews, standardized obsessive–compulsive symptom-based measures, and more idiographic process-oriented ratings of the appraisals and beliefs associated with targeted obsessions and compulsions. Together, data from diagnostic instruments, nomothetic questionnaires, and idiographic rating forms contribute to the formation of a working hypothesis about the situational, cognitive, emotive, and behavioral factors critical to the persistence of obsessive and compulsive phenomena. It is this formulation or working hypothesis that becomes the basis of the cognitive-behavioral intervention described in the following chapters.

APPENDIX 8.1. Situational Record and Rating Scales for Primary Obsession

Name of client: _____ Date: _____

Primary obsession: _____

Instructions: In consultation with your therapist, please record the obsessional thought, image, or impulse that is most troubling for you at this time. Then list the situations, objects, or circumstances that most often trigger the primary obsession. Please complete the rating scale associated with each situation.

List of triggering situations	Distress rating of situation (0 = none to 100 = extreme, panic-like)	Likelihood of provoking obsession (0 = never to 100 = certainty, always provokes)	Likelihood of avoiding situation (0 = never avoid to 100 = always avoid)
1.			
2.			
3.			
4.			
5.			
6.			
7.			
8.			
9.			
10.			
11.			
12.			
13.			
14.			
15.			

APPENDIX 8.2. Daily Record of Primary Obsession

Name of client: _____ Date: _____

Primary obsession: _____

Instructions: In consultation with your therapist, please record the obsessional thought, image, or impulse that is most troubling for you at this time. Record the approximate number of times you experienced the obsession on a particular day. Then complete the rating scales for each day, indicating your most typical experience of the obsession for that day. This form should be completed at bedtime each evening.

Day of week	Approximate frequency of obsession during the day	Average distress of obsession (0 = none to 100 = extreme, panic-like)	Intensity of effort to control obsession (0 = no effort to control to 100 = frantic effort to stop thinking the obsession)	Intensity of urge to engage in compulsion or neutralization (0 = no urge to 100 = irresistible urge)
Sunday				
Monday				
Tuesday				
Wednesday				
Thursday				
Friday				
Saturday				
Sunday				
Monday				
Tuesday				
Wednesday				
Thursday				
Friday				
Saturday				

Name of client: _____ Date: _____

Primary obsession: _____

Instructions: In consultation with your therapist, please record the obsessional thought, image, or impulse that is most troubling for you at this time. Then list the anticipated or feared consequences or outcome that you are concerned may occur if you continue to have the obsession in your mind. Please complete the rating scales associated with each outcome.

List of possible negative consequences or outcomes associated with obsession	Distress rating of outcome (0 = none to 100 = extreme, panic-like)	Likelihood that outcome will occur (0 = would never happen to 100 = most certainly would happen)	Importance of preventing outcome (0 = not at all important to 100 = critical to my survival)
1.			
2.			
3.			
4.			
5.			
6.			
7.			
8.			
9.			
10.			
11.			
12.			
13.			
14.			
15.			

Name of Client: _____ Date: _____

Primary obsession: _____

Instructions: In consultation with your therapist, please record the obsessional thought, image, or impulse that is most troubling for you at this time. Please complete the ratings below, on the basis of your experience of the primary obsession.

1. How guilty do you feel when you have the obsession? [GUILT]

   1 = not at all guilty
   2 = somewhat guilty
   3 = guilty
   4 = very guilty
   5 = extremely guilty

2. Does the obsession make you afraid for yourself or another person? [FEAR]

   1 = not at all afraid
   2 = somewhat afraid
   3 = afraid
   4 = very much afraid
   5 = extremely afraid

3. To what extent does the obsession make you uncertain about yourself or your actions? [DOUBT]

   1 = not at all uncertain
   2 = somewhat uncertain
   3 = uncertain
   4 = very uncertain
   5 = extremely uncertain

4. How disgusting or repulsive (immoral) is the obsession to you? [DISGUST]

   1 = not at all disgusting
   2 = somewhat disgusting
   3 = disgusting
   4 = very disgusting
   5 = extremely disgusting

5. Does the obsession make you feel more responsible for the well-being of yourself or others? [RESPONSIBILITY]

   1 = not at all responsible
   2 = somewhat responsible
   3 = responsible
   4 = very responsible
   5 = extremely responsible

6. Are you concerned that by thinking the obsession you may be more likely to act on it? [THOUGHT–ACTION FUSION]

   1 = not at all concerned
   2 = somewhat concerned
   3 = concerned
   4 = very much concerned
   5 = extremely concerned

(continued)

7. To what extent do you have to be precise and exact in response to the obsession? [INTOLERANCE OF UNCERTAINTY]

   1 = not at all exact

   2 = somewhat exact

   3 = exact

   4 = very exact

   5 = extremely exact

8. To what extent does the obsession indicate something important about you, the type of person you are? [IMPORTANCE]

   1 = not at all relevant to self

   2 = somewhat relevant to self

   3 = relevant to self

   4 = very relevant to self

   5 = extremely relevant to self

9. How important is it that you exercise strong control over the obsession? [CONTROL]

   1 = not at all important

   2 = somewhat important

   3 = important

   4 = very important

   5 = extremely important

Rating scales are based on items found in Part II of the Revised Obsessional Intrusions Inventory (Purdon & Clark, 1994b).

APPENDIX 8.5. Record of Control Strategies Associated with Primary Obsession

Name of Client: _____   Date: _____

Primary obsession: _____

Instructions: In consultation with your therapist, please record the obsessional thought, image, or impulse that is most troubling for you at this time. Below you will find a number of methods that people use to try to stop their obsessional thoughts, images, or impulses. Please indicate the frequency and success of each control strategy as it relates to your primary obsession. Use the rating scales provided with each category.

List of control strategies associated with primary obsession	Frequency that strategy is used (0 = never, 1 = occasionally, 2 = often, 3 = frequently, 4 = daily, 5 = several times a day)	Effectiveness of this strategy in stopping obsessional thinking (0 = never effective, 1 = occasionally effective, 2 = often effective, 3 = frequently effective, 4 = always effective)	Effectiveness of this strategy in reducing distress (0 = never effective, 1 = occasionally effective, 2 = often effective, 3 = frequently effective, 4 = always effective)
1. Engage in a behavioral compulsion (e.g., wash, check, repeat, etc.). [BC]			
2. Engage in a mental compulsion (e.g., say a particular phrase, repeat a prayer, think certain thoughts, etc.). [MC]			
3. Think about reasons why the obsession is senseless, unimportant, or irrational. [CR]			
4. Try to reassure myself that everything will be all right. [SR]			
5. Seek reassurance from others that everything will be all right. [OR]			
6. Distract myself by doing something. [BD]			
7. Distract myself by thinking another, possibly pleasant, thought or image. [CD]			
8. Try to relax myself. [R]			

(continued)

List of control strategies associated with primary obsession	Frequency that strategy is used (0 = never, 1 = occasionally, 2 = often, 3 = frequently, 4 = daily, 5 = several times a day)	Effectiveness of this strategy in stopping obsessional thinking (0 = never effective, 1 = occasionally effective, 2 = often effective, 3 = frequently effective, 4 = always effective)	Effectiveness of this strategy in reducing distress (0 = never effective, 1 = occasionally effective, 2 = often effective, 3 = frequently effective, 4 = always effective)
9. Tell myself to stop thinking the obsession. [TS]			
10. Get angry, down on myself for thinking the obsession. [P]			
11. Try to avoid anything that will trigger the obsession. [A]			
12. Do nothing when I get the obsession. [DN]			

Strategies adapted from Freeston and Ladouceur's Structured Interview on Neutralization (see Ladouceur et al., 2000), the Thought Control Questionnaire (Wells & Davies, 1994), and the Revised Obsessional Intrusions Inventory (Purdon & Clark, 1994b).

Coding key: BC, behavioral compulsion; MC, mental compulsion; CR, cognitive restructuring; SR, self-reassurance; OR, other reassurance; BD, behavioral distraction; CD, cognitive distraction; R, relaxation; TS, thought stopping; P, punishment; A, avoidance; DN, do nothing.

Name: _____ Date: _____

CONTRIBUTING FACTORS/EXPERIENCES	CHILDHOOD/FAMILY DETERMINANTS
_____	_____
_____	_____
_____	_____

OCD FEATURES TARGETTED FOR TREATMENT

_____

_____

_____

_____

OBSESSIONS   *COMPULSIONS*

Emotion Profile	Response Control Profile
_____	_____
_____	_____
_____	_____

Primary Appraisals	Appraisals of Control
_____	_____
_____	_____
_____	_____
_____	_____
_____	_____
	_____

Core Obsessional Beliefs	Core Control Beliefs
_____	_____
_____	_____
_____	_____

CHAPTER 9

Getting Started

Basic Elements and Rationale

At first glance cognitive interventions might seem quite ineffective, possibly even counterproductive, in the treatment of obsessional states. People with OCD usually recognize the irrational, even senseless, nature of their obsessions and compulsions. As a result, the use of finely tuned arguments about the improbability of an obsessional fear or the irrationality of a person's assumptions would be futile, because the patient already knows the fear is irrational (Salkovskis,1999; Steketee, Frost, et al., 1998). Even if you could convince a person with OCD that there is, for example, only a one-in-a-billion chance of catching a deadly disease by touching a doorknob, the individual would probably conclude that those slimmest of odds are enough reason to continue with compulsive washing and avoidance. Moreover, many individuals with OCD are particularly skilled at using intellectualization and rationalization to support their preoccupation with a primary obsession.

Despite justified skepticism about the utility of verbal therapies for the treatment of OCD, many prominent OCD clinical researchers are now advocating that cognitive strategies be added to standard exposure and response prevention (ERP) for obsessions and compulsions. The Expert Consensus Guidelines for the Treatment of Obsessive–Compulsive Disorder (March et al., 1997) recommended cognitive-behavioral therapy (CBT) alone for mild cases of OCD, and CBT plus medication for more severe obsessional states. Cognitive therapy was considered especially helpful for scrupulosity, moral guilt, and pathological doubt. The reasons for this shift toward a more cognitive orientation stems from considerable dissatisfaction with standard behavior theory and therapy of OCD (see Chapter 3 for a discussion of limitations).

This chapter discusses the basic elements and early stages of the cognitive-behavioral treatment of OCD. The CBT approach to obsessional states is a theory-driven intervention strategy derived from the cognitive-behavioral theories and research discussed in Chapters 5 and 7. The chapter begins with a definition and discussion of the main theoretical assumptions of CBT. The next section discusses the critical elements of a healthy therapeutic relationship and some of the pitfalls to avoid when offering CBT to individuals with OCD. The chapter concludes with a detailed presentation of the first phase of CBT, educating the patient to the cognitive-behavioral model of OCD. Specific intervention strategies, clinical resources, and therapist responses are presented that can facilitate the patient's acceptance of the therapeutic rationale.

FUNDAMENTAL ASSUMPTIONS OF CBT FOR OBSESSIONS

Definition

Cognitive-behavioral therapy (CBT) for OCD is a *psychological treatment that utilizes both cognitive and behavioral therapeutic change strategies to achieve reductions in obsessive and compulsive symptoms by modifying the faulty appraisals, specific core beliefs, and dysfunctional neutralization responses that are implicated in the etiology and persistence of obsessional complaints.* CBT is not defined by a particular set of therapeutic techniques, but rather is a treatment approach derived from cognitive-behavioral models of OCD. The basic cognitive-behavioral appraisal model of OCD illustrated in Figure 5.1 provides the theoretical framework for CBT of obsessions. In the early stages of therapy, clients are introduced to the cognitive-behavioral appraisal model as a framework for understanding their obsessions and as a rationale for various elements of the treatment. Thus, the cognitive-behavioral therapist should have a good understanding of cognitive-behavioral theory and research on OCD before offering CBT for obsessions.

Main Assumptions

CBT for obsessions and compulsions is based on a set of theoretical assumptions. These assumptions, which are summarized in Table 9.1, guide the selection and timing of intervention strategies.

Normalizing Unwanted Intrusions

As part of educating clients on the cognitive-behavioral model of obsessions, the therapist provides individuals with the information that unwanted, ego-dystonic intrusive thoughts, images, and impulses are univer-

TABLE 9.1. Main Assumptions of Cognitive-Behavioral Therapy for Obsessions

Normalization of mental intrusions. Obsessions are an extreme variant of normal unwanted intrusive thoughts, images, and impulses.

Role of faulty appraisals. Obsessions are highly persistent because exaggerated and erroneous importance is attached to the unwanted intrusive thoughts.

Differentiating appraisals. It is necessary to distinguish the intrusive (obsessive) thought from the personal meaning of the thought (i.e., the appraisal).

Neutralization strategies. Attempts to reduce the frequency and distress of obsessive thought through compulsions and neutralizing tactics will paradoxically contribute to a further escalation in the obsession.

Exaggerated mental control. Excessive effort at mental control inadvertently increases the salience of the obsession.

Core dysfunctional beliefs. Faulty "obsessogenic" appraisals are rooted in pre-existing maladaptive beliefs and assumptions about the nature and control of unwanted intrusive thoughts.

sal human phenomena. Thus, obsessions are an extreme variant of normal unwanted thoughts. Research on the frequency of obsessional content in nonclinical subjects can be used to support this point (see Chapter 2). Most individuals with OCD believe that it is the obsession itself that is the core problem and what defines their abnormal mental state. In CBT, education in the normality of obsessional content is important because it shifts attention to faulty appraisals of the obsession as the key element in the persistence of obsessional thinking. An important aim of therapy is for clients to realize that their distress is due to the meaning they attach to certain unwanted intrusive thoughts (obsessions), rather than to the occurrence of this thought content (Salkovskis & Wahl, 2003).

Role of Faulty Appraisals

The overarching aim of CBT is to modify the faulty appraisals of meaning that are considered a key element in the persistence of obsessional thinking. Although there is broad consensus among cognitive-behavioral researchers that a variety of appraisals are involved in obsessional thinking, there are differences concerning which appraisals should be the primary focus of treatment (see Chapter 5). Whatever the specific focus of the cognitive-behavioral therapist, clients' dominant ways of evaluating the importance of their obsessions are identified during assessment and treatment. These faulty appraisals or meanings are then tested by a variety of cognitive and behavioral intervention strategies.

Differentiating Appraisals from Obsessions

The modification of faulty appraisals is based on the premise that clients can be taught to distinguish between the obsession and their appraisal of the obsession. Whittal and McLean (1999, 2002) commented that clients often find it difficult to grasp the concept of appraisal. Many individuals with OCD are so focused on the obsessional content and whether it is true and likely to lead to dire consequences, that they find it difficult to examine the obsession from a metacognitive perspective ("how I think about the obsession"). Jakes (1989a, 1989b) warned that obsessions and appraisals are so closely linked that it is precarious to base treatment on the ability to distinguish the appraisal of the obsession from the obsession itself. However cognitive-behavioral therapists have had some success in communicating this distinction by explaining appraisal in terms of "the importance given to the thoughts" (Freeston & Ladouceur, 1997a), or what the person "thinks about the obsession," "its meaning" (Whittal & McLean, 1999).

Role of Neutralization

CBT for obsessions recognizes that compulsions, avoidance, reassurance seeking, mental control, and other neutralizing strategies must be eliminated in order to reduce the persistence and distress of the obsession. Exposure and response prevention will be most helpful, especially with overt compulsions and avoidance. However, unlike standard behavioral therapy, CBT also recognizes that treatment must focus on a wider range of mental control strategies that individuals use in response to their obsessions (see Chapter 2). The goal is to have the client "do nothing" in response to the obsession, or to purposefully attend to the obsession rather than engage in cognitive avoidance or dismissal tactics. Although the timing and relative emphasis placed on the modification of compulsions and other neutralizing responses will vary across clients, the importance of exposure and response prevention should not be overlooked. ERP is still the core therapeutic ingredient in CBT of obsessions and compulsions.

Excessive Mental Control

It is recognized that individuals with OCD place high premium on the control of unwanted thoughts, and so they try too hard to exert mental control over their obsessive intrusive thoughts (Clark & Purdon, 1993; Freeston et al., 1996; Rachman, 1998; Salkovskis, 1996a). This can lead to a preoccupation with attaining better mental control. The goal of CBT is to encourage the client to adopt a different stance toward the obsession and to relinquish any attempt to control his or her unwanted intrusive thoughts. Of course, this can seem to be entirely at odds with the client's reason for seeking treatment, which is to gain better control over the obsession. Individuals with OCD often believe that their main problem is "insufficient mental control," whereas the cognitive-behavioral therapist poses an alternative explanation—"that the problem is excessive mental control." In order to accept reduced mental control as a therapeutic goal, the client must embrace the CBT model of obsessions and its treatment rationale.

Core Dysfunctional Beliefs

A final assumption in CBT of obsessions is the fundamental role of specific dysfunctional beliefs and assumptions in the etiology and maintenance of obsessions. The beliefs implicated in obsessional thinking have been described by Freeston et al. (1996) and more recently in the edited book written by members of the OCCWG (Frost & Steketee, 2002). Although CBT emphasizes the need to change faulty appraisals and beliefs associated with obsessions, a clear distinction is not made between appraisals and beliefs (e.g., Steketee, Frost, & Wilson, 2002). The implicit assumption is that therapy that targets faulty appraisals will have an impact on the particular dysfunctional belief that supports an appraisal. This is in contrast with traditional cognitive therapy for depression, in which work at the core schema level is advocated later in therapy in order to improve long-term maintenance of treatment gains (Beck, Rush, Shaw, & Emery, 1979; J. S. Beck, 1995). At this point, treatment of obsession-related appraisals and beliefs occur simultaneously throughout the course of CBT.

THE THERAPEUTIC RELATIONSHIP

A successful trial of CBT for obsessions and compulsions requires a knowledgeable and caring therapist and a courageous, determined client. Overall the therapy must be offered in a collaborative, supportive atmosphere, with the client and therapist working together on the common goal of changing maladaptive reactions to obsessional intrusions (Salkovskis, 1999). Many of the guiding principles of standard cognitive therapy are applicable to CBT for obsessions (see Beck et al., 1979; J. S. Beck, 1995). Although a positive therapeutic relationship is not the primary catalyst for behavioral change, it is considered a necessary prerequisite for successful application of the cognitive and behavioral interventions that can produce change in obsessional complaints. Table 9.2 summarizes positive and negative elements of the therapeutic context that can make or break the effectiveness of treatment.

TABLE 9.2 Positive and Negative Characteristics of the Therapeutic Context

Positive elements	Negative elements
Collaborative empiricism	Focus on modification of obsessional
Shared treatment goals	content
Socratic questioning	Excessive reassurance seeking
Guided discovery	Therapy-induced neutralization
Therapist empathy and understanding	Highly didactic, rationalistic, or
Client motivation and positive	confrontational therapeutic style
expectations	Extreme rigidity, inflexibility; lack of
Homework assignment and completion	psychological mindedness

Positive Therapeutic Elements

Collaborative Empiricism

One of the most important positive elements in therapy is the attitude of collaborative empiricism that was first described by Beck et al. (1979). The therapist and client take shared responsibility for the success of treatment, working together as a team to discover the troubling thoughts, beliefs, and behaviors that lead to obsessive–compulsive symptoms. At the beginning of treatment the cognitive-behavioral therapist discusses the collaborative nature of therapy and illustrates how the therapist and client will together take an exploratory approach to problems. The client will provide the "raw material" of therapy (e.g., situations, problems, feelings, cognitions, behavior), and the therapist will provide structure and consultation on how to deal with problematic responses. Collaborative empiricism must be continually modeled by the therapist throughout the course of treatment.

A modified therapy excerpt illustrates a confrontational, didactic therapeutic style, followed by a more facilitative collaborative approach. The situation involves a 31-year-old Christian fundamentalist who suffers pathological doubt. She cannot make a decision to do even routine daily tasks (e.g., wash, get out of bed, etc.) because she is not sure whether she will make the right decision that pleases God.

DIDACTIC, CONFRONTATIONAL STYLE

CLIENT: God is continually putting me to the test to see if I will make the right decision that pleases Him.

THERAPIST: It is impossible to know whether one pleases a deity.

CLIENT: Well, it is important that I try to discern whether God is pleased with me or not.

THERAPIST: Your distress is caused by trying to answer an impossible question. You would feel less anxious if you give up trying to please God and focus more on your own personal needs.

CLIENT: But that would make me selfish. Pride is one of the most serious of sins.

THERAPIST: Your God appears harsh and judgmental. If you focused more on the loving, forgiving nature of God, you would not be so upset by thoughts of displeasing Him.

CLIENT: But the Bible tells us that God will judge our every deed and punish the sinner.

THERAPIST: You are striving to attain an impossible level of Christian obedience that is not humanly attainable. Each time you think about making a decision, you feel anxious because you search endlessly for signs that one decision or the next is the right one. Instead of this obsessive questioning, the next time you wonder if God is pleased I want you to take an immediate course of action, and then monitor your thoughts and feelings over the next few hours.

COLLABORATIVE, EMPIRICAL STYLE

CLIENT: God is continually putting me to the test to see if I will make the right decision that pleases Him.

THERAPIST: How does this thought make you feel?

CLIENT: Well, I feel very upset, frightened by the thought of not pleasing God by my decisions.

THERAPIST: So the question or doubt of whether or not you please God causes you a lot of anxiety, distress. This is obviously an important issue for you. What makes this doubting thought so important to you?

CLIENT: If I can't be certain that I've made the right decision that pleases God, then maybe I have displeased Him. If God is displeased, then I am not putting Him first, I'm not totally sold out to Him.

THERAPIST: What's so bad about that?

CLIENT: I have dishonored God; He will turn His back on me and condemn me to hell.

THERAPIST: This is obviously a terrible outcome, but especially for someone who is trying so hard to make the right decision that is honoring to God. Do you have any way of knowing when you may have made a right or wrong decision?

CLIENT: Well, when I feel at peace I think that my decision may have pleased God, but when I have doubts and turmoil I am convinced that my decision may be displeasing to God.

THERAPIST: I see. So you have a theological explanation for your distress. You believe that the problem (i.e., feeling distress) is due to not pleasing God, while the solution (i.e., peace of mind) is found in finding the right course of action that pleases God. Certainly, that is one way to look at your obsessional doubt. However, I wonder if we could explore to see whether there is another, possibly psychological, explanation for your distress and its remedy.

CLIENT: What might that be?

THERAPIST: Well, I was wondering whether there might be something in the way that you respond to your doubting thoughts that makes them more intense and upsetting. Would you like to take a look at this possibility and see what we can find?

CLIENT: (*with some reluctance*) I suppose we could take a look, but I am convinced that my problem is spiritual.

Shared Treatment Goals

It is important that the client and therapist agree on the main goals and direction of therapy. Without shared treatment goals, the therapist will have great difficulty in engaging the client in the therapy process. Salkovskis (1999) noted that there are two primary goals of CBT for obsessions: to help the client conclude that obsessions are irrelevant for further action and so should not be targeted for control because such strategies are counterproductive, and to adopt a less threatening interpretation of the occurrence and content of his or her unwanted intrusive thoughts. However, individuals with obsessional complaints most often seek treatment with a very different set of goals and expectations. Most individuals with OCD believe that the source of their anxiety is the obsession and that their core problem is poor control over its occurrence. Thus, they believe that the goal of treatment should be the reduction or elimination of the obsession through the provision of better mental control strategies. It may take the therapist a number of sessions to convince the client of the efficacy of focusing on appraisals and a reduction in mental control efforts.

The difficulty encountered in establishing shared goals is illustrated in the following case example in which a young man with a fear of vomiting prematurely terminated therapy after 10 sessions of CBT. The fear of vomiting took the form of a somatic obsession in which the client had frequent daily thoughts of "Am I getting sick?" In response to this anxiety-eliciting thought, he repeatedly checked his pulse or looked in mirrors to see if his face looked pale. He also avoided many different types of food and sat close to the door so that he could make a quick exit if he felt sick. However, his most prominent way to deal with his concern about getting sick was to seek reassurance from friends, and especially his spouse, on whether or not he looked sick. This created a serious problem, because he would ask, over and over again on a daily basis, whether he looked sick.

The client entered therapy believing that his anxiety stemmed from a fear of vomiting and that the best "cure" was evidence that he was not sick. Thus, he was hoping that therapy would provide him with the ultimate reassurance of his health. If a sense of wellness could be established, then he would no longer feel anxious. Over a series of sessions, the therapist proposed a different formulation, that his anxiety stemmed from "thoughts of getting sick." (In fact, the client had been sick a few months before without feeling traumatized by the incident. Moreover, he did not exhibit the typical profile of someone with a fear of disease or contamination.) It was his interpretation and response to these thoughts that escalated their frequency and distress. Thus, the goal of treatment was to reduce all efforts to obtain reassurance of his wellness and to develop a less threatening interpretation of the "could I be sick" thought. The client remained unconvinced of the counterproductive nature of checking or reassurance seeking, or that appraisals of the "getting sick" obsession were a core feature of his distress. Consequently, he soon became negative and pessimistic about the possibility of treatment success and so terminated therapy sessions. Despite the best attempts, some clients have great difficulty entertaining any alternative to their long held views about the cause and remedy of their obsessional fears.

Socratic Questioning and Guided Discovery

The previous therapy excerpt on collaborative empiricism also illustrates two other important features of the cognitive-behavioral therapeutic style: Socratic questioning and guided discovery. The concepts were introduced by Aaron T. Beck as a means to ensure the development of a collaborative therapeutic relationship between therapist and client (Beck & Emery, 1985). Socratic questioning involves a form of inductive questioning used by therapists to guide clients into discovering their own problematic thoughts, interpretations, and beliefs. Beck and Emery (1985) observed that good questioning expands the client's constricted thinking and helps establish structure, collaboration, and motivation.

Guided discovery is a process in which a series of Socratic questions are asked about the meaning of thoughts, so that through questioning the client becomes aware of underlying dysfunctional beliefs and subsequently evaluates the validity and functionality of these beliefs (J. S. Beck, 1995). Padesky (1995) noted that guided discovery involves (1) questions that identify information outside the client's current awareness, (2) concentrated listening and reflection, (3) statements that summarize the client's responses, and (4) a synthesizing question that requires the client to apply newly discovered information to the dysfunctional belief.

The therapist may need to modify Socratic questioning and guided discovery when interviewing clients with severe doubt. Individuals with obsessional doubt and indecision may find Socratic questioning particularly anxiety provoking as they search to provide the therapist with the "most correct" answer to each question. In such cases the therapist may have to use more summary statements and suggestive probes in order to avoid overwhelming the client or paralyzing the pace of therapy.

Motivation, Treatment Expectations, and Homework

A number of client characteristics are known to influence the effectiveness of cognitive therapy for depression and anxiety (see Dimidjian & Dobson, 2003, for review). There is no reason to believe that these same characteristics would not also affect the effectiveness of CBT for obsessions and compulsions. Poor motivation and low expectations for the effectiveness of treatment are two client characteristics that do not bode well for treatment success. In his review of cognitive therapy for depression, Whisman (1993) stated that "CT may be most effective when people are engaged, involved, and motivated for treatment and when there is a match between the cognitive model and clients' expectations of treatment" (p. 256).

Individuals with OCD can feel coerced into treatment because family and friends observe the debilitating effects of the disorder more than they themselves do. Others battling a long course of OCD may come to therapy particularly discouraged and demoralized, believing that nothing can possibly be effective in dislodging well-entrenched obsessive and compulsive symptoms. Or clients may have experienced a series of "treatment failures" and so can see no reason to believe that CBT will be different. Other individuals may be so convinced of the biological basis of their symptoms that it is hard for them to accept a psychologically based treatment. Whatever the reason, low client expectation and poor motivation must be acknowledged with the client and included as important topics for therapeutic intervention. Unless some change can be achieved early in treatment, the prospects for successful treatment are grim.

Dispositional resistance is another client characteristic that is often associated with poor treatment outcome. Beutler, Harwood, and Caldwell (2001) identified 10 characteristics of the high-trait resistant client, including resentment toward others, controlling, suspicious of other persons' motives, competitive, contrary-minded, and difficulty submitting to another person's authority. The authors note that therapy must be refined and modified to deal with the resistant client. They suggest that nondirective therapy interventions may be most effective, whereby the therapist uses more reflection, clarification, questions, support, paradoxical intention, and an approach–retreat strategy (difficult topics are introduced, followed by therapist's retreat into silence). Leahy (2001) published a most helpful therapy book on how to modify cognitive therapy to deal with the highly resistant client. Resistance in OCD is particularly challenging, because our most effective interventions against obsessions and compulsions (i.e., exposure and response prevention) are direct, therapist-initiated activities.

A final issue that deserves special mention is the importance of homework assignment and completion. Various studies have shown an association between compliance with homework assignments and positive treatment outcome (see Dimidjian & Dobson, 2003, for review). For example, Burns and Spangler (2000) found that homework compliance had a significant causal effect on the reduction of depression severity in cognitive therapy clients. In CBT for obsessions and compulsions, homework completion will be especially important, given the critical role of behavioral interventions.

Two issues are particularly important in assigning homework to individuals having obsessional complaints. First, it is important that the therapist work collaboratively to ensure that assignments are not overwhelming or too threatening for the client. Tasks must be finely tuned so that they represent a *moderate challenge* to the client. Even with a highly motivated client, a steady progression in behavioral assignments is central to maintaining strong motivation and compliance. Second, many individuals with OCD suffer from perfectionist tendencies. As a result, they may overdo homework assignments or be racked with anxiety about whether they completed the assignment correctly or thoroughly. Again, the therapist must remain vigilant for these issues and frequently question clients about their responses to homework assignments. "How difficult did you find that assignment?" "How long did it take you to do this each day?" "How did you feel while doing the assignment?" "Was there anything about the assignment that was difficult for you?" "Was there anything about it that you would do differently the next time?" The aim of this type of questioning is to identify any client responses to homework assignments that over the long term might undermine treatment motivation and compliance.

Avoiding the Pitfalls

Modifying Obsessional Content

Table 9.2 also lists a number of therapy characteristics that can undermine successful treatment of obsessions and compulsions. The first, a misplaced focus on the modification of obsessional content, is particularly important because it is an easy mistake when offering CBT for obsessions. Salkovskis (1985, 1989a) warns against trying to directly modify obsessional content by refuting the empirical basis of the fear or the truth of the obsession. He notes that this will have, at best, a transient therapeutic effect and, at worse, a negative impact because it may function as a form of reassurance and neutralizing. Furthermore, Salkovskis notes that it is useless to challenge the rational basis of obsessional thinking, as done in cognitive therapy of depression, because most people with OCD recognize that their obsessions are irrational. However, even the experienced cognitive therapist can fall into the trap of trying to refute the improbable basis of the obsessional fear, especially when the client may be seeking such support from the therapist (see Whittal & McLean, 1999, p. 394, for similar discussion).

Cognitive interventions intended to deal with the client's overestimated threat bias can tread close to the modification of obsessional content. An example is van Oppen and Arntz's (1994) suggestion that the therapist and client calculate the subjective probability of occurrence of each feared event in a sequence of events (e.g., "failed to extinguish my cigarette") leading up to the most feared outcome (e.g., "the carpet starts to burn, but I notice the fire too late to do anything about it"), and then calculate the cumulative chance that all these events will occur in the anticipated sequence of events. Whereas the estimated probability for the single event ("starting a fire") may be rated at 1/1000, the cumulative probability that a fire will start from a chain of events beginning with a spark from a partially extinguished cigarette would be much rarer (e.g., 1/10,000,000).

This exercise is a useful cognitive intervention because it illustrates how the client has an overestimated danger bias. In this example the exercise is directed toward the faulty threat appraisal related to the obsessive thought of causing an accidental fire. The exercise is not given to convince the client of the irrational or improbable nature of the feared event. This type of cognitive intervention will be counterproductive if the therapist uses it to refute the probable basis of the obsessional content (i.e., "You see, there is little chance that you will cause a fire by not extinguishing your cigarette") rather than using the exercise to highlight the faulty appraisal of threat overestimation (e.g., "As you can see from this exercise, when you get the thought 'maybe I could cause a fire,' there is a bias to overestimate the threatening nature of the thought by focusing on the probability of the catastrophe as a single event rather than focusing on the cumulative probability of the sequence of events"). The aim of this exercise is to help clients reach the conclusion that they tend to overestimate threat when they have the thought "I could cause a fire," rather than to provide them with reassurance that the chance of causing fire is extremely low.

The problem of modifying obsessional content is clearly illustrated in the following case example. A married woman with two young children had obsessional thoughts of disturbing sex and violence. In the early phase of treatment she was plagued with obsessive doubts about her sexual orientation. Later this fear changed to concerns that she might have latent tendencies toward sexual perversion and violence, eventually leading her to rape an innocent victim, especially a child. The only evidence that she might have violent or perverted tendencies was an incident of playing with a female friend when she was 10 years old. She recalled that while playing a game, she pretended to take her friend hostage and then somewhere in the sequence of events felt sexually aroused. She remembered feeling intense pleasure, but afterward terrible guilt for what she had done. After the onset of OCD a few years later, the client became preoccupied with this incident of childhood sexual arousal and wondered whether it meant that she was sexually perverted and attracted to violence. The obsessional content was "Did I engage in childhood masturbation because I am a pervert who is sexually aroused by being physically aggressive to victims?"

Assessment and case formulation revealed that the client's primary obsession was the childhood masturbation incident. Many sessions of standard cognitive therapy were provided in which the therapist focused on contrary evidence that childhood masturbation was abnormal or a sign of perversion. The therapist questioned whether her memory of the incident was accurate and whether there might be other explanations for her feelings and behavior at that time other than sexual arousal to aggressive stimuli. She was also given educational material on childhood sexuality, and both logical persuasion and behavioral experiments were used to test whether there was more evidence for or against the belief that she might be a sexual deviant. After many sessions of cognitive therapy, the client reported that she was much improved and that the frequency and distress of her obsessions had subsided significantly. This was counted as a successful treatment outcome.

Within a couple of years, the client returned for treatment, indicating that her obsessional concerns about sexual deviance and violence had returned with even greater frequency and intensity. It was discovered that she was slavishly using cognitive restructuring to look for evaluative evidence that she did or did not have tendencies for violence and sexual perversion. In this case the cognitive intervention had become transformed into a reassurance-seeking strategy. In addition, the primary obsession had changed slightly to "Maybe I will lose control and rape an innocent person, particularly a child." This time therapy focused on her reactions to the thought—that is, her faulty appraisals and control strategies. She was encouraged to cease cognitive restructuring responses to the obsession and, instead, to complete homework assignments in which she purposefully exposed herself to the "sex and violence" obsession.

Cognitive and behavioral intervention focused on her faulty appraisals of the overimportance, significance, and need to control the "sex and violence" obsession. The concept of thought–action fusion bias was introduced (e.g., "If I think about rape, I am more likely to lose control and do it"). The most helpful intervention was the juxtaposition of two possible explanations for why she was so distressed by the "sex and violence" thoughts. One possibility was that she had latent deviant and violent tendencies that had to be held back at all cost. The other possibility was that she was a tender, caring, and compassionate person at heart who became very upset with this type of unwanted intrusive thought. A behavioral experiment was prescribed in which the client was asked to persuasively initiate sex with her husband. ("Try to have sex when you know he really doesn't want it.") In the following session the client reported that she just could not bring herself to do the experiment. She had absolutely no desire to force sex on her husband. This was taken as evidence that the distress caused by the obsessive thought was due to her reaction to it; that she is a tender, nonviolent person who reacts to such thoughts because they are entirely contrary to the type of person she really is. Just 10 sessions of this focused CBT approach with its emphasis on appraisals and control strategies proved highly effective for the client.

Excessive Reassurance Seeking

A number of authors have warned that therapists must guard against inadvertently providing reassurance to the client with OCD (Freeston & Ladouceur, 1999; Salkovskis, 1985; Whittal & McLean, 1999). Reassurance seeking is a control strategy employed to reduce distress or diffuse perceived responsibility. Clients who experience harming obsessions, for example, may frequently ask family members for reassurance that they have not committed, or would not commit, some injurious act against others. Most often people with OCD turn to friends or family members for reassurance, but the therapist can also be drawn into this process. In all cases the reassurance focuses on establishing a sense of safety, that the client either has not or will not experience the feared outcome. A good example of this is the man mentioned previously who continually asked for reassurance that he was not getting sick. Even during therapy sessions, most of his conversation dealt with evidence that he was or was not feeling sick. It was clear that he was also hoping that therapy would provide him with some type of "perfect reassurance" that he was well, and then he could use this reassurance whenever he felt anxious about getting sick. When he discovered that therapy would not focus on the issue of whether he was a "sickly" or "perfectly healthy" person, he lost motivation to continue in treatment. For him, the only solution to his anxiousness was to find proof that he was not sick.

　　Reassurance seeking is countertherapeutic because it is a neutralizing strategy that will increase the salience of the obsession (Freeston &

Ladouceur, 1999). Moreover, the provision of reassurance focuses therapy on obsessional content rather than on the faulty appraisals and control responses associated with the obsession. It is important that therapists recognize the occurrence of reassurance in a therapy session. The therapist needs to remind the client that providing reassurance on whether or not the obsessional content is true (e.g., "Could I ever lose control and seriously harm someone?") will have little lasting impact on the client's distress and will, in fact, increase the intensity of the obsession. The therapist needs to redirect therapy back to the person's appraisals and responses to the obsession in a gentle, supportive fashion.

"Therapy-Induced" Neutralization

A related problem to reassurance seeking occurs when tried-and-true cognitive interventions, such as logical persuasion or evidence gathering, are transformed by the client into a covert compulsive ritual or other form of control strategy aimed at neutralizing the anxiety elicited by the obsession. Sometimes a client with OCD will embrace "cognitive analysis" with such commitment and enthusiasm that verbal interventions become stereotypic, repetitive responses to the obsession. This can occur in a couple of ways. In some cases individuals with strong perfectionistic tendencies may become unduly preoccupied with finding the single best cognitive challenge to the obsession. Here the right or perfect cognitive response is judged in terms of the amount of anxiety reduction experienced, so the person is constantly striving to perfect his or her "cognitive restructuring skills." In other cases clients may discover a cognitive response that appears to relieve their anxiety and then use this response over and over again in a stereotypic, compulsive fashion. Freeston and Ladouceur (1999) suggested that if a client repeats the same cognitive analysis again and again, uses the analysis in a stereotypic way, and/or finds that it takes increasing effort to convince him- or herself of the response, then it is likely that the therapeutic intervention has become a neutralizing strategy. Obviously, it is important that the therapist recognize such an occurrence and deal with it in the therapy session.

Two clinical examples illustrate the problem of "therapy-induced neutralization." One concerns the woman described previously who suffered from the harming obsession. When she discovered that intentionally exposing herself to the harming obsession (i.e., forcing herself to attend to and dwell on the harming thoughts) led to a reduction in anxiety, she began using exposure in a compulsive manner. Of course, with time the exposure became less effective because it changed into a compulsive mental control response (i.e., a need to think the "right harming thoughts" for a specified period of time). Once it was realized that the exposure exercise had become a neutralizing strategy, therapy refocused on her appraisals and beliefs about the importance of gaining mental control over the obsession. She was asked to cease doing the exposure exercise, which had included reading a written imagery script.

In a second case a man was successfully treated for sex and harming obsessions with a combination of audiotaped habituation training and cognitive restructuring. Years later he returned with a new primary obsession that his wife had had her first experience of sexual intercourse "with another guy," and now his concern was whether she enjoyed it or felt sufficient guilt and remorse for her past behavior. In response to this obsessive rumination, he interrogated her over and over again until she was brought to tears. He also wrote copious notes, using the evidence-gathering technique to test the rationality or irrationality of his thinking. In the end both responses led to an increase in the frequency, intensity, and distress of the obsessional rumination. His response to the obsession could be seen as an attempt to neutralize anxiety through reassurance. In the case of evidence gathering, he could never find the evidence, the right argument that effectively reduced his distress, despite feeling compelled to engage in long periods of cognitive restructuring.

Confrontational Style and Client Readiness

Occasionally individuals with obsessional complaints are argumentative, particularly when seeking reassurance from the therapist (Salkovskis, 1989b). Given that individuals with OCD often exhibit excessive rigidity, meticulousness, intolerance of uncertainty or ambiguity, and perfectionistic strivings when it comes to their obsessional complaints, it is not surprising that therapy sessions can degenerate into arguments between the client and therapist. This is most likely to happen when therapy is misdirected to the obsessional fear itself, rather than the client's response to the fear.

To avoid arguments in a therapy session, the therapist must maintain a calm, supportive, and caring attitude toward the client. It is important to remember that no matter how absurd the obsession, most individuals afflicted with OCD suffer greatly from their obsessive–compulsive symptoms. The therapist must ensure that the spirit of collaborative empiricism and the principle of guided discovery characterizes each therapy session. Clients' perspectives or beliefs about their obsessions or an avoided situation should be respected and acknowledged by the therapist as a distinct possibility that needs to be tested in therapy. The point that must be continually reinforced throughout therapy is that all beliefs and appraisals should be investigated through cognitive and behavioral interventions.

As a case example, suppose a client believes that she will feel more distress if she does not give in to her "need to know" urge and so reads and rereads the printed material in front of her. The therapist should not attempt to confront this belief with verbal refutation. Instead, the therapist should summarize this view as one possible belief and explore with the client other possible perspectives for understanding "the urge to know." Then a behavioral task can be designed, such as response prevention of the urge, in order to test whether distress is worsened by not giving in to the urge. The whole orientation of CBT is to adopt an open-minded, exploratory approach to the client's problematic thoughts, feelings, and behavior.

There is no empirical research on which client characteristics are associated with poor outcomes in CBT for obsessions. As noted in Chapter 3, comorbid personality disorder, low motivation, lack of compliance, and possibly severe depression and overvalued ideation, may impede or interfere with the effectiveness of ERP. It is unclear whether these same factors may undermine the effectiveness of CBT. However, clinical experience indicates that individuals with extreme rigidity, inflexibility, and poor psychological mindedness may not do as well in CBT. The therapy assumes that individuals have the capacity to entertain the possibility of more than one perspective. In addition, individuals must demonstrate an ability to report on their reactions to thoughts, that is, to think about thinking. If a client has difficulty grasping this "metacognitive" level of abstraction, then CBT for an obsession will be very difficult to implement.

GETTING STARTED: THE INITIAL SESSIONS

A number of primary therapy ingredients are found in CBT for obsessions and compulsions. These ingredients or components of therapy are not different stages but, rather, are evident to a greater or lesser degree throughout the course of treatment. Table 9.3 summarizes the main components of CBT. Each of these components is discussed in the following chapters with clinical examples of their implementation.

Assessment and Case Formulation

The previous chapter provided a detailed account of a cognitive-behavioral approach to assessment and case formulation. Although diagnosis, assessment, and treatment planning represent the entry points to therapy, this type of work will continue throughout treatment. Treatment goals and planning will be revised and the case formulation refined as the therapist gains new insights into the client's OCD. Moreover, obsessional complaints are not static and can be expected to change across a course of treatment.

The assessment orientation presented in Chapter 8 is derived from

TABLE 9.3. Therapeutic Components of Cognitive-Behavioral Treatment for OCD

Education on the appraisal model. A cognitive explanation based on the role of faulty appraisals and neutralization is presented for the persistence of obsessive–compulsive symptoms and associated distress. This provides the client with a rationale for the treatment that follows.

Identification and differentiation of appraisals and intrusions. Individuals are taught to identify the primary way they misinterpret the importance or significance of their obsessions. It is critical that clients learn to distinguish between the obsession or intrusion itself, and their cognitive reaction to the intrusion (i.e., their appraisal of the unwanted thought).

Cognitive restructuring strategies. Individuals are taught how to use standard cognitive techniques to question the maladaptive appraisal of the obsession.

Alternative appraisals of the obsession. Emphasis is placed on the development of a more adaptive, less anxiety-provoking interpretation of the occurrence and/or content of an unwanted intrusive thought.

The role of compulsive ritual, neutralization, and avoidance. Clients are given instruction in exposure and response prevention in order to reduce the impact of compulsions, neutralization, and avoidance on the persistence of the obsession.

Behavioral experimentation. Behavioral assignments are given that test the faulty appraisals and beliefs associated with the obsession. The aim of these experiments is to provide the client with experiences that will lead to an abandonment of maladaptive reactions to the obsession and the acceptance of healthier responses.

Modifying self-referent and metacognitive beliefs. Core beliefs about the significance and control of unwanted intrusive thoughts must be addressed as part of treatment maintenance.

Relapse prevention. Before treatment is terminated, response to symptom relapse and recurrence is addressed.

---

the cognitive-behavioral theory of obsessions and compulsions (see also Steketee, 1993, for a detailed description of behavioral assessment of OCD). Thus, the measures recommended in that chapter are designed to provide the type of information needed to implement a course of CBT for OCD. In particular, the forms found in Appendices 8.1–8.5 provide valuable information necessary for treatment planning. The assessment will culminate in the development of a cognitive-behavioral case formulation (Appendix 8.6), which plays a major role in the educational component of CBT.

Educating the Client

The importance of the educational component in CBT is emphasized by a number of clinical researchers and practitioners (Freeston & Ladouceur, 1999; Rachman, 1998, 2003; Salkovskis, 1996a; Steketee, 1999; Whittal &

McLean, 1999). There are two main objectives of the educational component: to normalize the experience of unwanted intrusions and to provide a treatment rationale.

Normalizing Unwanted Intrusions

Having identified the primary obsession during the assessment, the therapist then begins the process of changing the client's interpretation of his or her obsession by *normalizing* the experience of unwanted intrusive thoughts, images, and impulses (Salkovskis & Wahl, 2003). Individuals enter therapy believing that they are abnormal because of the bizarre, disturbing thoughts that preoccupy their minds. The therapist explains that 90% of people report that they have unpleasant, even quite disturbing, unwanted intrusive thoughts of contamination, dirt, sex, aggression, mistakes, dishonesty, religion, making rude or embarrassing remarks, causing accidents or injury to self or others, or losing control. Sometimes these thoughts come out of the blue, but at other times they are triggered by particular situations, such as seeing a knife and then having the thought of stabbing someone, or handling money and then thinking of dirt and contamination (Freeston & Ladouceur, 1999).

At this point it can be helpful to provide clients with a list of common unwanted intrusive thoughts with obsessive themes that have been reported by nonclinical subjects. Appendix 9.1 provides a list of the most common unwanted obsessive-like intrusive thoughts, images, and impulses reported by university students. This is based on two different studies conducted by the research group of which I am a member at the University of New Brunswick in Canada. The first study, by Purdon and Clark (1993), involved 293 participants, and the second study, by Byers et al. (1998), is based on a sample of 169 students. Note that the percentages refer to the number of women and men who reported that they had had a particular type of unwanted mental intrusion. Overall, 99% of the individuals in the Purdon and Clark (1993) sample reported at least one type of obsessive intrusive thought, image, or impulse, and 84% of those in the Byers et al. (1998) study reported at least one of 20 unwanted intrusive sexual thoughts.

Similar lists can be found in the study by Rachman and de Silva (1978), as well as in publications by Rachman (1998, 2003) and Steketee and Barlow (2002). In regard to Appendix 9.1, it is important to explain that the current list is only a sample of the different types of unwanted intrusive thoughts reported by nonclinical subjects. Steketee and Barlow (2002), for example, list more than 70 different types of nonclinical obsessions and mental intrusions. Even though some of the percentages for individual intrusions may seem quite low, the important point is that many people who are nonclinical subjects report even more unusual or disturbing cognitive intrusions (i.e., items 13–15).

Normalizing the experience of obsessions can have a very positive therapeutic impact. Clients often believe that they are abnormal or that they suffer a serious "brain chemistry imbalance" because they have these obsessions. Hearing that many people have similar mental experiences may be one of the first hopeful messages they have heard about obsessions. Yet clients will no doubt quickly point out that these "normal" people do not have obsessions of the same frequency, intensity, and distress that they experience. This, of course, is a correct observation and leads into the second aspect of the "normalizing phase of treatment." Salkovskis and Wahl (2003) suggest that the therapist explore with the client the idea of who is most likely to have obsessional thoughts, whereas Rachman (2003) focuses on the difference between a trivial unwanted intrusion and an intrusion of great personal significance.

I suggest that the therapist take the list of intrusions in Appendix 9.1 and ask the client to select two or three different unwanted intrusive thoughts that they themselves have not experienced, or have at least experienced infrequently. Using Socratic questioning and guided discovery, the therapist should then inquire of the client, "Who is most likely to be bothered by this particular thought, and under what circumstances?" "What do you think might be so upsetting about this thought for a person bothered by it?" The aim of this inquiry is to introduce the client to the key point of CBT: that distress is not caused by the obsession itself but, rather, by how it is interpreted. This exercise also makes the point that obsessions usually deal with issues that are most sensitive to a person's main concerns. It is important to begin educating the client on the appraisal model by selecting unwanted mental intrusions that are not currently troubling to him or her. It is easier to see the role of appraisal in a "hypothetical" intrusive thought than in one the client is currently experiencing.

Explaining the Role of Appraisals

The "normalizing exercise" leads naturally into the second part of the educational component of treatment—presentation of the CBT model and treatment rationale. A good transitional question may be, "Now that we have seen that practically everyone has unwanted intrusive thoughts, how is it that for some people certain intrusive thoughts become so frequent and distressing, but for other people they remain infrequent and benign?" This time the therapist should select an unwanted intrusive thought that the person has experienced only occasionally but is not particularly upsetting nor likely to lead to neutralizing responses.

Using the CBT model illustrated in Figure 5.1, the therapist and client work collaboratively to explore possible reactions to the selected negative intrusive thought that may lead to increased persistence and distress. Appendix 9.2 presents a CBT diagram that is useful in eliciting client reactions to the low-frequency intrusive thought. The goal of this exercise is to further promote the idea that a person's interpretations and attempts to control unwanted intrusive thoughts are critical in their persistence. It is important that the client see how his or her cognitive and behavioral reaction to a low-frequency, nondistressing negative intrusive thought can turn it into a highly frequent and disturbing cognitive phenomenon. Moreover, by selecting a low-frequency, nondistressing negative thought, the therapist can point out that the client also experiences many negative thoughts that evoke very healthy responses that result in low frequency.

Salkovskis and Wahl (2003) suggest that the therapist discuss how a positive thought can become distressing if interpreted in a threatening manner. Appendix 9.2 can be used to facilitate this exercise. The following example illustrates how this expercise might proceed: You are having a pleasant restaurant dinner with your partner. You are thinking how much you are enjoying the dinner. Instead of being comforted by this thought, you immediately think to yourself how selfish, and irresponsible, to be enjoying this meal when your mother is lying in the intensive care unit of the local hospital (the pleasant thought is interpreted as a sign of irresponsibility and selfishness). You begin to feel guilt and shame for your behavior and find that you cannot get your mother's precarious medical condition off your mind. You leave the restaurant before dessert, feeling distraught and upset with yourself.

Having worked through the appraisal exercise a couple of times with nonthreatening intrusive thoughts, the exercise can now be repeated with the client's primary obsession (see also the demonstration described by Rachman, 2003). Once again Appendix 9.2 may be used to facilitate the process. No doubt, clients will find this exercise more difficult because of their emotional involvement with the obsession. Identifying the triggers and control strategies associated with the obsession can probably be done quite easily. Much of this information has already been obtained during the assessment. In fact, the monitoring forms in Appendices 8.1–8.6 can be reviewed to facilitate completion of the appraisal exercise.

The Role of Neutralization

Another important step in the educational phase of CBT is to introduce the client to the counterproductive effects of neutralization and other mental control strategies (Rachman, 1998, 2003). Freeston and Ladouceur (1997a) describe an exercise they call the "camel effect" to demonstrate the futility of trying to intentionally remove or suppress unwanted intrusive thoughts or obsessions. The client is asked to close his or her eyes and to think about a camel for 2 minutes. Each time the camel thought disappears, the client raises his or her hand. Next, the client tries *not* to think about a camel for 2 minutes and to indicate each time the thought recurs.

Clearly, few people are completely successful in maintaining or dismissing the target thought. Discussion then centers on the difficulty of maintaining and suppressing "camel" thoughts. The therapist can ask what it would be like to try hard not to think of a camel for hours on end. "What would happen if some dire consequence occurred if the camel thought recurred, such as if you lost $100 each time you allowed your mind to drift toward a camel?" The aim of this exercise is for the client to experience the negative impact that intentional mental control and other neutralizing responses have on the frequency and distress of unwanted thoughts.

Summing Up the Appraisal Explanation

A number of practitioners have noted that clients often find the concept of appraisals difficult to grasp (Freeston & Ladouceur, 1997a; Whittal & McLean, 1999). Strategies for assisting clients in the identification of their faulty appraisals are presented in the next chapter. In the meantime, I suggest that the term *appraisal* be avoided at this stage of treatment, and that the therapist refer to "the reasons that the primary obsession is important to you." Once the exercise in Appendix 9.2 is completed for the primary obsession, the therapist should summarize, emphasizing how "the importance given to the obsession" (appraisals) and attempts to control the obsession and its distress (neutralization) can actually cause an increase in the frequency and intensity of the obsession. The client should be given a copy of Appendix 9.2 as well as the standard diagram of the CBT model (Figure 5.1). Every attempt should be made to discuss the CBT model (Figure 5.1) in terms of the client's experience with the primary obsession (Appendix 9.2). The following points about the model should be stressed:

- All people have unwanted thoughts that intrude into their minds against their will. It is not possible to live a life free of unwanted intrusive thoughts.
- Most of the unwanted negative thoughts people experience do not bother them because they do not consider the thoughts important or threatening. In fact, even people suffering from obsessions have other potentially troubling intrusive thoughts that do not bother them.
- It is the importance that a person attaches to an unwanted thought that determines whether it becomes more frequent and upsetting.

Thoughts that are viewed as leading to some terrible negative consequence are more likely to be interpreted as highly significant.

• Once an unwanted thought is considered personally significant and threatening, then a person takes action to deal with the thought. However, as seen in the "camel" exercise, we have very little control over unwanted thoughts. In fact, the harder we try to control the thought, the worse it gets.

Treatment Rationale

The final element of the educational component is an explanation of the treatment approach. Once individuals understand the cognitive-behavioral explanation for the persistence of their obsessions, the therapist should explain the treatment rationale. Clients are informed that therapy will focus on helping them change their reactions to the obsessions. The following illustrates a possible treatment rationale that can be given to clients.

"As you have seen from the work we've done so far, how a person reacts to his or her unwanted intrusive thoughts and obsessions has a major impact on their frequency and distress. Treatment will involve a variety of intervention strategies that will be used to explore different ways to interpret or understand the obsession so that you assign less importance or personal significance to whether or not it occurs. One goal of therapy is to help you see the obsession as less threatening. A second major goal is to develop different ways to respond to the obsession, to reduce the use of compulsive rituals, neutralization, and other mental control strategies. Based on the cognitive-behavioral model, we should see significant reductions in the frequency of the obsession and in your level of distress once the thought has become less important to you and you have learned different ways to respond to it other than mental control, neutralization, or compulsive ritual. You can expect treatment to take another 15–20 sessions. In addition to the work we will do in the weekly therapy sessions, there will be a variety of self-help tasks that you can do between sessions. These are designed to help you develop better responses to the obsession. Do you have any questions about the treatment?"

Although exposure and response prevention (ERP) will play a critical role in the treatment plan, if feasible it is suggested that discussion of ERP be reserved for a later session. Kozak and Foa (1997) offer a very nice explanation of ERP that therapists can use with clients. Because ERP initially involves an increase in anxiety level, this procedure can be quite threatening to clients in the early stage of treatment. Further work on beliefs and appraisals may improve client compliance with ERP. However, with certain subtypes of OCD, such as washing and checking compulsions, ERP plays such a fundamental role that discussion of this intervention should be included when providing the initial treatment rationale.

SUMMARY AND CONCLUSION

As evident in the central tenets of CBT for obsessions and compulsions, this is a theory-driven approach to treatment. The rationale for CBT of OCD is derived from the cognitive appraisal theories of Salkovskis, Rachman, the OCCWG, and others. Although the efficacy of cognitive-behavioral treatment for obsessions must be demonstrated in its own right, negative findings for the cognitive appraisal models would weaken the case for a cognitive approach to the treatment of OCD.

The first few sessions of CBT lay the foundation for an effective treatment strategy. Often a failure to respond to CBT can be traced to problems in the early stage of treatment. A positive therapeutic relationship is necessary, characterized by collaborative empiricism, shared treatment goals, and strong motivation for change. Certain pitfalls must be avoided, such as a misguided focus on obsessional content, the provision of reassurance, the unnecessary use of confrontation, or the unintended occurrence of "therapy-induced" neutralization.

An important part of the cognitive-behavioral approach to OCD is the provision of education on the cognitive-behavioral model of obsessions. This educational phase of treatment can take two or three sessions. It is important that the therapist not rush too quickly into the cognitive restructuring and behavioral intervention components of the treatment. Clients must understand and accept the cognitive-behavioral explanation for the distress and persistence of their obsessions. If clients continue to raise serious doubts about the central role of faulty appraisals and neutralization in the maintenance of their obsessions, it is unlikely that they will comply with cognitive and behavioral exercises aimed at modifying cognitive appraisals and control responses. However, if a client accepts the cognitive-behavioral model, then heightened motivation and expectation for change will lead to better engagement in the therapeutic enterprise.

APPENDIX 9.1. Endorsement Rates for the Most Common Unwanted Obsession-Relevant Intrusive Thoughts, Images, and Impulses Reported by Nonclinical Subjects

Unwanted thought	% women	% men
1. Did I leave heat, stove, or lights on that could cause a fire?	79	62
2. Left the door unlocked, and an intruder could be inside.	77	65
3. While driving, an impulse to run the car off the road.	64	53
4. I could get a sexually transmitted disease from touching a toilet seat or handle.	60	40
5. Even though the house is tidy, an impulse to check that absolutely everything is put away.	52	40
6. Feel sudden impulse to say something rude or insulting to a friend even though I'm not angry at him.	59	55
7. Impulse to say something rude or insulting to a stranger.	50	55
8. While driving, the impulse to swerve the car into oncoming traffic.	55	49
9. The thought of having sex in a public place.	55	67
10. The thought of having sex with an authority figure (e.g., minister, boss, teacher).	51	62
11. While driving, the thought of running over pedestrians or animals.	46	51
12. When talking to people, intrusive thought of their being naked.	44	63
13. Impulse to indecently expose myself by lifting my skirt or slipping down my pants.	14	24
14. Impulse to masturbate in public.	11	18
15. When I see a sharp knife, the thought of slitting my wrist or throat.	20	22
16. When in a public place, the thought of becoming dirty or contaminated from touching doorknobs.	35	23

Data from Purdon and Clark (1993) and Byers et al. (1998).

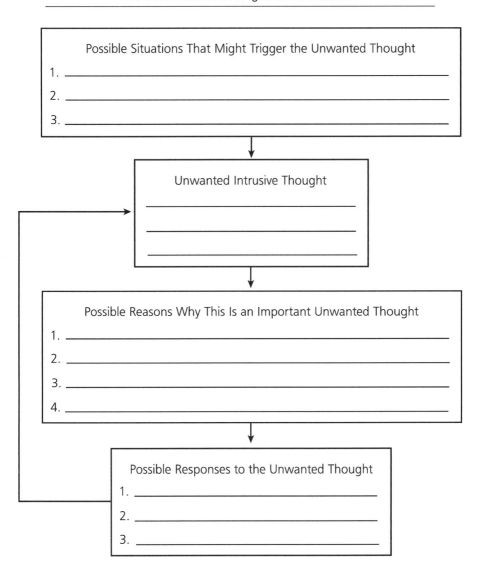

CHAPTER 10

Cognitive Restructuring and Generating Alternatives

Education on the cognitive-behavioral model is critical to treatment effectiveness, because client compliance and motivation in large part depend on embracing the model and treatment rationale. The education phase begins during assessment and continues over the first two or three treatment sessions. Another important element of the education component is teaching the client how to distinguish appraisals from obsessions, the different types of faulty appraisals, and the presence of neutralization, mental control strategies, compulsive rituals, and avoidance in his or her cycle of obsessive–compulsive symptoms.

This chapter continues the education phase of CBT with a focus on teaching clients how to distinguish their appraisals from their obsessions. As noted earlier, individuals with OCD often find this distinction difficult because of their excessive focus on the obsession itself. Shifting attention from the obsession to "how you think about the obsession," "your interpretation of it," can be a challenging part of the therapy (Whittal & McLean, 1999). However, it is not possible to proceed with the cognitive or behavioral interventions unless clients are able to identify their faulty appraisals and neutralization responses.

Once clients are aware of their cognitive and behavioral reactions to the obsessions, cognitive restructuring exercises are introduced in order to modify the erroneous appraisals and beliefs. There is some disagreement among cognitive-behavioral therapists on when cognitive interventions should be introduced. Freeston and Ladouceur (1999) and Steketee (1999) start with ERP and then introduce cognitive restructuring in the later sessions, whereas Salkovskis (1999) and Rachman (2003) begin with cognitive tactics aimed at modifying faulty appraisals and then introduce ERP later in therapy. I tend to agree with the latter therapy progression because the cognitive interventions are usually less threatening than ERP and so can prepare the client for more challenging behavioral work to follow. Moreover, cognitive restructuring and generating alternative explanations help to reinforce the educational phase of treatment by directly focusing on the faulty appraisals and beliefs associated with the obsessions.

IDENTIFYING NEUTRALIZATION AND APPRAISALS

Neutralization

Most individuals are quite aware of their compulsions and avoidance patterns. Early in treatment the therapist should work on constructing a fear hierarchy, similar to the example found in Chapter 3 (Table 3.2). This will include situations that are more or less likely to trigger the obsession and cause varying levels of anxiety. Many of these situations, especially those toward the top of the hierarchy, will be actively avoided. The fear hierarchy is the basis for ERP that occurs in the middle phase of treatment. Steketee (1993, 1999) provides a helpful discussion and illustrations on constructing fear hierarchies and dealing with avoidance. Her format for "listing obsessive fears" (Steketee, 1993, p. 77) can be used for planning ERP. The client workbook developed by Foa and Kozak (1997) has some excellent forms that can be used to identify ritualizing and behavioral avoidance (see pp. 23–27). Their accompanying explanation is written for clients and explains the role of situational triggers, avoidance, and rituals in the persistence of obsessions.

Clients are likely to be much less aware of the neutralization and other mental control strategies used in response to an obsession. The therapist can discuss neutralization, reassurance seeking, and thought control, using Tables 2.5 and 2.6 from Chapter 2 to explain and illustrate each of these concepts. If the client completed the Record of Control Strategies (Appendix 8.5) during the assessment, this will provide valuable information on the primary responses to the obsession. In some cases it might be necessary to elicit the obsession during the therapy session and then discuss how individuals normally reduce their anxiety or cancel out the negative effects of the obsession. In most cases it will be important to assign a self-monitoring homework task in order to gather additional information on the variety of ways that clients deal with the obsession. This will help them become more aware of the role of neutralization in the persistence of the obsession. The Record of Control Strategies can be assigned for this task.

Appraisals

To help clients understand the difference between appraisal and the intrusive thought, a number of authors have suggested that appraisal be described as "your interpretation of the obsession," "what the obsession means to you," "what you think about the obsession," or "the importance given to the thoughts" (Freeston & Ladouceur, 1997a; Whittal & McLean, 1999). In addition, appraisals can be probed with questions like "What makes this a significant thought for you?" "What's so upsetting about this thought?" "What are the reasons this thought is important to you?" or "What is it about the thought that grabs your attention (makes it difficult to ignore)." Such explorations with the client will result in verbal material that does not perfectly map onto the specific types of faulty appraisals discussed in Chapter 5 (e.g., responsibility, personal significance, overimportance, need for control, thought–action fusion, etc.).

Once a client has explained his or her view on the importance of the intrusive thought or obsession, the therapist must then focus on identifying the different types of faulty appraisals involved in the client's understanding of the importance of the thought. Table 10.1 provides some clinical examples of obsessional content, the client's interpretation of the obsession, and the various faulty appraisals involved in the interpretation.

As can be seen from Table 10.1, clients' interpretations of their obsessions will most likely involve a number of the faulty appraisal styles discussed in cognitive-behavioral theories (see Chapter 5). The therapist should first focus on obtaining a detailed description of the client's interpretation of the obsession. This will also most likely involve some appraisal of the compulsive ritual if one is present. Once the interpretation of importance is obtained, the therapist then works on breaking down the interpretation into the various faulty appraisal patterns. This might be introduced to the client in the following way:

"Now that you've told me why this unwanted intrusive thought (obsession) is so important to you, I would like to look at this much more closely to see if there are some themes or ways of evaluating the obsession that make it so important. The cognitive–behavioral model assumes that there are certain ways we tend to evaluate our thoughts that can make them more frequent and distressing. I would like to see if these problematic evaluations are evident in your interpretation of the obsession."

Appendix 10.1 provides a description and an example of the main faulty appraisals proposed in cognitive-behavioral models of obsessions. A copy of this table can be given to clients to assist in their understanding and application of the appraisal concept to their own symptomatology. An entire session will be needed to fully explore the faulty appraisal patterns evident in clients' "interpretations of importance." A useful homework assignment is to ask clients to self-monitor their obsessions and appraisals using the form in Appendix 10.2. Obviously, the client cannot record every occurrence of the obsession. Instead, the therapist should

TABLE 10.1. Clinical Examples of Faulty Interpretations and Specific Appraisals Associated with a Primary Intrusive Thought or Obsession

Intrusive thought or obsession and compulsion	Client's interpretation of obsession	Types of specific faulty appraisals
"I have a strict routine and sequence of activities that must be followed before going to bed. If this routine is not followed, I will redo until correct."	"The thought of following a strict bedtime routine is important because if I don't, I become quite anxious and can't fall asleep. If I don't get my sleep, then I am more likely to get sick and vomit. If I'm sick, then I'll miss a lot of school and be a burden on others."	1. *Overestimation of threat.* "If I lose sleep, I'll get sick." 2. *Perfection.* "Specific bedtime routine must be followed." 3. *Responsibility.* "I need to avoid getting sick so as not to burden others." 4. *Intolerance of anxiety.* "I can't let myself get anxious."
Thought that the client's boyfriend could be harmed. Would engage in repeating rituals.	"If something were to happen to him, it would be my fault for thinking that he would be harmed. Also these thoughts make me feel so anxious. In the past I worried a lot about people getting hurt, so it's important I don't let my thoughts get that bad again."	1. *Thought–action fusion.* "Thinking about harm seems to make it more likely to happen." 2. *Responsibility.* "I need to do something to ensure that harm does not occur to my boyfriend." 3. *Need for control.* "I need to control these thoughts so they don't get worse."
Thought of sexual touch by a teenage babysitter when the client was a preschooler. In response, the client would repeat verbal phrases over and over or redo activities again and again (e.g., retrace his steps).	"The thought makes me suffer great anxiety, and so I need to repeat whatever I am doing at the time I have the thought. By repeating the action over and over until I can do it without thinking the obsession, I will break the connection between the thought and my action. If I don't do this, more and more things will trigger the thought, causing me to have more obsessions. Eventually, I'll become so absorbed in the obsession and overwhelmed with anxiety that I'll have a nervous breakdown."	1. *Overimportance.* "A thought of the possibility that I was touched sexually as a child becomes my most important thought." 2. *Need for control.* "I need to ensure that the thought does not become more frequent." 3. *Neutralization.* "I need to cancel out the effects of the thought by repeating the action associated with it." 4. *Overestimated threat.* "The thought will escalate until I have a nervous breakdown." 5. *Intolerance of uncertainty.* "I have to repeat a phrase or action over and over until I'm certain that I've done it perfectly without having the obsession."

suggest that three to four times a day, the client tries to capture an occurrence of the obsession and the associated interpretation. The aim of this exercise is to heighten clients' awareness of their faulty appraisals of unwanted obsessive intrusive thoughts.

COGNITIVE RESTRUCTURING STRATEGIES

Once the client is well aware of his or her reaction to the obsession, the next step in the therapy process is to provide cognitive skills in challenging the "interpretations of importance" associated with the obsession. Generally, cognitive interventions are less effective in modifying faulty appraisals and neutralization responses to the obsession than behavioral strategies like ERP. However, cognitive intervention strategies are usually less threatening for clients, and so these interventions are introduced first as a way of easing the client toward more challenging behavioral work. One of the advantages of CBT is that treatment compliance may be improved by structuring a range of interventions that proceed from least to most demanding.

There are three objectives to the cognitive intervention element of CBT for OCD:

- To help clients realize that their "automatic" appraisal or interpretation of an unwanted thought is one of *several possible ways* to react to the thought.
- To demonstrate that appraisals of the importance or significance of the obsession are based on a *possibility inference* (O'Connor & Robillard, 1999). That is, the obsession is considered important not because of "what will happen" but "what could happen."
- To highlight for the client that the faulty appraisal and overcontrol of the obsession is a *highly selective* approach to a particular type of unwanted thought(s). If it can be shown that the client reacts to low-frequency, nondistressing unwanted intrusive thoughts one way, and to high-frequency, distressing obsessions in another way, then the cognitive strategies have paved the way to consider alternative ways to deal with the obsession.

The following discussion considers some specific cognitive interventions that can be used with the primary appraisals implicated in the persistence of obsessions. Although cognitive-behavioral therapists may start with these cognitive interventions, they should quickly integrate them with behavioral tasks and experiments. Discussion of specific cognitive interventions for obsession-relevant beliefs and appraisals can be found in Freeston et al. (1996), O'Connor and Robillard (1999), Rachman (2003),

Salkovskis (1999), Salkovskis and Wahl (2003), Steketee (1999), van Oppen and Arntz (1994), and Whittal and McLean (1999, 2002).

Challenging Overestimated Threat Appraisals

Van Oppen and Arntz's (1994) exercise, described previously, involves comparing the probability of single threat events with the cumulative probability based on an analysis of the sequence of events leading to the imagined catastrophe associated with the obsession. This is a good exercise for focusing on the tendency to make abnormal estimates of risk concerning obsessional fears (see also illustration in Steketee, 1999). However, the point of this exercise is to demonstrate the presence of an overestimated threat appraisal and not to debate the relative likelihood that the feared event could happen.

The "downward arrow technique" described by Beck et al. (1979) and J. S. Beck (1995) can be used to cognitively challenge all the faulty appraisals of obsessions (Salkovskis, 1999; Steketee, 1999). In this exercise the client begins with the obsessional thought, and then the therapist probes with the question, "For you, what's so bad about that?" As the client responds to each probe, the therapist is able to peel back the layers, to uncover successively more basic dysfunctional appraisals and beliefs associated with the obsession. Once the therapist exposes the basic core fear, then he or she can summarize by stating, "So your fear is that if the obsession is true, then this awful outcome will occur." The therapist should explore with the client whether this might be an example of overestimated threat. The therapist can say, "As you look at this way of thinking, do you think this is an example of overestimating the severity of the danger and maybe the probability that it will occur?"

Figure 10.1 illustrates the use of the downward arrow technique to expose faulty threat appraisal by a person with a washing compulsion. As can be seen in this illustration, the critical point is the summary "that handling books will increase risk of contracting AIDS." The client may even be asked to generate a probability estimate that "handling books will lead to AIDS." The objective of this exercise is for clients to accept the idea that they are making faulty (overestimated) threat appraisals when they assume that the obsession is terribly threatening or dangerous. If, at this point, the client agrees that the appraisal of threat is biased and unrealistic, then the therapist can propose a series of ERP tasks that involve handling books. The ERP would be introduced as a way to further test the dangerousness of handling books.

If clients will not consider the possibility that the threat estimation is biased or exaggerated, then they are not ready to accept ERP. Instead, further cognitive work is necessary to deal with the overestimated threat appraisal. One approach is to use the double-column evidence-gathering

When I handle books at the store I feel so dirty.
[Therapist: What's so bad about feeling dirty?]
↓
I get uncomfortable at the thought that my hands are dirty.
[Therapist: What's so bad about being uncomfortable about dirty hands?]
↓
Well, when I get anxious I'm reminded that other people have touched this book.
[Therapist: What's so bad about other people touching a book you've just touched?]
↓
Maybe one of these people who touched the book is dirty or has some disease.
[Therapist: What would be so bad if the person did have a disease?]
↓
The person would contaminate the book. The book might have germs on it.
[Therapist: What would be so bad about a book covered with germs?]
↓
When I handle the book, I would become infected from the germs.
[Therapist: If you did get infected, what do you fear could happen next?]
↓
I would then get horribly sick.
[Therapist: For you, what would be the worst type of sickness you could get?]
↓
I would end up getting AIDS and dying.
[Therapist summarizes: So if we follow the sequence of your thoughts, you are basically saying that you could die of AIDS by handling a book that other people have touched. Do you think you are overestimating the risk involved in touching books?]

FIGURE 10.1. Example of downward arrow technique for demonstrating overestimated threat appraisal in person with washing compulsion.

technique (i.e., reality testing) introduced by Beck et al. (1979) and popularized by Christine Padesky (e.g., see *Mind Over Mood* by Greenberger & Padesky, 1995). Steketee (1999) and Rachman (2003) also discuss how the evidence-gathering approach can be used to challenge interpretations of significance or threat.

    In the case example illustrated in Figure 10.1, the therapist can explore with the client evidence for and against the proposition that a person can get AIDS from handling books. "How many people have died from AIDS because they handled books?" "How often do people handle books without getting AIDS?" "How often have you [the client] handled books without getting AIDS?" Another intervention strategy can involve having the client gather information on how the AIDS virus is transmitted. The therapist can then ask the client to generate probability and threat severity estimates concerning certain known risk factors for the disease such as having unprotected sex, sharing needles, or handling human blood. These estimates can be compared with the estimates associated with "handling books." The client may then be asked, "If you had to choose between handling a book or working in a pathology lab without protective clothing, which would you select?" No doubt, the client would choose the book. The therapist can explore the reasons for the client's choice, one of which will be that handling books is really less risky. This can then be used to point out whether the client initially overestimated the threat of handling books. "In light of the real risk factors for AIDS, do you think that you tend to automatically overestimate the risk of handling books?"

Thought–Action Fusion Bias

TAF Likelihood Bias

Cognitive interventions for Likelihood TAF bias will be very similar to the strategies discussed in regard to overestimated threat because Likelihood TAF involves the erroneous view that the obsession increases the probability that a feared outcome will occur. Freeston et al. (1996) illustrate use of the downward arrow technique to expose Likelihood TAF associated with a harm and accident obsession. Once the therapist has clarified and explicitly stated the client's belief that the obsession increases the likelihood of a negative outcome (e.g., "If I think that my boyfriend will have an accident, he is at greater risk of being in an accident"), a belief rating should be obtained to determine how strongly the person believes that this is true. Assuming that the Likelihood TAF bias is firmly held, the therapist should then obtain a specific and detailed account of how the obsession increases the likelihood of a negative event.

For example, the therapist might ask, "In your mind, how does thinking about an accident cause the accident to happen?" "Do you think the accident could happen immediately when you think about it, or is there a time delay?" "When you think about the accident, does it increase the chances of accidents over a short or long period of time?" "Does it increase the likelihood of just a certain type of accident or any accident in general?" "Does the length of time you have the accident thought, or the number of accident thoughts, further increase the likelihood of the accident?" "Do you think you could be held legally responsible for harm or death to someone because you thought about it?" "How many people do you think are killed each year by someone else's thoughts?" Again, the objective with this line of questioning is to highlight the faulty nature of individuals' thinking so that they can identify the presence TAF bias. Once clients are willing to accept the idea that Likelihood TAF may be present, then the behavioral experiments described by Freeston et al. (1996) and Whittal and McLean (2002) can be assigned to challenge this line of thinking.

TAF Moral Bias

Moral TAF, in which the obsessional thought is considered as morally reprehensible as its behavioral counterpart, can be quite resistant to cognitive intervention. Freeston et al. (1996) again recommend the downward arrow technique to expose the core dysfunctional thinking that underlies Moral TAF (e.g., "that I am an evil person, a 'pervert,' for having thoughts that maybe I would sexually touch a child"). Once the highly critical self-judgment is clearly articulated with the client, the therapist proposes to test the view that "the way we think determines our true moral character." Socratic questioning can be used to introduce doubt in the client's global, rigid, and absolutistic belief that having "bad thoughts" is the basis of "bad character."

"Have you ever changed your mind about someone you at first thought was highly moral (a good person) but now you find is not so moral? What happened that caused you to change your mind? Was it what that person thought or what the person did?" The therapist could give an example from news reports of clergy accused of sexually assaulting children. "If morality is mainly determined by what we think, how many bad thoughts must a person have to be immoral?" "Is one terribly immoral thought equal to 100 slightly immoral thoughts?" "Is it the number of different types of immoral thoughts, or frequency with which a person thinks a single immoral thought that brings into question that person's moral character?" These questions are intended to suggest that judgments of morality cannot be rigid and absolutistic and that a person's behavior is a more valid measure of moral character than his or her thoughts.

To highlight the presence of Moral TAF, Whittal and McLean (2002) suggest that the client be presented with a continuum, with one end labeled "best person ever" and the other "worst person ever" (see also Steketee, 1999). Clients are asked to think of someone who would fit either end of the continuum; then they are asked to indicate where they would place themselves on the continuum. The therapist provides examples of people who have either had bad thoughts or have done bad deeds, and they are placed on the continuum (e.g., a person who had a thought of shoplifting but didn't, versus another person who is charged with shoplifting). Discussion then focuses on why one person is placed closer to the immoral end of the continuum than the other person. Again, this exercise reinforces the view that "bad deeds" are more important criteria of immorality than "bad thoughts."

The therapist can also explore whether a person's will plays any role in moral value. Consider a person who intentionally runs down a pedestrian versus a person who accidentally runs over someone who has run out in front of traffic. Freeston et al. (1996) suggest that the client can be asked to talk to close friends or family about their "strange thoughts" as a way of normalizing unwanted, even abhorrent, intrusive thoughts. The purpose of this cognitive intervention is to help clients (1) to be aware of when they engage in the faulty appraisal of Moral TAF, (2) to realize that moral value is not primarily determined by our thoughts, and (3) that morality is based on a deliberate choice of action.

Inflated Responsibility

A number of authors recommend pie charting to directly challenge excessive responsibility appraisals (Salkovskis & Wahl, 2003; van Oppen & Arntz, 1994; Whittal & McLean, 2002). The client is asked to identify a situation involving personal responsibility and to give a rating as to how responsible he or she felt for causing this situation (e.g., "A boy in my class got sick. I am 95% responsible for this because I wore fingernail polish, and the last time I did this someone also got sick"). The client is then asked to think about all the possible contributors to this situation (e.g., number of different possible causal factors for the boy's getting sick). A circle is drawn (i.e., pie chart), and the client is asked to place all of the possible contributors in the pie, with an estimate of the percentage of importance or responsibility of each contributor for the situation. Van Oppen and Arntz (1994) suggest that the client's own contribution should be placed last as the leftover part of the pie. The therapist can then compare the client's initial responsibility estimate with the final estimate represented in the pie chart after taking all other possible factors into account.

   This exercise is a useful cognitive intervention for (1) drawing attention to the client's automatic tendency to exaggerate his or her personal responsibility in negative situations associated with the obsession, (2) emphasizing the multifaceted and dimensional nature of responsibility, and (3) highlighting the difficulty in partitioning overall responsibility for any negative situation because of multiple interacting contributors (see discussion by Salkovskis & Wahl, 2003). Rachman (2003) also suggests that clients list their main responsibilities and then give examples of how they overstep realistic bounds of responsibility. Discussion can center on examples of main responsibilities (e.g., getting to work on time), partial or shared responsibilities (e.g., shared parenting duties), and minimal responsibilities (e.g., picking up sharp objects in your neighbor's driveway). Again, the purpose of this intervention is to sensitize clients to their tendency to exaggerate their perceptions of responsibility.

   Freeston et al. (1996) and Rachman (2003) describe another cognitive intervention for highlighting the faulty nature of a client's exaggerated responsibility appraisals. In the "transfer of responsibility" exercise, a situation in which the client feels a moderate level of distress might be chosen. For example, the young woman who assumed that others might get sick from her fingernail polish may rate this as a moderately distressing concern. The client is then asked to temporarily transfer responsibility for others getting sick to the therapist for 1 week. In that week the client self-monitors the frequency, distress, and reactions associated with wearing fingernail polish. This can be compared with a week when the client assumes the usual high level of responsibility. The aim of this exercise is to demonstrate the negative consequences associated with inflated responsibility appraisals.

A courtroom role play can also be used, in which a client assumes the role of prosecuting attorney, who must find evidence of his or her own guilt or responsibility for some negative event (Freeston et al., 1996; Steketee, 1999). The individual then assumes the role of defense attorney, who must prove that he or she cannot be found guilty "beyond a reasonable doubt." Clients find that they have little evidence to convict themselves of their guilt or responsibility. Notice that the point of such exercises is to emphasize that responsibility appraisals of obsessions tend to be exaggerated. The therapist should be careful to avoid debating with the client over the actual amount of personal responsibility for the negative situation.

In the following clinical example, cognitive restructuring was used to modify exaggerated responsibility appraisals involving a 52-year-old man with obsessional ruminations about harm. The client was quite preoccupied and anxious over whether thinking about the possibility of an accident made him responsible to prevent the possible occurrence of the accident. For example, he had thought that a railway crossing near his home was dangerous and that someone could get killed. Ten years later someone was killed at that crossing, and now he felt tremendous guilt because he was irresponsible and did not warn the authorities that the railway crossing was dangerous. A cognitive restructuring exercise focused on one aspect of his inflated responsibility appraisals, "that bad thoughts can cause bad events to happen" (Likelihood TAF bias). First, an alternative view to this proposition was posed, "that the association between a bad thought and action might be coincidence." We then examined evidence that bad things happen to people even when he does not have thoughts about the accident or misfortune beforehand, and evidence that he has had thoughts about possible misfortunes and nothing has happened. Evidence gathering took place in the session and also as a homework assignment (i.e., he was asked to record times when he thinks about possible misfortune and to note whether the misfortune occurs). At this point the therapist can compare the number of times a bad thought led to a bad event and the number of times when there was no connection between thinking and outcome. Is the evidence more supportive of the "causal hypothesis" or the "coincidence hypothesis?" This cognitive intervention was useful in demonstrating that the client's reasoning involved Likelihood TAF bias as well as an exaggerated appraisal of his own responsibility for the cause of accidents to complete strangers.

Overimportance of Thoughts

Any cognitive interventions focused on challenging TAF bias or responsibility appraisals will also have relevance to the overimportance of thought appraisal. While implementing the previously described cognitive exercises, the therapist should point out that once an unwanted thought is considered important because it signifies personal responsibility or the increased possibility of some imagined threat, then the person dwells on the thought. Dwelling on the thought leads to further appraisals that the thought must be important, and so on. What must be highlighted in therapy is that overimportance appraisals are both a *cause* and a *consequence* of thought frequency. "I interpret certain unwanted thoughts as highly important and so they occur more frequently, and vice versa."

Whittal and McLean (2002) suggest that Socratic questioning on this theme can be used to point out the circularity of the client's thinking and the presence of a faulty overimportance appraisal. Therapeutic work on an overimportance appraisal can proceed by discussing the client's experience with "thoughts considered important" versus "thoughts not considered important." The client is asked to give examples of important non-obsessive–compulsive thoughts (e.g., thinking about an impending medical test, not having an income tax return completed, the outcome of a job interview) and to discuss whether there is a tendency to dwell on these thoughts. A second list of unimportant non-obsessive–compulsive thoughts can be listed, and the extent to which one tends to dwell on these thoughts should be noted. A final list of obsessive–compulsive thoughts is produced, and the client is encouraged to evaluate their importance in light of the previous lists. The point of this exercise is to show that the frequency of a thought is not the sole determinant of its importance.

Freeston et al. (1996) refer to this circular thinking as "distorted cartesian reasoning" and illustrate this with the example of "people buy more of a particular brand of sausage[s] because they are fresh and they are fresh because people buy more" (pp. 437–438). Another objective of these exercises is to emphasize that appraisals of importance cause a preoccupation with the thought, and not the reverse. The exercise also reveals that faulty circular reasoning is involved in the assumption that preoccupation with a thought means that it must be important. It is critical that these within-session cognitive exercises be followed with behavioral experiments (discussed in Chapter 11, under "Overimportance of Thought") that test the appraisal, "It must be an important thought because I dwell on it."

Another key element of the overimportance appraisal that should be the focus of treatment is "dwelling on the thought means it signifies something important about me." This aspect of the overimportance appraisal can be subjected to cognitive restructuring. This is illustrated with the young woman who interpreted her frequent, upsetting obsessions of disgusting sex and violence as important because these thoughts meant that she had the potential to rape an innocent person. The therapist first isolates the overimportance appraisal "because I am so preoccupied with thoughts of sex and violence, I must have latent desires to rape." Through Socratic questioning, the therapist then draws out the circularity involved in overimportance appraisals: "Does being a latent rapist *cause* you to have frequent thoughts of sex and violence, or is the concern about being a latent rapist a *consequence* of frequent thoughts of sex and violence?" The therapist can then explore with the client evidence from her past showing that she was concerned about being a rapist before—or after—she started having the sex and violence obsessions.

Obviously, any evidence that "concern about being a rapist" was a consequence of preoccupation with sex and violence thoughts would highlight the presence of a faulty overimportance of thought appraisal. The therapist can then explore other times when high-frequency thoughts were misinterpreted as indicating something significant about the person (e.g., being preoccupied with not knowing material for an exam and then wondering if she is not very smart, thinking a lot about whether people like her and then wondering if people really don't like her, thinking a lot about whether her partner loves her and then doubting his love, etc.).

The client can also be asked to provide examples of incidents that were revealing about the type of person she is and whether or not these were connected with her thoughts (e.g., overcoming obstacles in her life, compliments or criticisms from other people about her actions, observations about her frequent patterns of behavior). The objective of this cognitive restructuring exercise is to challenge the overimportance of thought appraisal by providing evidence of the circularity of high thought frequency and importance (i.e., cause vs. consequence) and to demonstrate that the frequency of an individual's unwanted intrusive thoughts is not an accurate indicator of his or her inner motives and values.

Intolerance of Uncertainty/Perfectionism

Two aims of cognitive interventions focused on faulty appraisals of uncertainty and perfectionism are: (1) to demonstrate the negative consequences associated with both types of appraisal, and (2) to show that a state of certainty (complete absence of any doubt) and perfection is rarely, if ever, achieved. Once intolerance of uncertainty or perfectionism has been identified in a client's interpretation of the importance of the obsession, Freeston et al. (1996) propose, the therapist and client should together work on a list of advantages and disadvantages to the high need for certainty and perfection (see also Steketee, 1999).

Clients are asked to recall the most memorable times in which they were certain of an action or decision, or when they acted perfectly. Each certain and perfect incident is evaluated in terms of the advantages and disadvantages of such appraisals. In other words, "What was the consequence or outcome of certain or perfect performance?" "How much effort was involved to achieve the certainty or perfection?" "In retrospect, was it worth the effort?" "What advantage or positive outcome was associated with the certainty or perfect state?" "Were there any costs or disadvantages associated with striving for certainty or perfection in this specific situation?"

Clients can then be asked to recall important occasions on which certainty or perfection was not achieved and they had to live with doubt. Again using Socratic questioning, the therapist probes the positive and negative consequences of tolerating uncertainty and imperfection. The therapist should also explore the frequency with which certainty and perfection are achieved, as well as how much effort is involved in striving for these difficult goals. The point of this line of questioning is to highlight how infrequently certainty and perfection are achieved. The cognitive restructuring exercise should conclude with a cost/benefit analysis: "Is striving for certainty and perfection really worthwhile?" "On balance, do the costs far outweigh the benefits?" If clients agree that the appraisals of uncertainty and perfection are not beneficial, then the therapist can explore alternative ways of thinking that are not so dichotomous and absolute.

Control of Thoughts and Neutralization Appraisals

Cognitive-behavioral therapists readily acknowledge that cognitive interventions must also focus on challenging clients' beliefs and appraisals of the need to control their obsessions, as well as their more specific appraisals about the importance and effectiveness of compulsive rituals, neutralization, and other mental control strategies (Freeston & Ladouceur, 1997a; Salkovskis, 1999; Salkovskis & Wahl, 2003; Whittal & McLean, 2002). Freeston et al. (1996) concluded that "need to control" appraisals usually occur at an intermediate level, at which further questioning leads to "deeper" beliefs about TAF, responsibility, or overestimated threat. However, the cognitive control theory of obsessions proposed in Chapter 7 suggests that secondary appraisals and beliefs of control play a more prominent role in the pathogenesis of obsessions than previously acknowledged. Because the modification of secondary appraisals of control is considered so vital to an effective cognitive-behavioral treatment program, an extended discussion of these interventions is presented in Chapter 12.

Intolerance of Anxiety/Distress

Although appraisals and beliefs about the experience and consequences of anxiety or distress are not specific to OCD, they do play an important role in the persistence of obsessions and so should be targeted for treatment (Freeston et al., 1996; Rachman, 1998). Freeston et al. (1996) noted that faulty appraisals of the intolerance of anxiety can undermine compliance with ERP. Three elements of the intolerance of anxiety appraisals can be identified: (1) that anxiety will lead to serious or threatening consequences, (2) that one cannot function or perform while anxious, and (3) that anxiety or distress must be kept to an absolute minimum level. Rachman (1998) noted that intolerance of anxiety often involves "ex-consequentia reasoning" (Arntz, Rauner, & van den Hout, 1995) in which a person deduces the presence of threat or danger from the feeling of anxiousness (e.g., "I'm feeling anxious so there must be something threatening about this situation").

The most effective interventions for intolerance of anxiety/distress are behavioral tasks such as ERP, which involve direct exposure to higher levels of anxiety. However, in order for these exercises to be effective in challenging intolerance appraisals, the therapist must specifically explore the client's thoughts and appraisals about his or her heightened anxiety and the outcome. "So when you left the house and felt anxious about whether the door was truly locked or not, what were your concerns about being so anxious?" "Did the anxiety last as long as you expected?" "How did the anxiety affect your ability to function?" "Was there any direct consequence for allowing your anxiety to remain elevated longer than normal?" "What were you like 2 hours after leaving the house (4 hours, etc.)?" The therapist can also have clients keep records and compare their experience and interpretations of anxiety when they worked hard to control anxiousness and at other times when they let the anxiety dissipate on its own. The downward arrow technique can also be used to identify the core catastrophic belief about the consequences of the anxiety (Steketee, 1999). The aim of this intervention is to use behavioral exposure and response prevention as a way to challenge the client's belief that anxiety will lead to more serious negative consequences, or that he or she cannot function when anxious.

People with chronic anxiety can be quite resistant to the notion of intentionally elevating their anxiety level via exposure to fear situations because of their belief that anxiety is intolerable and must be reduced at all costs. Consequently, cognitive strategies may have to be introduced before behavioral work can proceed. One approach is to explore the client's experience with anxiety in obsessive–compulsive-relevant situations. First, the therapist should obtain a description of the anxiety and a rating of its intensity. "What was the worst thing about that feeling of anxiousness?" "Was there a particular sensation, physical symptom, or feeling that bothered you most?" "How intense was the anxiety on a scale from 0 to 100?" "How long did the anxiety last?" Then the therapist should explore the client's interpretation of the anxiety in order to identify faulty appraisals of intolerance. "Were you afraid that the anxiety would do something to you if it continued?" "What were you afraid might happen if you couldn't get your anxiety level down?" "What effect did the anxiety have on you?" "How concerned were you to get the anxiety under control?" "What did you do to reduce the anxiety?" "How effective was it?" This line of Socratic questioning should culminate in a summary statement in which the therapist emphasizes the client's conclusion that he or she could not tolerate the anxiety for the reasons identified in the questioning.

Once the faulty appraisal of intolerance is identified, Socratic questioning then shifts to explore evidence that the anxiety was more tolerable and less threatening than the client had assumed. "I would like to go back over this anxious situation again, and see whether there is any evidence or indication that you had some control or were able to perform at some minimal level." "Is there any evidence that you could have tolerated a little more anxiety, or that you could have tolerated the anxiety a little longer?" "Have you ever been in that anxious situation when you were prevented from reducing the anxiety [e.g., a person with washing compulsion feels contaminated but cannot wash because another person is present]?" "What was that like?" "What was the outcome, the short- and the long-term consequence?" The therapist should direct this line of questioning so that clients can consider whether they might have a tendency to overestimate the negative aspects of anxiety and therefore to assume that it is intolerable. If clients accept this possibility, then they may be prepared to expose themselves to higher levels of distress.

A *cognitive reframing* exercise can be used for clients who continue to believe that anxiety must be avoided or reduced, because it is intolerable. The therapist obtains examples of non-obsessive–compulsive experiences in which the client felt high levels of anxiety. Examples may be narrowly avoiding a fatal car accident, undergoing medical tests for a life-threatening illness, having one's employment terminated, threats of losing a valued relationship (i.e., marriage), an unexpected large expense, or the like. The therapist then obtains a description of the anxiety associated with the situation, a rating of its intensity, and interpretations of the anxiety and its consequences. A comparison can then be made between the person's anxiety rating for the obsessive–compulsive situation and his or her anxiety rating for the non-obsessive–compulsive situation.

Normally, a client with OCD will rate the obsessive–compulsive-related anxiety higher than the non-obsessive–compulsive anxiety. This can be pointed out, and then the therapist explores whether this is a realistic appraisal of the obsessive–compulsive-relevant anxiety. "I notice that you rated your anxiety level higher when you were worried about whether the door was locked than when you were told that your employment was terminated." "Which of these situations was more important in your life?" "Which had more immediate and long-lasting negative consequences?" "What is it about the obsessive–compulsive-related anxiety that makes you think it is worse than upset over a life stressor?" "In light of some of the significant threats to your health and well-being, do you think you might be overreacting to the obsessive–compulsive anxiety?" "Given how you coped with worry and anxiety in other areas of your life, does this cause you to reconsider your ability to tolerate a little more anxiety in obsessive–compulsive-relevant situations?" "Is it possible that you can tolerate more anxiety than you give yourself credit for?"

With this exercise, anxiety experienced with major life events is used to "reframe" the obsessive–compulsive-relevant anxiety in a more realistic light. It would be rare to find a person with OCD who has not experienced a major life event. However, if such is the case, hypothetical life events can be used, but this would be much less effective than using a real-life experience. In the end, the purpose of cognitive work on intolerance of anxiety or distress is to prepare the client for the exposure exercises that are so critical for the success of CBT for obsessions and compulsions.

GENERATING ALTERNATIVE APPRAISALS

Because so much emphasis is placed on cognitive and behavioral interventions that challenge the faulty appraisals and beliefs involved in obsessions and compulsions, the importance of working collaboratively with the client to develop alternative, more functional and adaptive interpretations is often overlooked in CBT (Clark, 1999). However, the development of alternative interpretations for the persistence of obsessive and compulsive symptoms is critical to treatment success. If clients are to accept the idea that their faulty appraisals and beliefs of obsessions are erroneous, then they must develop a different framework for understanding the persistence of their symptoms.

Salkovskis and Freeston (2001) emphasized that systematic restructuring of faulty obsessive–compulsive assumptions should result in a new, less threatening understanding of the obsession, which will encourage healthier responses that, in turn, support the new account and disconfirm the old perspective. Moreover, this alternative perspective should be in direct opposition to the faulty interpretation so that accepting one view means rejection of the other. Table 10.2 illustrates the primary faulty interpretations and possible alternative perspectives associated with each of the obsessive–compulsive appraisal patterns.

The more functional interpretations offered in Table 10.2 are meant only as a guide for developing alternative interpretations for particular clients. There are a number of aspects in generating alternative beliefs and appraisals that must be considered. First, the alternative interpretation must be tailored to the specific idiosyncratic content and meaning of the person's obsession. Standard explanations will be much less effective in countering the client's faulty appraisals of the obsession. For example, the young woman with harming obsessions believed that her frequent thoughts about whether she could lose control and rape an innocent person were evidence that she might be a "latent rapist" (overimportance of thought appraisal). The alternative explanation developed was that she had frequent "rape-related thoughts" because she was an over sensitive and conscientious person who was especially offended by these types of thoughts and so paid more attention to them. Notice that the alternative interpretation fits with the explanation offered in Table 10.2, but is tailored to the client's obsessional content.

Second, it is important that the alternative interpretation be developed through the process of guided discovery (see Padesky, 1995). The client is less likely to consider alternative interpretations that are presented by the therapist without collaborative work. In this regard, it may be useful to do some cognitive and behavioral intervention on the faulty appraisals and beliefs prior to introducing an alternative interpretation. However, at least some of the interventions should involve a test between the adaptive and maladaptive appraisals. In the aforementioned example, a behavioral experiment was set up to gather evidence that the woman had "unconscious motives to rape" versus that she was "hypersensitive to thoughts of hurting another person." Rachman (2003) provides guidelines on how to collect new information that therapist and client can use to construct alternative interpretations of the significance of obsessions.

Finally, the underlining theme to the more adaptive appraisals and beliefs is that the persistence of obsessive–compulsive symptoms and anxiety is due to faulty appraisals of the importance or significance of the obsession and secondary appraisals of the need to control the obsession through neutralization, avoidance, and compulsive rituals. If a person can accept the idea that his or her unwanted thoughts, images, or impulses are harmless, irrelevant, even silly phenomena that require no particular response, then a more adaptive perspective is developed that will counter future obsessional tendencies.

TABLE 10.2. Illustrative Faulty Interpretations and Alternative, More Adaptive Explanations for Each of the Primary Obsessive–Compulsive Appraisals

Type of appraisal	Faulty interpretation	Adaptive alternative interpretation
Overestimated threat	Anything that elicits the obsession will increase the possibility of highly undesirable consequences.	Situations are safe unless there is external, real-life evidence of actual threat or danger. Having thoughts and feelings about the possibility of imagined negative consequences does not mean that real-life negative outcomes are more certain.
Thought–action fusion (TAF)	*Likelihood TAF.* The occurrence of the obsession increases the probability that a negative event will happen. *Moral TAF.* Having "bad" thoughts is as immoral as acting on these thoughts.	*Likelihood TAF.* Thoughts cannot have a direct causal influence on events in the real world. *Moral TAF.* Moral character is based on what we do and not on what we think.
Inflated responsibility	Because one thinks about the possibility of the occurrence of harm, that person is primarily responsible to prevent the possible harm occurring to self or others.	All real-life negative events involve multiple factors that cause them to happen. As a result, responsibility is distributed across many contributing factors, with a person's own contribution to the event often playing a very minor, practically insignificant role. Because an individual's influence over a possible negative event is so limited, his or her responsibility to prevent that event is minimal, if not practically nonexistent.
Overimportance of thought	Persistent obsessions must be very important, because they signify some undesirable inner motive or potential.	Because obsessions involve themes that are completely contrary or alien to a person's cherished values and inclinations, a person tends to give them undue attention. Just dwelling on a thought can raise its perceived importance.

230

Control of thoughts	Failing to exert strong and effective control over the obsession will lead to highly undesirable negative consequences.	Great effort at controlling an unwanted thought will cause an increase in its frequency, salience and associated distress. By relinquishing effort to exert mental control over the obsession, ultimately less attention is devoted to the thought and the personal importance of the thought is downgraded.
Intolerance of uncertainty	One must strive to achieve absolute certainty in thought and/or action in order to reduce doubt, ambiguity, and the possibility of negative outcomes, which, in turn, elicit anxiety or distress.	Uncertainty is an unavoidable aspect of human experience and cannot be completely eliminated. It is the striving for certainty (or the complete eradication of doubt) that elevates anxiety and perceived dangerousness rather than the presence of some degree of uncertainty.
Perfectionism	One must strive to achieve a perfect response or solution to every problem or situation in order to avoid the serious consequences that occur because of minor mistakes and inaccuracies.	Minor mistakes, inaccuracies, or flaws are an inevitable aspect of all human endeavors that do not result in serious negative consequences. Anxiousness and distress are products of striving for that which cannot be attained–absolute perfection. The alternative is a person's best performance that meets the requirements of a situation.
Intolerance of anxiety/distress	If anxiety or distress is not reduced or eliminated, it will lead to harmful consequences.	Anxiety and fear are natural human emotions that are integral to being alive. A person can adapt to varying levels of short-term anxiety without harmful long-term consequences.

SUMMARY AND CONCLUSION

What distinguishes CBT from a strict behavioral approach to the treatment of OCD is the heavy emphasis on cognitive tactics to directly challenge faulty obsessive–compulsive appraisals and beliefs. Clients must be taught to distinguish their faulty appraisals or interpretations of importance from the obsession itself. Once this skill is achieved, cognitive restructuring strategies are introduced to directly challenge faulty appraisals of threat, TAF, inflated responsibility, overimportance, control, intolerance of uncertainty, perfectionism, and intolerance of anxiety/distress. Cognitive restructuring is introduced early in treatment in order to improve the client's acceptance of more potent but distressing behavioral exercises. Moreover, cognitive restructuring encourages the client to adopt a more inquiring, less restrictive and absolutistic perspective on firmly held obsessive–compulsive beliefs. With such an attitude the client will gain more benefit from later exposure-based exercises.

It is important that clients start working on alternative explanations for the persistence and frequency of their obsessions early in the treatment process. Explanations that emphasize faulty appraisals and excessive control or neutralization as the cause of the frequent obsessive thinking will provide a solid rationale for the behavioral interventions that follow. Ultimately, it is important that clients learn to view their unwanted intrusive thoughts as meaningless, insignificant "mental chaff" that deserves no response.

APPENDIX 10.1. Types of Appraisals Involved in the Persistence of Unwanted Intrusive Thoughts and Obsessions

Type of appraisal	Explanation of the appraisal	Examples of the appraisal
Overestimated threat	To overestimate the severity and/or likelihood that a highly negative, even catastrophic, consequence of the obsession could occur. As a result, the obsession represents a serious threat to personal well-being.	1. "If I shake a stranger's hand, then I will contract a fatal disease." 2. "If I left the car unlocked, then someone will steal it." 3. "If I feel even a little physical discomfort, this means I must be getting seriously sick."
Thought–action fusion	To assume that thinking about a negative event increases the likelihood that the negative event will happen, or that "bad" thoughts are morally equal to "bad" deeds.	1. "If I think something evil, it is more likely to happen." 2. "If I think (or imagine) that a person is having an accident, he or she is more likely to have one." 3. "Thinking that I might have sexually touched a child is almost as bad as doing it." 4. "If I think I've made a mistake, it is more likely that I really have made a mistake."
Inflated responsibility	To hold oneself responsible to prevent a perceived negative outcome that could have a real or imagined consequence for the self or for others. The person believes that he or she has influence over the negative outcome and therefore is responsible for that outcome.	1. "If I see a piece of broken glass on the road, I must pick it up. If I don't, it would be my fault if a car ran over the glass and had an accident." 2. "If I do something wrong, God will punish me by making other people sick." 3. "I must make sure that I don't contaminate other people."
Overimportance of thought	To assume that a highly persistent unwanted thought must have some significance for the self because it occurs so frequently against one's will.	1. "I must be very susceptible to disease and illness because I am preoccupied with avoiding contamination." 2. "If I have violent and aggressive thoughts against people, maybe deep down I want to harm them."

(continued)

Type of appraisal	Explanation of the appraisal	Examples of the appraisal
Overimportance of thought (cont.)		3. "Because I so frequently have blasphemous thoughts against God, I must be an evil person or demon possessed." 4. "If I continually wonder if I've done things right and correct, maybe it is because I have to be extra concerned about carelessness."
Control of thoughts	To assume that it is possible and highly desirable to have near perfect control over unwanted thoughts in order to avoid negative consequences.	1. "If I don't get better control over these obsessions, I will become overwhelmed with anxiety." 2. "If I do a better job controlling my obsessions, this means I am less likely to act on them." 3. "If I don't control these thoughts, they will eventually drive me 'crazy'."
Intolerance of uncertainty	To assume that it is critical to achieve almost absolute or perfect certainty in thought or action in order to maximize predictability and control. Ambiguity, newness, change, or not knowing should be avoided because they can increase anxiety and stress.	1. "If I feel any doubt about a decision, I must keep going over and over it until I am convinced beyond doubt that the decision was the right one." 2. "I must have proof, a guarantee that I am a peaceful person and not capable of rape." 3. "I need to be certain that I did not make a mistake on that form." 4. "It is critical that there is no possibility of contamination in my house (or apartment)."
Perfectionism	To assume that it is possible and highly desirable to strive for the one best response to each problem or situation. Even minor mistakes and inaccuracies must be avoided, because they can lead to serious consequences.	1. "It is important that I find the 'perfect' gift for every special occasion." 2. "I can answer 'yes' to a questionnaire item only if it describes me perfectly in every situation." 3. "I should never have a bad or sinful thought against God or other people." 4. "I must ensure that there is not even a speck of dirt in my room that could contaminate me."
Intolerance of anxiety or distress	To assume that anxiety or distress is bad because it may have harmful consequences. Therefore, every effort should be made to avoid feeling anxious or to reduce anxiety as soon as it occurs.	1. "I can't stand this anxiety much longer." 2. "If I am bothered or upset by an unwanted intrusive thought, then I have to do something to relieve the anxiety." 3. "I'm afraid the anxiety and distress will get worse if I don't deal with distress when I first feel it."

Instructions: Please use the form below to record three or four daily occurrences of your main unwanted intrusive thought or obsession. In four or five words note what you think triggered the obsession, the obsessional content, and then your interpretation of its importance. That is, write down what made the unwanted thought so important to you at the time it occurred. In the last column see if you can pick out any of the appraisal patterns we've gone over in the last therapy session. You will probably need to use the sheet that explains the appraisals to assist you in this task (Appendix 10.1). Don't worry if you can't seem to identify the appraisal patterns in your interpretation of the obsession. We can do this together at the next session.

Date/ time	Situational trigger	Obsession	Interpretation of importance	Main appraisal patterns

CHAPTER 11

Empirical Hypothesis Testing

Behavioral interventions are critical to the effectiveness of CBT for obsessions and compulsions. It is unlikely that significant reductions in obsessive–compulsive symptoms can be achieved solely by verbal techniques such as logical persuasion, evidence gathering, or hypothesis testing. Exposure and responsive prevention are still the central therapeutic elements in CBT for OCD. In addition, behavioral experiments that are tailored to the specific faulty appraisals and beliefs of the obsessional client are essential for creating significant therapeutic change. This chapter discusses refinements that must be made to standard ERP so that it can directly modify the dysfunctional cognitive basis of OCD. In addition, various behavioral experiments are proposed that are used to empirically challenge the faulty obsessive–compulsive appraisals and reinforce alternative explanations for the obsession. In fact, a large proportion of therapy time is spent on developing, evaluating, and consolidating clients' experiences of within-session and between-session behavioral exercises.

EXPOSURE AND RESPONSE PREVENTION (ERP)

ERP for obsessions and compulsions is described in a number of behaviorally oriented treatment manuals, as well as in Chapter 3 of this book (Kozak & Foa, 1997; Steketee, 1993, 1999). The current discussion focuses more specifically on the use of ERP within a cognitive-behavioral context.

Both within-session and between-session ERP should be introduced within the first 5–10 sessions of treatment. It will then become the primary method for behaviorally challenging faulty appraisals and beliefs and for developing healthier responses to the obsession. The application of ERP within CBT is illustrated in the following example involving treatment of compulsive washing. In addressing one of the moderately anxiety-provoking situations in her fear hierarchy, a client is encouraged to use the toilet in a public washroom at least once or twice a day. She is asked to refrain from washing her hands for at least 1 hour after each exposure. This particular ERP exercise challenges a number of faulty appraisals and beliefs, such as overestimated threat ("I'll get some terrible disease from using a public toilet"), inflated responsibility ("I'll become contaminated from the washroom and then spread this to others"), intolerance of uncertainty ("I need to feel clean and be certain there is no chance that I could be dirty or contaminated"), and intolerance of anxiety ("I can't stand the anxiety because it will escalate and get much worse").

In order for ERP to effectively challenge faulty appraisals and beliefs, the exercise must be introduced and evaluated within a cognitive context. That is, the therapist introduces ERP as a task that will test specific appraisals and beliefs about the importance and dangerousness of certain thoughts or situations. During ERP, clients record their thoughts and feelings, the outcomes of the exercise, and their interpretation of the outcomes (e.g., "I was really quite surprised that my anxiety declined fairly quickly even though I did not wash my hands").

At the following session, the therapist spends a considerable amount of time going over the client's self-monitoring record. Emphasis is placed on drawing out aspects of the ERP experience that are contrary to the faulty appraisals and beliefs, as well as data that support the alternative interpretation. Naturally, ERP must be repeated in a variety of situations at increasing anxiety levels in order to produce stable changes in obsessive–compulsive appraisals and beliefs. Moreover, depending on the OCD subtype and the personal obsessional content, behavioral intervention may primarily involve repeated exposure to the obsession itself, as in the use of habituation training for obsessional rumination.

BEHAVIORAL EXPERIMENTATION

Behavioral experimentation, or empirical hypothesis testing, is the backbone of CBT for OCD. Beck et al. (1979) noted that behavioral techniques are designed as mini-experiments that test the validity of dysfunctional thoughts and beliefs in order to bring about cognitive change. In CBT for obsessions and compulsions, behavioral experiments are introduced once the faulty primary and secondary appraisals and beliefs have been identified. Table 11.1 summarizes 26 different behavioral experiments that can be used to test the validity of the faulty appraisals associated with obsessions.

Behavioral exercises should be introduced as early in the treatment process as possible, because they will prove the most effective in producing cognitive and behavioral change. Although primarily cognitive inter-

TABLE 11.1. Typical Behavioral Experiments Used to Evaluate Faulty Appraisals of Obsessions

Type of appraisal	Behavioral experiment
Overestimated threat	*Risk assessment.* The client gathers "real-life" evidence of increased risk after threat exposure.
	Threat survey. The client interviews people or collects "archival" evidence of real-life harm or danger resulting from his or her primary obsessional concerns.
	Atypical exposure. The client engages in an exposure task that involves some unusual behavior outside normal activity in order to test a specific belief about negative consequences.
Thought–action fusion (TAF)	*Premonitions experiment.* The client thinks about people and records every time he or she hears from these individuals.
	Intrusions survey. The client surveys trusted friends and family on the types of unwanted ego-dystonic intrusive thoughts they experience.
	Power of thoughts. Begin by having the client form a specific thought about a positive or neutral event and record whether the event occurs. The client then proceeds to thinking about bad things happening to therapist, friends, or self, and records the outcome.
	Cognitive risk. The client increases the frequency and duration of ruminating on unwanted thoughts and records any evidence of increased tendency for negative outcomes.
Inflated responsibility	*Responsibility manipulation.* The client records the frequency and distress of the obsession during a week in which he or she focuses on his or her personal responsibility for any negative consequences of the obsession (high responsibility condition). In the following week responsibility is temporarily shifted to the therapist through a written contract, and the client records frequency and distress of the obsession for a week, during which the client reminds him or herself that the therapist is responsible for the possible negative outcome (low responsibility condition).
	Responsibility gradient. The client is exposed to a hierarchy of successively greater responsibility for tasks involving the primary obsessional concern.
Overimportance of thought	*Artificial importance.* The client is asked to pay particularly close attention to some innocuous external stimulus (e.g., house for sale signs) for one week and then to refrain from attending to the target stimulus in the following week.
	Importance manipulation. The client selects an intrusive thought that is not an obsessional concern, forms it for 30 seconds, and then rates its perceived importance and distress. The client repeats the exercise but this time inflates the thought's significance, again rating its importance and distress.

(continued)

TABLE 11.1. *(continued)*

Type of appraisal	Behavioral experiment
Overimportance of thought *(continued)*	*Inflated significance.* The client deliberately thinks about the obsession for a short interval (10 seconds) and rates its perceived importance and distress. The client thinks about the obsession a second time for a longer interval (60 seconds) and rates its perceived importance and distress.
	Attentive days task. On alternative days the client is to attend closely to the obsession, recording its frequency, associated anxiety, and any other outcomes; on the remaining days the client is to let the obsession go as if it were an unimportant thought.
Control of thoughts	*Thought suppression effect.* The client tries to suppress a neutral thought for 2 minutes, and the therapist records each time the client signals a thought occurrence. The client is then asked to suppress a non-obsessive–compulsive important thought (e.g., current worry) for 2 minutes and thought recurrences are recorded. Finally, the client tries to suppress the primary obsession for 2 minutes and the thought recurrences are recorded.
	Alternate suppress days. Similar to the previous exercise, except that the client is instructed to deliberately suppress the obsession on alternate days and simply record the obsession on the remaining days. Ratings of frequency and distress are recorded and graphed for the suppression and monitor-only days.
	Alternate control days. On alternate days the client refrains from intentionally trying to control the obsession and compares these with the other days when engaged in obsessive–compulsive control responses.
Intolerance of uncertainty	*Certainty survey.* The client interviews friends, family, and work colleagues on their certainty of remembering whether routine actions were performed (e.g., stove turned off, door locked, etc.).
	Certainty manipulation. The client records level of certainty and remembering for routine non-obsessive–compulsive activities (e.g., brushed teeth, vacuumed house completely). The client selects one of these tasks and increases attempts to be certain; records frequency and distress throughout the exercise.
	Uncertainty exposure. Tasks are performed or decisions made in a way that results in varying levels of uncertainty for obsessional concerns. The client records the level of doubt or uncertainty and distress over a waiting interval of hours or days. The person then checks to see if any negative consequences occurred as a result of the prior actions or decisions.
Perfectionism	*Cost/benefit analysis.* The client selects a number of key tasks at work or in the home that are associated with perfectionistic concerns. These tasks are completed, and the client rates the level of perfectionism, effort, and distress associated with each task. How much extra time and effort would be involved to increase the perfection rating? What were the costs/benefits of attaining "additional perfection" of the task?

(continued)

TABLE 11.1. *(continued)*

Type of appraisal	Behavioral experiment
Perfectionism *(continued)*	*Perfectionism observation.* A friend or work colleague is selected whom the client admires for his or her high performance. This person's level of perfection in performance of key tasks is observed and rated. How often is "absolute perfection" achieved? What mistakes or flaws were evident? What effect did this have on the final outcome? Did the person focus on absolute perfection or simply on meeting the requirements of the situation?
	Intentional errors. Certain tasks are selected that involve varying levels of obsessional concerns. These tasks are performed with the client intentionally including some minor flaw or inaccuracy. The consequences of the flawed performances are recorded.
Intolerance of anxiety or distress	*Anxiety survey.* The client interviews friends about their experiences with being anxious, nervous, or fearful. How common is anxiety? What was it like? How did they cope and what was the outcome?
	Anxiety monitoring. The client observes people in a variety of situations and rates their anxiety levels. How did the client know he or she was anxious? How intense was the anxiety? What effect did it have on his or her performances or the outcome of the task?
	Anxiety comparison. The therapist has the client perform a nonobsessional anxious task and an obsessional task, and records the different experiences of anxiety.
	Anxiety prediction. During exposure exercises the client makes predictions about his or her anxiety and its effects. The client then completes the exposure task and records actual anxiety and its effects. Comparisons are made between predicted and actual levels of anxiety.

Note. Material based on Freeston and Ladouceur (1997a), Freeston et al. (1996), Rachman (1998), Salkovskis (1999), and Whittal and McLean (2002).

ventions may be initially introduced, in practice the cognitive and behavioral elements of treatment should be well integrated and used together to effect therapeutic change. All behavioral interventions must be introduced in a collaborative manner and tailored to the client's idiosyncratic obsessional concerns. Behavioral experiments that provide disconfirming evidence for the faulty appraisal and support for the alternative explanation will be the most effective intervention. It is important that the therapist evaluate the outcome of the behavioral assignments at the following session in order to highlight evidence against the faulty appraisals and beliefs. The therapist should continue, in future sessions, to reinforce with the client the significant insights that have been gained through behavioral experimentation (e.g., "Recall the experiment you did a few weeks ago, in which you tried to suppress the obsession on some days and not on other days. Do you remember the outcome of that experiment?"). The behavioral exercises summarized in Table 11.1 are briefly described in the following sections. In addition, Rachman's (2003) treatment manual for obsessions describes a number of behavioral experiments for inflated responsibility, TAF bias, control of thoughts, and neutralization.

Overestimated Threat

Exposure-based interventions are best suited to test the tendency to exaggerate the probability and severity of negative consequences associated with obsessional concerns and to determine whether obsessive–compulsive situations are safer than assumed. Table 11.1 describes three types of behavioral interventions that may be particularly effective with this type of faulty appraisal. The *risk assessment exercise* involves having the client look for real-life evidence of increased risk of danger after completing an exposure task. For example, individuals with a washing compulsion could be asked to use public telephones and not wash their hands afterward. They then record any indication of feeling sick or unwell that might suggest contamination (e.g., sore throat, coughing, aches or pains, etc.). The absence of real-life indicators of danger can be used as evidence that they tend to assume an excessively high level of risk and danger in obsessive–compulsive situations when safety is the more likely outcome.

A *threat survey* is very useful for individuals with harm and injury obsessions and checking compulsions (see also Rachman, 2003; Steketee, 1999). For example, the client can be asked to interview acquaintances and/or search for statistics or other recorded information on the number of houses burglarized because of unlocked doors, houses that catch fire as a result of leaving lights on, cancer that is contracted by using public toilets, children who are stabbed while their mother uses a kitchen knife, children or strangers who are sexually assaulted by persons who suddenly lose control of themselves, and the like. Even if the client does find evidence that on very rare occasions an obsessional concern led to the feared outcome, data can be collected on the most likely route to the negative event (e.g., most frequent cause of house fires, etiology of cancer, characteristics of sexual predators). Evidence can also be gathered on the frequency with which the obsessional concern does not lead to the negative outcome (e.g., number of times people shake hands without getting a disease, etc.). It is important that the therapist use this evidence to test the client's tendency to overestimate threat and to avoid any "debate" on whether the obsessional concern is realistic or rational.

Atypical exposure involves performing an exposure task outside the normal sphere of one's behavior in order to test a specific obsessional belief. For example, a businessman suffered from harming obsessions, one of which involved the upsetting thought of attacking his wife with a hammer. He sincerely loved her, and there was absolutely no hint of domestic violence or abuse of any kind (a necessary assessment before assigning this exercise). In this case, the therapist could suggest that the carpenter's hammer, which was normally kept in the basement, be moved to different locations in the house. The client could be asked to rate "urge to engage in violent behavior" associated with varying levels of accessibility to the hammer (e.g., when the hammer is moved to the kitchen, living room, bedroom). By increasing exposure to the hammer, the person is testing the exaggerated threat belief "I have to avoid hammers because I might snap, lose control, and become violent." Specific exposure tasks can be designed to test whether negative outcomes are as likely as the client assumes, even when going slightly beyond the usual bounds of normal behavior (e.g., leave the house unlocked for an hour, have a speck of dog feces on your pant leg, leave the trunk of the car open and then shut it without looking).

Thought–Action Fusion Bias

Whittal and McLean (2002) describe a *predictions* or *premonitions experiment* in which clients are asked to think about a specific person or situation and then record the number of times they hear from that friend or the number of times the situation occurs in the following week or two (see also Rachman, 2003). The point of this exercise is to test the Likelihood TAF belief that merely thinking about things can influence whether they happen. A variation on this exercise is to test whether the more one thinks about an event, the more likely it is to happen. For example, a client can be asked one week to only occasionally think about his mother phoning, and on an alternative week to think a great deal about his mother phoning. Predictions can be made about the number of times she will phone each week, and then a record kept on the actual number of phone calls.

Clients can be asked to conduct an *intrusions survey* in which trusted people are interviewed on the types of "strange thoughts" they experience (Freeston et al., 1996; Rachman, 2003). The client may use a list of typical unwanted ego-dystonic intrusive thoughts, such as those in Appendix 9.1, to prime individuals' recollection of their own mental intrusions. Freeston and colleagues (1996) note that this can be a useful exercise for normalizing obsessions and challenging the basis of Moral TAF, that having certain types of thoughts is an indication of immoral character. The client can also be asked to discuss the basis of moral character and the role of unwanted thoughts with individuals that the client highly respects for their moral standing.

Both Whittal and McLean (2002) and Rachman (1998, 2003) discuss variations on the *power of thoughts exercise* to demonstrate that the probability of an outcome is not influenced by thinking about that outcome (i.e., Likelihood TAF). The therapist can begin with a positive event, such as winning the lottery, or even more mundane things such as number of compliments on the person's physical appearance. The client is asked to record a baseline occurrence of these events (winning the lottery would probably have a baseline of zero). Over the subsequent week the client is asked to begin each day by imagining the positive event and then to frequently think about the outcome during the day. Predictions are made on whether there will be an increase in the occurrence of the event during the "mentation week." All occurrences of the target event are recorded during the baseline and mentation weeks. The therapist then discusses the outcome and whether there is any evidence that thinking about the event caused an increase in its occurrence.

The *cognitive risk exercise* is a natural extension of the power of thoughts experiment. As Rachman (1998) noted, if the client notices no increase in the targeted outcome when thinking positive or neutral thoughts, then the assignment can progress to negative thoughts and events. The therapist can start with a nonobsessional negative thought and record whether increased mentation results in greater likelihood of the event (e.g., thinking about being criticized at work results in more criticism). If this exercise goes well, then the therapist can progress to mild, and then moderate, obsessional concerns (e.g., thinking more about feeling sick and noting whether the person actually gets sick, thinking more about friends in minor mishaps and noting whether they have such mishaps, etc.). Not only can these exercises be used to challenge Likelihood TAF, but they can also reinforce the alternative explanation that thoughts do not have direct causal effects on real-life events. Completing these exercises may also improve the client's acceptance of more threatening exposure and response prevention tasks.

Inflated Responsibility

Lopatka and Rachman (1995) developed a responsibility manipulation that can be used to demonstrate the negative effects of assuming excessive personal responsibility for the prevention of highly improbable negative outcomes to self or others. Rachman (2003) describes the application of the *transfer of responsibility* task to the therapy setting. First, a primary obsessional concern is identified, such as "I will expose my family to increased risk of contamination if I wear my work clothes around the house." Because inflated responsibility is most typical for this client, the procedure begins with a "high responsibility" week, for which the client is given written instructions to frequently remind herself that she is responsible to prevent contamination from entering the house. Records are kept on the frequency of the obsession and associated distress during the week. The following week, a "low responsibility" condition is introduced, in which the client transfers responsibility to the therapist. Written instructions are developed as a reminder that the client is following the therapist's instructions and that the therapist will assume all responsibility for any ill effects to the family resulting from the client's doing the exposure exercise (e.g., wearing work clothes in the house). At a subsequent session the therapist compares obsession frequency and distress during the periods of high and low responsibility, for evidence that obsessive–compulsive symptoms declined under conditions of low responsibility.

Once clients realize that they erroneously assume inflated personal responsibility in obsessive–compulsive situations, therapy should then focus on correcting the faulty responsibility appraisals. A behavioral exercise effective in this regard is to use the *responsibility gradient*. Here, clients are exposed to a hierarchy of obsessional situations that involve assuming successively higher levels of responsibility for previously avoided or anxiety-provoking tasks. For example, a person with a checking compulsion can be asked to leave the house, lock the door, and check the handle once for no more than one second. Initially, the client's spouse might stand beside him as he locks the door, observing that the door is locked but not reassuring the client that the door is secure. Next, the spouse may stand at the bottom of the steps as the door is locked. Then the spouse can sit in the car and watch the client lock the door. Finally, the client locks the door but the spouse purposely looks away so as not to attend to the task. Notice that as the assignment progresses, more responsibility for the locked door is shifted from the spouse to the client. Not only is this a good exercise for directly modifying faulty responsibility, but it is also a useful modification of ERP that may improve client compliance.

Overimportance of Thought

The primary objective of the behavioral exercises directed at this faulty appraisal (overimportance of thought) is to demonstrate that the more a person attends to an unwanted thought, the greater its perceived importance and significance for that person. Whittal and McLean (2002) describe a behavioral exercise for overimportance (or control) appraisals, which I have labeled the *artificial importance task*. In this exercise clients are first asked to estimate the number of times in a week they see an innocuous target stimulus, such as a sign advertising "house for sale." Then, for a 1-week period they are to attend closely to the target stimulus and record the number of sightings. In the following week clients no longer seek out the stimulus but simply record the number of times the target is sighted. The usual finding with this exercise is that merely attending to a neutral stimulus increases its frequency, even in the week when attention to the target stimulus is discontinued. This task highlights the circularity of overimportance and attention by indicating that the more we attend to or think about an unwanted topic, the greater its perceived importance.

Another exercise that directly addresses faulty overimportance appraisals is the *importance manipulation* described by Rachman (1998). Clients are asked to select from a list of unwanted intrusive thoughts a statement that is not their current obsessional concern. They focus on this intrusive thought for 2 minutes and then rate its subjective importance and associated distress. Both should be rated quite low at this point. The therapist and client then explore how a person could think about the intrusive thought that would increase its level of importance. The following example is a possible therapist intervention:

> "I can tell from your ratings that you are not particularly bothered by the thought 'Maybe I will become terribly sick from using this public toilet.' Obviously, this is not an important thought to you, but some people become very upset by thoughts like this. What do you imagine they think about that makes this an upsetting thought? Let's write down some ideas of how a person might inflate the importance attached to this thought."

Once an "inflated importance scenario" is developed, the client is again asked to form the intrusive thought for 2 minutes and to use the "importance scenario" to obtain a more complete formation of the intrusive thought. Importance and distress ratings are again completed after the 2-minute interval. Ratings from the first and second thought formation intervals are then compared to determine the effects of artificially inflating the perceived importance of the thought. This exercise not only highlights the negative effects of overimportance appraisals, but also demonstrates how perceived negative implications for the self are central to this faulty appraisal.

Rachman (1998) suggests that if manipulation of the significance of a nonobsessional thought goes well, then the therapist can progress to deliberate formation of the obsessive thought. The *inflated significance task* listed in Table 11.1 is a variation on Rachman's suggestions. Clients are asked to form the obsession for a short interval (i.e., 10 seconds) and then again for a much longer interval (i.e., 60 seconds). Ratings of the perceived importance and distress of the obsession are completed after each interval and compared. The aim of this exercise is to test whether more sustained attention to the obsession increased its perceived importance.

Salkovskis (1999), Rachman (1998, 2003), and Whittal and McLean (2002) discuss variations on an *attentive days task* that emphasizes the negative effects of overimportance and control appraisals. On alternate days clients are instructed to pay close attention to their obsession, recording its frequency, associated distress, and any other significant outcomes. This would represent the client's usual obsessive–compulsive symptom pattern.

On the remaining days, clients are instructed to let "the thoughts come and go as if they were unimportant" (Whittal & McLean, 2002, p. 424). Prior to the exercise clients are asked to predict on which days the obsessions will be more frequent and distressing. Findings that the unwanted thoughts are less problematic on the "low attention" days is strong evidence of the negative effects of overimportance appraisals and the positive therapeutic benefits of paying less attention to the obsessions.

The common objective of all of these behavioral exercises is to provide evidence that an obsession persists not because it represents something significant about a person, but because the person devotes too much attention to the thought.

Control of Thoughts

Three behavioral exercises are presented in Table11.1 that challenge appraisals and beliefs about the need to control unwanted intrusive thoughts and obsessions via neutralization, compulsive ritual, or thought suppression. Because these intervention strategies are most relevant to modifying the faulty secondary appraisals of failed thought control, as proposed by the cognitive control model, further discussion of these exercises is reserved for the next chapter.

Intolerance of Uncertainty

The behavioral exercises listed for faulty appraisals in regard to intolerance of uncertainty all target the belief that one can and must eradicate all doubt and uncertainty about the accuracy and correctness of one's actions and decisions in order to avoid an imagined negative outcome. Whittal and McLean (2002) recommend that clients conduct a *certainty survey* among trusted friends. Individuals can be interviewed on whether they actually remember instances of doing certain routine tasks like locking the car or house door, washing their hands, turning off the stove burners, and the like. Before doing the interviews, clients make predictions about how much confidence people have in their memories. As Whittal and McLean note, clients are often surprised that most people do not remember doing these routine tasks and that even though uncertainty is common, it rarely results in increased danger.

The *certainty manipulation* is a possible follow-up exercise to the survey. Clients select a number of daily activities that are not the focus of obsessional concerns (e.g., brushing teeth, vacuuming the house, coming to a full stop at stop signs, putting stamps on envelopes, returning e-mail or telephone messages, etc.). Estimated ratings are made of the certainty that these activities are performed correctly and completely on a daily basis. One of these activities is selected, and the client is asked to keep detailed records on level of certainty that the activity was performed completely over the coming week. Again, the client is to make ratings of confidence and distress while performing the task, as well as 1–2 hours after completing the behavior.

There are a number of findings that can be drawn from this exercise. Individuals with OCD learn that they perform many "nonobsessional" tasks on a daily basis with some level of uncertainty that does not lead to negative consequences. In addition, the exercise highlights the near impossibility of maintaining a level of absolute certainty over an extended period of time. The task also demonstrates that striving for certainty increases distress even for nonobsessional activities. In addition, the therapist can discuss whether there was any benefit or reduced risk associated with being more certain about performing the nonobsessional task.

A more direct therapeutic intervention involves exposing clients to varying levels of uncertainty for obsessional concerns. *Uncertainty exposure* involves completing various obsessive–compulsive-related activities in a manner that generates moderate levels of doubt and uncertainty. The client is instructed to wait a few hours or days and then check to determine whether there were any negative consequences associated with the behavior. For example, a person with checking compulsions may be instructed to quickly (impulsively) buy a friend's birthday card. The client then writes a couple of lines of greetings in the card without rereading what is written. The card is placed in the envelop, sealed, stamped, and mailed without checking. A few days later the client is to call the friend and ask to see the card to determine the outcome. This is a useful intervention for providing evidence that tolerance of uncertainty, even with obsessional tasks, does not necessarily increase risk of negative consequences, threat, or danger. However, it is also important for the therapist to ensure that "delayed checking" does not become entrenched as a type of ritualistic checking or reassurance-seeking behavior.

Perfectionism

Because appraisals of perfectionism and intolerance of uncertainty overlap, behavioral exercises listed under each appraisal are mutually applicable to the other appraisal construct. The *cost/benefit analysis* that Whittal and McLean (1999) used to challenge "need for certainty" appraisals can be modified to deal with perfectionism. Various obsession-related tasks at work or home can be selected, and the client rates level of perfection achieved in performing these tasks, effort to perform, and associated distress. In the following week the client is asked to attempt to improve his or her performance of the task, thereby increasing the perfectionism rating. The therapist then discusses the costs and benefits associated with putting extra effort in doing the task even better.

For example, a person with compulsive checking indicates that he achieves 85 out of a 100 on a perfectionism scale when he writes letters because he rereads and rewrites them over and over. In the following week, the client is asked to try to boost his letter-writing perfectionism rating to 95. Effort and distress are noted, as well as time taken to write letters and the outcome. The therapist can use data collected from this exercise to determine whether striving for perfection is associated with significant increased cost (i.e., delayed task completion, more distress) and only slight, if negligible, benefits.

Often, individuals with perfectionistic tendencies assume that their perfectionism is admirable or an adaptive characteristic that will lead to greater success in life. They may erroneously focus on the perceived benefits of perfectionism and overlook the negative consequences associated with pathological perfectionism. To address this issue, the therapist can suggest that the client engage in a systematic *perfectionism observation exercise*, in which a friend or work colleague is selected who is admired for his or her high performance level. In the following week the client can be asked to record various tasks completed by this person and the outcome of the tasks, and to give the performances a perfection rating. Strengths and weaknesses of the performances should be noted. For example, a client may indicate that she is particularly impressed with how well the director in her office chairs departmental meetings. The client could be asked to observe the director's performance at the next meeting and rate the level of perfection. The aim of this exercise is to demonstrate that even people we admire can perform imperfectly and yet achieve very positive outcomes. Thus, perfectionism is not necessary to ensure good performance or a desired outcome.

Once less threatening perfectionism exercises are completed, the therapist can progress to a more direct challenge to perfectionism using a modification of the uncertainty exposure task. Certain obsession-related tasks are selected, and the client is instructed to perform the tasks in a way that includes a minor flaw or inaccuracy. The consequences of these *intentional errors* are recorded for discussion at the following session. A client with obsessional doubts about whether he might have said something embarrassing while conversing with a friend could be encouraged to say something that has potential for slight embarrassment. For example, the client could say to the friend, "I'm sorry, my mind wandered and I wasn't paying attention. Would you please repeat what you just said to me?" The client would later record the outcome of this "flawed conversation," including the friend's reaction to the request and any long-term perceived or actual consequences. The aim of this exercise is to test the belief that minor mistakes must be avoided because they will lead to serious negative consequences.

Intolerance of Anxiety or Distress

The behavioral exercises listed under faulty appraisals in regard to intolerance of anxiety or distress, focus on providing evidence that anxiety is common and that individuals can tolerate and function quite well under anxious conditions. Once again, a *survey method* can be used in which clients interview trusted friends about their experiences with feeling anxious, nervous, or fearful. Most individuals will report anxious symptoms at varying levels of intensity in situations such as giving a speech, going for a job interview, taking an exam, going to the dentist, and the like. This information should help clients realize that feelings of anxiety are common even among nonanxious individuals and that these individuals experience some of the same anxious symptoms that the client feels in obsessive–compulsive-related situations.

A complementary *anxiety monitoring exercise* can also be used, in which clients are asked to observe people at work or in public settings for signs of anxiety. Notes should be made on the situation and the specific behaviors that indicated a person was anxious. In addition, an anxiety rating should be made and the outcome of the person's anxious performance noted. These exercises are intended to show that anxiety is common, that people function even when they are anxious, and that negative consequences resulting from anxious performances are rarely significant.

The final two behavioral exercises focus on the client's own experience of anxiety. An *anxiety comparison task* can be used to provide evidence that the client can tolerate anxiety in nonobsessional situations. Data can be collected on the experience of anxiety in a non- obsessive–compulsive anxious situation (e.g., preparing for an exam, taking a trip to a new city, making a speech, going to the dentist, etc.) and in an obsessive–compulsive-relevant context. Similarities and differences in the anxiety in both contexts should be discussed. ERP exercises can also be modified to directly challenge the belief that one cannot stand anxiety. An *anxiety prediction* element can be added to ERP, in which a comparison is made between predicted level of anxiety before exposure and actual anxiety level after exposure (Rachman, 2003). Often, individuals with anxiety disorders like OCD anticipate a higher anxiety level than is actually experienced in the fear situation.

SUMMARY AND CONCLUSION

This chapter presented a detailed discussion of the behavioral interventions used in CBT for obsessions and compulsions. Many of these intervention strategies are modifications of standard ERP. They are specifically designed to directly challenge the faculty appraisals and beliefs of patients with OCD. And yet, for treatment to be effective, individuals with OCD must have repeated opportunities to face their obsessional fears without engaging in compulsions or other neutralizing responses. Symptomatic improvement is possible only through cognitive change, that is, when individuals learn that the dreaded consequence associated with the obsession will not occur and that their efforts to control their obsessional thinking are futile. The most effective way to achieve this change in the cognitive basis of obsessional states is through the exposure-based strategies discussed in this chapter.

CHAPTER 12

Modifying Secondary Appraisals of Control

As discussed in Chapter 7, a person with OCD is usually preoccupied with the control of unwanted thoughts, feelings, and behavior in an effort to avert the possibility of certain feared negative outcomes if control should fail. OCD is characterized by excessive effort to control obsessions, compulsive urges, and, often, even the performance of routine activities like deciding when to stop washing or determining whether a light switch is really off (Salkovskis & Forrester, 2002).

CBT for OCD has always included intervention strategies that target compulsive rituals and neutralizing behaviors (Freeston & Ladouceur, 1997a, 1999; Rachman, 1998; Salkovskis, 1999). More recently clinical researchers have recognized that treatment must also focus on faulty appraisals and beliefs of control (Clark & Purdon, 1993; Freeston et al., 1996; OCCWG, 1997; Purdon & Clark, 2002; Rachman, 1998; Salkovskis et al., 1995; Whittal & McLean, 2002). Although some cognitive–behavioral theorists argue that beliefs and appraisals of control are secondary to more basic cognitive constructs like thought–action fusion, responsibility, or overestimated threat (Freeston et al., 1996; Salkovskis et al., 1995), Chapter 7 emphasized the importance of mental control appraisals and beliefs in the pathogenesis of obsessions.

The cognitive control model proposes that individuals with OCD are highly motivated to establish extreme, rigid control over the obsession, not only because of primary appraisals of importance, but also because of secondary appraisals involving misinterpretations of the nature of mental control and the imagined consequences of failure to establish control (see Figure 7.1). An important goal of treatment, then, is to guide the client toward termination of all activities that are aimed at reducing the frequency of the obsession and its associated distress (e.g., compulsive rituals, neutralization strategies, thought suppression, avoidance, reassurance seeking). According to the cognitive control model, it is not sufficient to target only the primary appraisals of the obsession; the secondary appraisals of control and coping ability must also be addressed to effectively treat obsessional ruminations.

This chapter details intervention strategies directed at modifying the secondary appraisals of control. This treatment approach is based on the cognitive control model discussed in Chapter 7 and on interventions recommended by other cognitive–behavioral therapists for treatment of "need to control" beliefs and appraisals. Because this treatment approach is so recent, these recommendations are based on clinical experience rather than empirical investigation.

In any intervention, long-term maintenance of gains is an important aspect of a treatment's effectiveness. Two issues relevant to maintenance of treatment gains are discussed in this chapter: modification of core beliefs and relapse prevention. Two types of core beliefs particularly important to obsessional states are negative self-referent beliefs and metacognitive beliefs. Core belief issues, as well as specific relapse prevention strategies, should be introduced in later sessions in order to ensure maintenance of treatment gains.

INITIAL PHASE OF INTERVENTION

Although Figure 7.1 suggests a particular sequence with primary appraisals leading to secondary appraisals of control, a cognitive-behavioral treatment plan would not necessarily follow this strict order. Intervention will move freely between the primary and secondary levels, and many of the same therapy exercises will have an impact on both cognitive levels. Thus, modification of secondary appraisals should be viewed as an integral part of standard CBT and not a distinct or later stage of treatment. As Salkovskis and Wahl (2003) noted, the primary appraisals of threat and the secondary appraisals of coping ability involve a complex process in which they occur virtually simultaneously. As a result, many of the specific cognitive and behavioral interventions described in the last chapter are relevant for the modification of control beliefs and appraisals. In addition, the following specific treatment strategies are also essential for modification of secondary appraisals of control.

Education on Secondary Appraisals

Chapter 9 emphasized the importance of educating the client on the cognitive appraisal model of obsessions in order to provide a rationale for treatment and to normalize the experience of unwanted, ego-dystonic intrusive thoughts or obsessions. An important part of this educational component is demonstrating the counterproductive effects of neutralization and other attempts to control the obsession. It was suggested that the therapist introduce the "camel exercise" described by Freeston and Ladouceur (1999) to demonstrate the role of neutralization and intentional mental control in the persistence of obsessions (see Chapter 9). As Freeston and Ladouceur (1999) note, most clients are readily able to see that keeping a thought is difficult, but keeping it totally away is next to impossible. The client should also immediately recognize the relevance of the camel exercise for understanding the persistence of obsessions. If this does not happen, the exercise may be repeated with a more personally relevant negative thought, such as a worry (e.g., "whether I will get an expected job promotion"). After the client tries to think and then not to think about the worry, the therapist can focus discussion on the difficulty of maintaining strict mental control.

Educating the client on the deleterious, counterproductive effects of neutralization, compulsive rituals, and other mental control or safety-seeking strategies is an important treatment element also emphasized by Salkovskis (1999) and Rachman (1998, 2003). Two points must be drawn from the "camel demonstration" (Freeston & Ladouceur, 1999). To accept the treatment rationale, the client must understand that the occurrence of obsessions and the ineffectiveness of neutralization (i.e., the camel effect) are beyond voluntary control. Consequently, therapy does not focus on preventing the obsession or improving mental control because these processes are involuntary. However, there are three other processes that are partially under a person's control: (1) the importance the person gives to an unwanted thought, (2) the strategies employed to control the thought, and (3) the importance placed on exercising mental control over the obsession. The following example suggests how the role of neutralization and secondary appraisals of control can be explained to clients.

"As you have seen from the camel exercise, it is very difficult to maintain strong mental control over unwanted thoughts. When you want to focus on a particular thought, it is hard to keep your attention on the thought, and when you don't want to think about a thought, it is even harder to shift your attention away from the thought. As soon as you tell yourself not to think about a thought, your mind seems to be drawn even more forcefully to that very thought, kind of like iron filings drawn to a magnet. Do you think this has any relevance to why you continue to have these obsessional thoughts even when you don't want them? [Therapist discusses parallels between camel exercise and the persistence of the client's obsessions.] There are two other, more specific, conclusions that can be drawn from this exercise. First, there are some things that are outside our personal control. We can't stop certain thoughts from popping into our minds, and we can't overcome the camel effect (i.e., have perfect control over our thoughts). As a result, it would be ineffective, even unfair, to focus therapy on preventing obsessions or improving ways to dismiss (remove) these unwanted thoughts, because this is beyond our human ability. However, there are mental processes over which we do have some control. We can control how much importance we place on a thought, we have control over how we react or respond to the thought, and we have control over how much importance we place on mental control itself. Thus, it makes sense to focus treatment on things over which we have partial control. Each of these processes, the importance placed on the obsession and its control and attempts to neutralize the obsession, makes an important contribution to the persistence of the obsession. [Therapist can illustrate by reference to Figures 5.1 and 7.1.] By modifying these processes, the frequency and intensity of the obsession is reduced."

The preceding treatment rationale can be integrated with the rationale presented in Chapter 9. Together, these explanations should lead the client to clearly understand the goal of CBT for obsessions and compulsions. After providing the treatment rationale, the therapist should question how this approach to treating obsessions and compulsions matches with the client's treatment expectations. It is likely that the client entered therapy expecting a focus on improving control strategies in order to reduce the frequency and distress of obsessive–compulsive symptoms. Instead, clients are presented with a contrary viewpoint, that the persistence of obsessive–compulsive symptoms is reduced by relinquishing efforts to control or neutralize the obsession and downgrading the importance of the unwanted intrusive thoughts. Therapists may have to devote additional therapy time dealing with differences between clients' prior expectations and the cognitive-behavioral treatment rationale. Whatever the case, it is important that clients clearly understand and accept the goals and rationale of CBT before proceeding further with treatment.

Identifying Secondary Appraisals

In the process of teaching clients how to identify appraisals and distinguish them from the obsession itself (see Chapter 9), it is also important to introduce the concept of secondary appraisals of control. This can be accomplished by referring to clients' evaluation of their ability to control the obsession and its associated distress. "We have identified a number of reasons why you think the obsession is important. I would now like to shift our attention to your ability to cope with the obsession." "How important is it for you to control the obsession?" "How effective are your thought control efforts?" "What worries you most if you can't get control over the obsession?" The aim of this line of questioning is to focus on how clients evaluate their coping ability and the consequences of failed control over the obsession.

As noted in Chapter 10, the Record of Control Strategies (Appendix 8.5) can be used to highlight the types of neutralization, compulsions, and mental control strategies used to cope with persistent obsessions. However, it is important to focus on clients' interpretation of their mental control efforts in order to understand the persistence of these response strategies. The therapist can explore secondary appraisals by presenting the table in Appendix 12.1 and inquiring as to whether any of these ways of thinking about control apply to the client. It is important to recognize that there is a high degree of overlap across the various types of secondary appraisals. Thus, the therapist should avoid trying to make fine distinctions between appraisals and instead use Appendix 12.1 as a guide to how a client might misinterpret the importance and consequences of controlling the obsession.

On occasion, a behavioral demonstration may be necessary to identify the role of secondary appraisals of control in the pathogenesis of obsessions. Salkovskis (1999), Whittal and McLean (2002) and Rachman (1998, 2003) describe a homework assignment in which the client is asked to try to control the obsession in the usual way on alternate days and to let the obsession come and go on other days. In this context, clients are asked to record their reactions to the obsession on "control" and "noncontrol" days. "What was the outcome of control and noncontrol?" "What bothered you most about letting the obsession come and go?" "What was the worse thing about the recurrence of the obsession on control days?" "What concerned you most about not being able to control the obsession?" "Were these concerns different on 'control' and 'noncontrol' days?" The client might use Appendix 12.1 to assist in the identification of faulty control appraisals. In addition, the therapist might use the downward arrow technique to explore the client's appraisals and beliefs about "What is the worst that could happen if you could not get the obsession out of your mind?"

INTERVENTION STRATEGIES FOR SECONDARY APPRAISALS

There are three main objectives of cognitive and behavioral interventions at the secondary appraisal level. First and foremost, it is critical that treatment focus on the elimination of all neutralization and other control strategies. Exposure and response prevention will be most helpful in this regard. Second, faulty appraisals and beliefs of control that are responsible for the persistence of neutralization must be challenged. If this is not done, the client may be less motivated to comply with response prevention instructions. And third, decreases in the frequency and intensity of the obsession due to the elimination of mental control responses will reinforce a more positive view on the control of unwanted thoughts, images, and impulses.

Cognitive Treatment Strategy

Cognitive interventions at the secondary appraisal level focus on challenging the client's assumption that reduction in the frequency and distress of the obsession can be achieved only by exercising greater control over the obsession. One way to highlight the importance of control appraisals is to have the client write out a *control appraisal script* associated with his or her primary obsession. For example, a client with an obsessive fear of getting sick could be asked the following: "We have been discussing why the thought 'maybe I am getting sick' is important and why you believe it is so crucial that you stop dwelling on this thought. In four or five sentences, can you write out why it is so important that you achieve better control over this thought?" A sample control appraisal script might be as follows:

"Whenever I think that I might be getting sick, I get really anxious. If I don't do something about this thought, the anxiety will get so bad that I might really work myself up to the point of vomiting. If I can do something about the thought, like convince myself that I am not sick, then I'll stop thinking this way and then I will be able to get on with my work. Also, the sooner I stop thinking about getting sick, the less likely I am to get sick. Most people don't constantly question their physical health. I should be able to stop thinking like this."

Once the control appraisal script is written, the therapist can explore with the client whether there is evidence of faulty secondary appraisals of control. In this example, evidence can be seen of exaggerated appraisals of threat, misperceived consequences of failed control, the possibility and desire for greater control, and faulty inferences of control (e.g., "If I keep thinking about getting sick, I will get sick"). Appendix 12.1 can be used to help the client identify dysfunctional control appraisals. The client can also be asked how long he or she tried not to think about getting sick. "Have you noticed whether you are getting more or less of these thoughts since you've tried so hard not to think about them?"

After generating their maladaptive control appraisal scripts, the therapist can ask clients to imagine how a person not bothered by the thought of getting sick would react when he or she has this thought. Depending on how long clients have been bothered by this obsession, it may be difficult for them to come up with a healthier control appraisal script. However, it is important that clients try to think through a healthier response rather than have the therapist write out a script for them. As a homework assignment, clients could be asked to interview a close friend or family member on that person's response to thoughts that he or she might be getting sick. The following is a clinical vignette that illustrates this intervention.

THERAPIST: We've seen how important it is for you to do something about the thought of getting sick. Now I would like to turn our attention to how other people might respond to thoughts of getting sick. What do you think other people do when they think they might be sick?

CLIENT: Well, I suppose they don't worry too much about it.

THERAPIST: Let's say a person is at work and he has the thought "I don't think I'm feeling well." What do you imagine happens next? What does he do with that thought?

CLIENT: I guess he probably looks for evidence that he feels sick or feels well.

THERAPIST: OK. But let's assume that after looking for the evidence, he still remains uncertain; he can't seem to decide if he feels well or not.

CLIENT: I suppose at this point he decides not to worry about it and gets on with his work.

THERAPIST: How do you suppose he convinces himself that the thought of getting sick is not important, that it is safe to ignore the thought? Could you write out a four- or five-line script that individuals might use to convince themselves not to be concerned with the thought of getting sick?

By generating an alternative, more adaptive control appraisal script, clients are given a clear alternative to their faulty appraisals of control. Rather than focus on the importance of controlling the obsession, individuals are provided with an interpretation that emphasizes ignoring the obsession. This script, then, becomes the treatment goal. As a way of reinforcing the alternative control script, the therapist might explore how the client appraises the control of other important nonobsessive thoughts. In sum, the objective of this cognitive intervention is to contrast the deleterious impact of appraisals of overcontrol with the more beneficial effects of relinquishing intentional control over unwanted thoughts.

Exposure and Response Prevention

ERP will be the most effective intervention for reducing neutralization and challenging faulty appraisals and beliefs about control. ERP was described in Chapter 3, and its role in modifying maladaptive cognition was discussed in Chapter 11. To specifically modify secondary appraisals of control, it is important that the therapist elicit the client's interpretation of an ERP task.

For example, a client with a checking compulsion is instructed to press the automatic key once in order to lock her car doors. She is to walk away from the car without checking whether the doors are really locked. In standard ERP the therapist obtains ratings on degree of distress or anxiety, urge to engage in compulsion, and length of exposure (see Steketee, 1993, 1999). However, in order to use ERP as an intervention for restructuring secondary appraisals of control, it is important that the therapist use Socratic questioning to inquire about interpretations of control. "When you first walked away from the car and didn't check, what were you afraid would happened?" "After an hour had passed, what were you thinking and feeling?" "What did you find when you returned to the car?" "It sounds as though you've learned that when you have worries that you didn't lock the car and you just let those worries come and go, eventually they disappear—and the anxiety with them. What does this experience tell you about trying to control or deal with thoughts of not locking the car door?" Using guided discovery, the therapist helps the client come to the realization, through ERP experiences, that just letting the obsession go, not reacting or trying to control it, will lead to less anxiety and fewer obsessive intrusive thoughts in the long term.

Behavioral Experimentation

More direct behavioral experimentation can also be effective in challenging secondary appraisals of control. Table 11.1 presents three experiments that are useful for modifying these appraisals and beliefs. Wegner's (1987) classic *thought suppression experiment* can be modified to test the effects of intentional mental control (see also Rachman, 2003). In the first instance the client is instructed to suppress a neutral thought for 2 minutes and to signal each occurrence of the unwanted thought. The therapist records the number of thought intrusions and explores with the client his or her perceived self-efficacy and outcome of the mental control efforts. The experiment is repeated a second time with a nonobsessional worry (e.g., failing an exam) as the to-be-suppressed thought. Again discussion centers on perceived success and efficiency of control. A third trial of thought suppression is finally attempted with the primary obsession. It is expected that the client will have greater difficulty suppressing the primary obsession than the nonobsessional thoughts. This experiment is useful for highlighting the deleterious effects of exaggerated appraisals of significance for controlling unwanted intrusive thoughts.

Another variation on the thought suppression experiment described by Rachman (2003) could be labeled the *thought traffic controller*. The client is asked to examine every thought that occurs in a 5-minute interval and to respond to each of these thoughts. In this instance the "thought traffic controller" is on duty. The client is then questioned on the costs and benefits of "being on duty." "Did you feel safer, and how effective were you in directing all your thoughts?" Next the therapist instructs the client to take a 5-minute break, to let his or her thoughts come and go because the thought traffic controller is off duty. After this interval the therapist inquires about the client's success and other related effects due to "taking a break from one's thoughts." This exercise gives the client experience with the deleterious effects of overvigilance and control of unwanted thoughts, as well as the possible benefits of "letting go of one's thoughts."

A number of other experiments can be devised to highlight the consequences of effortful control versus "noncontrol" of obsessions (Rachman, 2003; Salkovskis, 1999; Whittal & Mclean, 2002). In an *in vivo alternative thought suppression* task, clients are instructed to engage in exceptionally strong efforts to control their unwanted thoughts or obsessions on alternate days and then to react to the obsession in their usual way on other days. Records are kept on the frequency of the obsession, as well as ratings on level of distress, amount of control effort, and urge to neutralize. After several days, the therapist can collect this data and plot it on a graph (for illustration, see Salkovskis, 1999). The graph can provide a powerful visual demonstration that frequency of obsession was not substantially lower on days when extra effort was expended in mental control. This experiment provides a useful cost/benefit analysis of devoting so much effort to controlling unwanted intrusive thoughts. Again, the therapist uses Socratic questioning and guided discovery of clients' experiences in this exercise to challenge faulty appraisals and beliefs about control of obsessions.

A variation on this experiment is the *in vivo alternative thought control exercise*, whereby days in which the client engages in his or her usual neutralization response are compared with days on which the client simply records each occurrence of the obsession without any attempt to neutralize the thought. Again, by graphing the data collected over a number of days, the therapist can illustrate the benefits of "letting go of the obsession" (i.e., refraining from any intentional mental control) versus use of neutralization and other control strategies to suppress the obsession. A related behavioral experiment is proposed by Rachman (2003) to test the perceived benefits of thought suppression. In a *prediction of control* exercise, clients predict whether they will feel safer if they suppress an obsession for an entire day. They then attempt to suppress the obsession for the day and report back on their findings. Next, they predict the effects of "not suppressing" for a day, implement the exercise, and report their findings. The therapist then focuses on whether clients' beliefs that they are safer when they suppress the obsession are supported by the evidence or not.

In order to incorporate the benefits of relinquishing thought control into the client's daily life, the therapist can encourage *"thought holidays"* (Rachman, 2003). Just as people take vacation time from work, so individuals with OCD can be encouraged to take a holiday from trying to control their obsessions. Data can be collected to determine whether any anticipated negative consequences occurred as a result of not engaging in efforts to control an obsession. Once again, any evidence that efforts to control or neutralize the obsession are futile or unnecessary can be used to challenge the faulty secondary appraisals and beliefs about control. As can be seen, these behavioral experiments play an important role in the effectiveness of CBT for OCD.

SELF-REFERENT AND METACOGNITIVE BELIEFS

Certain recurring cognitive themes will eventually emerge from cognitive-behavioral treatment of specific faulty obsessive–compulsive appraisals and beliefs. These themes represent broader, more generalized ideas and assumptions about the self and the significance of unwanted intrusive thoughts or obsessions. Some of these generalized themes are *self-referent,* reflecting core beliefs about the self, the world, and the future. Beck et al. (1979) defined faulty assumptions as "basic beliefs that predispose the person to depression" (p. 244). J. S. Beck (1995) characterized negative core schemas as global, overgeneralized, unarticulated, and absolute fundamental beliefs about the self, others, and the world that are rooted in childhood and remain latent until activated by psychologically distressing situations (see also the discussion in Clark & Beck, 1999).

Other recurring cognitive themes reflect *metacognitive beliefs* about the importance and significance of thoughts, especially unwanted intrusive thoughts or obsessions, and their control. Chapter 7 discussed the nature and role of metacognitive beliefs as possible vulnerability factors for persistent intrusive thoughts and obsessions. Table 12.1 lists a number of self-referent core schemas and metacognitive beliefs that underlie the specific faulty appraisals and beliefs that characterize OCD.

The core schemas and metacognitive beliefs listed in Table 12.1 illustrate the types of cognitive themes that may emerge during CBT for obsessions and compulsions. Naturally, the specific content of core schemas and metacognitive beliefs will be idiosyncratic to the values and concerns of clients. However, it is suggested that most of these schemas reflect basic ideas or assumptions about the self, the world, and others, as well as the significance of unwanted thoughts and their control, that are stable over time and pervasive across various situations. Thus, maladaptive core schemas and metacognitive beliefs emerge from interventions such as the downward arrow technique, in which the same theme or idea occurs over and over again

TABLE 12.1. Sample of Core Self-Referent and Metacognitive Beliefs Associated with OCD

- "I must be a terrible person because I have awful thoughts that I cannot control."
- "I must be a mentally or emotionally weak person who could lose complete control at any moment."
- "Unwanted intrusive thoughts [obsessions] reflect one's true inner character."
- "It is important to exercise strict control over unwanted intrusive thoughts."
- "I lack adequate mental control."
- "I am prone to carelessness and mistakes."
- "I can easily become overwhelmed with anxiety or distress."
- "I am responsible to minimize any perceived risk of harm to self or others."
- "My personal world is full of risk and danger."
- "I have to be certain that my actions and decisions are correct."

in a variety of situations or with different unwanted distressing cognitions (e.g., "I have to work hard in exercising mental control over intrusive thoughts because my mind is fragile; I am on the verge of going insane.")

Most of the core beliefs listed in Table 12.1 fall within one of the six belief domains proposed by the OCCWG (see Chapter 5). Basic ideas that reflect an overimportance of thought and thought–action fusion, overestimated threat, inflated responsibility, need for thought control, intolerance of uncertainty, and perfectionism will be evident in fundamental views about the self and the mind. After years of struggling with disturbing obsessions and compulsions, individuals with OCD become convinced that they must be inherently terrible or weak because they have such poor control over their thoughts and behavior. They live in a personal world dominated by fear, risk, and the possibility of some imagined danger or catastrophe. Because of such threat, they feel personally responsible to minimize risk to self or others in a variety of situations. They view anxiety as a nemesis in which they are engaged in a titanic struggle for survival. The persistence of disturbing, even tormenting, obsessions is viewed as the reason for their "emotional breakdown," and so they believe that better mental control is the way to recovery. Temporary relief from the obsession is better than nothing at all. The longer the obsession persists, the more likely the imagined catastrophic ending.

The existence of core schemas and metacognitive beliefs becomes evident in therapeutic work on specific faulty appraisals and beliefs. There is not a distinct point in therapy when the focus shifts to this more fundamental level. Instead, throughout the course of treatment the cognitive-behavioral therapist should be vigilant for more basic, generalized cognitive themes that repeatedly emerge in clients' interpretations and reactions to their obsessional concerns. The following is a hypothetical exchange between therapist and client that illustrates the identification of core schemas and metacognitive beliefs.

THERAPIST: We have looked at a number of different situations in which you feel anxious because you have unwanted thoughts about harming other people. Each time, you believe these unwanted thoughts are important because they might cause you to actually harm someone [i.e., Likelihood TAF, overestimated threat, overimportance of thoughts, inflated responsibility].

CLIENT: Yes, that's what I worry about. I'm afraid that eventually I will "snap" and actually attack someone. These thoughts are so powerful and persistent.

THERAPIST: OK, but there seems to be a common theme that runs through these different situations. Do you think that your worry about harming other people suggests anything about what you think of yourself?

CLIENT: Not sure what you're getting at.

THERAPIST: Well, in a variety of situations, and even with different types of thoughts, it always seems to come back to feeling anxious that you might harm other people. What kind of person goes around harming people?

CLIENT: Criminals, immoral, evil, and uncaring people.

THERAPIST: So is that how you see yourself? An immoral or evil person?

CLIENT: No, I don't think I'm that bad. But I worry that I could become like that.

THERAPIST: OK, you're not convinced you are a terrible or evil person, but you worry that you have the potential for evil. But every day for months and months you have been preoccupied with this worry that "maybe I have the potential for harm." What do you think of someone who has the potential for harm? What would you think of a person you knew who would eventually murder his wife but has not done it yet?

CLIENT: I would think that man is evil, a terrible person.

THERAPIST: So the potential for harm suggests to you a terrible person. Do you suppose that by reminding yourself day after day, "maybe I could harm someone," that you are subtly convincing yourself that you are a terrible person, that you are the type of person who really could do this awful thing?

CLIENT: Yeh, deep down I've always felt like I was terrible, a bad person. I've had to work so hard all my life to be good, but I always end up feeling like I'm still bad.

Once core schemas and metacognitive beliefs have been identified, the therapist can use the evidence gathered from the previously described cognitive and behavioral exercises to challenge these fundamental assumptions. Thus, sustained therapeutic work on specific appraisals and beliefs can be used to modify core schemas and metacognitive beliefs as long as the therapist also focuses the intervention at this deeper level. For example, in reviewing the outcome of a thought suppression exercise, the therapist might summarize as follows: "So you discovered that even though you had more harm and aggression thoughts, you did not feel a greater inclination to harm people. What does this experience tell you about your belief that you are a terrible person who has the potential to harm other people?" In sum, modification of core schemas and metacognitive beliefs is achieved through cognitive and behavioral interventions that repeatedly challenge the more specific faulty appraisals and beliefs that are rooted in these fundamental assumptions. Intervention at the core schema level is considered critical to treatment maintenance and relapse prevention (e.g., Beck et al., 1979; J. S. Beck, 1995).

RELAPSE PREVENTION

As in psychological interventions for other disorders, it is important that relapse prevention be integrated into CBT for obsessions and compulsions early in treatment. As noted in Chapter 1, OCD is a chronic disorder that tends to take a fluctuating course. Symptoms can be reactivated by life stress, deterioration in mood state, or exposure to a life experience that rekindles obsessional concerns. Thus, specific steps must be taken to ensure long-term maintenance of treatment gains and symptom remission.

This was clearly demonstrated in a study by Hiss et al. (1994). Twenty patients with OCD who showed at least 50% improvement with ERP treatment were randomly assigned to a 1-week relapse prevention program or a control condition called associative therapy. Relapse prevention involved four 90-minute sessions of training in self-exposure, cognitive restructuring, expectation of setbacks, and planned lifestyle changes. Over a 6-month follow-up period, individuals who completed the relapse prevention program experienced significantly fewer relapses than those assigned to the control condition. Other authors have also discussed the importance of building relapse prevention into the treatment plan (Freeston & Ladouceur, 1997a, 1999; Steketee, 1993, 1999).

Emmelkamp, Kloek, and Blaauw (1992) found that poor cognitive strategies (distress reduction, avoidance of problems, and denial), life events, daily hassles, and expressed emotion were all significantly associated with relapse in 21 individuals with OCD treated with standard ERP. The authors recommended that individual booster sessions be provided to clients at high risk of relapse, and cognitive therapy and problem-solving strategies be included for their possible prophylactic benefits.

From the early stages of educating the client on the nature of OCD and the CBT model of obsession and compulsions, any erroneous expectations that treatment will "cure" obsessive–compulsive symptoms should be challenged. The client must be prepared for the eventuality that obsessive and compulsive symptoms will re-emerge after treatment. In addition, treatment should be presented as a focused, time-limited intervention that emphasizes the acquisition of skills for coping more effectively with obsessive and compulsive complaints. The goal of treatment must be continually clarified to help the client develop a healthier attitude and coping responses to obsessions and compulsions in order to reduce their frequency and severity. Unrealistic expectations that treatment can lead to a permanent eradication of all obsessive–compulsive symptoms must be corrected from the outset. Table 12.2 presents some therapeutic elements that should be included in treatment to foster relapse prevention (see also specific relapse prevention tactics recommended by Steketee, 1999).

It is important that clients adopt a "chronic illness model" of OCD. That is, they should realize that they will continue to have obsessional tendencies, residual symptoms, and possible episodes of "full-blown" obsessions and compulsions. Treatment should be seen as a new approach for dealing with their obsessive–compulsive proclivities. Treatment goals and expectations should be clearly identified so that clients are fully prepared for setbacks or the return of symptoms after treatment termination. Cli-

TABLE 12.2. Therapeutic Elements Used to Promote Relapse Prevention in CBT

- Educate client on the nature and course of OCD.
- Ensure realistic treatment expectations, including presence of residual symptoms.
- Identity situations that trigger obsessions and compulsions.
- Ensure a clear understanding of the CBT model.
- Provide written instructions on response to a relapse of obsessions.
- Instruct client to be vigilant about re-emerging avoidance, reassurance seeking, or other compulsive and neutralizing responses.
- Instruct client to take a problem-solving approach to episodes of unwanted intrusive thoughts or obsessions.
- Teach coping skills for stress and other life difficulties.
- Fade therapy sessions, providing continued access and support.

ents should also have a clear understanding of the triggers to their obsessions and compulsions. In this way, they can be prepared for a resurgence of symptoms when they are in high-risk situations. The therapist should also ensure that clients have a good understanding of the cognitive-behavioral model of obsessions. Of course, educating clients in the model is necessary for treatment success, but it is also critical for relapse prevention. If clients adopt the CBT framework for the persistence of obsessions and compulsions, they will be more likely to utilize the cognitive and behavioral strategies taught in therapy to deal with recurring obsessions and compulsions.

Freeston and Ladouceur (1999) recommend that clients be given written instructions on what to do in the case of relapse. Strategies include the following: (1) Use the cognitive-behavioral model to understand the re-emergence of obsessional thinking, (2) identify the faulty appraisals of the obsession ("how you are attaching importance to the thought"), (3) refrain from neutralizing, avoiding, engaging in reassurance seeking, and the like, (4) reinstate exposure exercises, (5) use cognitive strategies to challenge the importance of the thought, (6) problem solve ways in which stressful situations can be handled better, and (7) view relapse not as a setback or failure of treatment, but rather as an opportunity to practice newly learned coping skills. Before termination there should be evidence that the client is able to engage in these strategies without the support or prompting of the therapist.

Steketee (1993, 1999) discusses the importance of teaching clients how to manage stress and other life difficulties in order to promote relapse prevention. Financial problems, employment difficulties, martial discord, parenting issues, major physical illnesses, and the like are only a few of the additional problems that may face a person with OCD. Some of these problems may be a consequence of the OCD. Whatever the case, life stressors and daily hassles can trigger obsessive–compulsive symptoms, so efforts to teach clients better life management skills should have a positive effect on relapse prevention.

In the latter phase of treatment, therapy sessions should be increasingly spaced in order to fade out therapist contact. Three-month, 6-month, and 1-year booster sessions can be scheduled as a means of easing treatment termination and reinforcing relapse prevention strategies. The therapist can also provide occasional brief telephone consultations as part of phasing out treatment. Throughout the termination process, the client should be reassured of quick access to the therapist and continued support. Knowing that one can have a brief telephone consult or a single booster session when self-initiated relapse prevention strategies appear to fail will encourage the acceptance of treatment termination and efforts at self-therapy.

SUMMARY AND CONCLUSION

Cognitive and behavioral treatment strategies that challenge faulty secondary appraisals and beliefs about the need to control or neutralize obsessions are an important part of CBT for OCD. The treatment rationale and interventions described in this chapter are derived from the cognitive-behavioral formulation of obsessions presented in Chapter 7 (see Figure 7.1). Behavioral exercises based on exposure to obsessional concerns and the prevention of compulsions and other neutralizing responses are used to test faulty appraisals and beliefs of control. Behavioral experiences that challenge the client's belief that obsessional thinking must be controlled and that reinforce the alternative perspective of "letting go of the obsession" (i.e., refrain from control or suppression) play a critical role in the effectiveness of cognitive-behavioral treatment of obsessions. In summary, treatment protocols that include interventions for both the primary and secondary appraisals of the obsession and its control should have a stronger therapeutic impact on OCD than therapies that define the cognitive dysfunction in OCD more narrowly.

To improve treatment maintenance, underlying core self-referent beliefs and metacognitive schemas must be addressed. In addition, the later therapy sessions should focus on termination issues and introduce specific relapse prevention strategies. Clients are encouraged to be vigilant for any urge to slip back into the "control mentality" when re-experiencing a resurgence of obsessional thinking.

APPENDIX 12.1. Appraisals of Control Associated with the Persistence
of Unwanted Intrusive Thoughts and Obsessions

Type of secondary appraisal	Explanation of the appraisal	Examples of the appraisal
Inflated significance	To interpret any failure to control the obsession as a highly significant shortcoming.	1. "I must stop thinking about the obsession immediately." 2. "The obsession must be important because I can't seem to control it." 3. "My inability to control the obsession is a sign of weakness."
Exaggerated threat	To believe that failure to control the obsession increases the probability of certain dreaded outcomes.	1. "If I lose control over thoughts of violence, I might end up harming someone." 2. "If I don't stop the obsession, I will become more and more anxious." 3. "I could eventually lose even more control if I don't stop thinking this way."
Possibility appraisal	To believe that it is entirely possible to exercise effective control over unwanted thoughts.	1. "I should be able to completely shut my mind off to the obsession." 2. "If I don't control the obsession, it will control me." 3. "Most people are much better at controlling their thoughts than I am."
Unrealistic expectations	To expect oneself to achieve such a high level of control that there are no reoccurrences of the obsession.	1. "I have to get to the point where I don't think this way." 2. "If I try hard enough, I should never have the obsession."
Inflated responsibility	To hold oneself accountable for maintaining effective control over unwanted thoughts and their imagined consequences to self or others.	1. "I blame myself for allowing such disgusting thoughts to enter my mind." 2. "God will judge me for the types of thoughts that I dwell on." 3. "It is my fault for allowing these thoughts to take over my mind."
Faulty control inferences	To assume that failure in mental control has a causal influence on real-life experience.	1. "If I can't control my thoughts, then I might lose control of my behavior." 2. "If I can stop the obsessions, then I will feel more comfortable." 3. "Because I continue to think that I might have made a mistake, it is more likely that I did make a mistake."

CHAPTER 13

Empirical Status
and Future Directions

The phenomena of obsessions and compulsions have perplexed clinical researchers and diagnosticians and confounded the intervention efforts of mental health practitioners of all theoretical persuasions and professional training. Even though some of the greatest minds in psychiatry have grappled with the problem of obsessions and compulsions, advances in research and treatment of OCD have lagged behind the progress made in other psychiatric conditions. In fact, psychological contributions to the disorder were meager and uninspiring until the late 1960s with introduction of the behavioral theory and treatment of OCD.

Behavioral research and intervention resulted in a substantial advance in our understanding of the disorder and offered the first empirically verified psychological treatment of OCD. However, further progress, from a behavioral perspective, stagnated in the 1980s. Salkovskis's (1985) proposal of a cognitive-behavioral approach to obsessions and compulsions based on the behavioral research of Rachman and the cognitive theory of Beck revitalized psychological research on OCD. In the last decade, clinical researchers have shifted their attention to the cognitive basis of the disorder with new theoretical models and experimental paradigms that offer new insights into OCD.

Innovative cognitive interventions for obsessions and compulsions emerged simultaneously with the new cognitive-behavioral formulations. Clinical researchers advocated that cognitive assessment and treatment strategies should be combined with standard behavioral practices like ERP in order to modify the maladaptive cognitive basis of OCD. The new cognitive-behavioral approach to OCD is a theory-driven treatment that combines a practical clinical perspective with an empirical orientation.

This final chapter examines the empirical status of CBT for obsessions and compulsions. Although considerable theoretical, empirical, and clinical evidence has been presented in this volume in support of CBT (see also Rachman, 2003; Salkovskis, 1999; Steketee, 1999), a number of fundamental issues remain unresolved concerning the efficacy of this new treatment approach. How significant are the new cognitive strategies to the effectiveness of CBT for obsessions and compulsions? Is CBT more appropriate for some subtypes of OCD than others? What therapeutic processes account for the effectiveness of CBT? Does CBT increase treatment acceptance and compliance? Has the adoption of a more cognitive treatment strategy for OCD improved treatment maintenance and lowered relapse rates? These issues are addressed in the following review of the emerging psychotherapy research on CBT for OCD. The chapter concludes by considering the key issues that remain for the future direction of cognitive-behavioral theory and therapy for OCD.

EMPIRICAL STATUS OF COGNITIVE-BEHAVIORAL THERAPY FOR OCD

Is CBT an Effective Treatment for Obsessions and Compulsions?

Given that ERP is an effective intervention for OCD, one would expect that behavioral treatments that include a cognitive component should also be at least as effective as ERP alone. However, it is possible that the addition of a cognitive emphasis dilutes the quality and amount of ERP (Kozak, 1999). Moreover, different types of cognitive therapy have been applied to obsessional problems. Thus, it is incumbent upon cognitive-behavioral therapists to first demonstrate that CBT can significantly reduce obsessive and compulsive symptoms.

Self-Instructional Training and RET

Early reports on the effectiveness of cognitive therapy for OCD involved noncontrolled single-case and group studies. The interventions were based on self-instructional training, rational–emotive therapy (RET), or some variant of Beck's cognitive therapy for depression. In some studies cognitive therapy alone was administered, whereas other studies added cognitive interventions to behavior therapy, primarily exposure and response prevention. In many cases, the treatment approach was not compared with a control condition, so little can be drawn from these studies about the effectiveness of CBT for OCD.

Later research involved controlled treatment outcome designs in which a sample of patients with OCD were randomly assigned to CBT, another comparison treatment or a wait list control. These studies are better able to tease apart the specific effectiveness of cognitive interventions, especially when compared with another treatment approach. This section focuses on controlled studies that compared CBT against a wait list control condition. Studies that compared CBT against another treatment, mainly ERP alone, are discussed in the next section. However, I begin with a controlled comparison study because it is one of the only studies to investigate self-instructional training in OCD.

Emmelkamp, van der Helm, van Zanten, and Plochg (1980) published one of the first controlled studies to examine the effectiveness of adding a cognitive intervention to exposure and response prevention. *Self-instructional training*, in which patients with OCD were taught to verbalize more productive self-statements for handling anxiety, plus ERP was compared with ERP alone in 15 patients with OCD randomly assigned to either treatment condition. Both treatments produced statistical and clinically significant improvement at posttreatment, with gains maintained over a 6-month follow-up period. With a finding of no significant difference between treatment conditions, Emmelkamp et al. (1980) concluded that self-instructional training did not improve on the effectiveness of ERP alone. However, Robertson, Wendiggensen, and Kaplan (1983) reported that a type of cognitive restructuring based on Meichenbaum's (1977) writings plus ERP was effective in treating three patients with severe OCD. Nevertheless, van Oppen and Emmelkamp (2000) concluded in their review that self-instructional training may not be an appropriate treatment strategy for individuals who already engage in excessive self-talk and rumination.

A number of early single-case and group treatment studies investigated the effectiveness of RET in alleviating obsessive and compulsive symptoms. As discussed in the next section, Emmelkamp, Visser, and Hoekstra (1988) and Emmelkamp and Beens (1991) found that RET was equally effective as ERP in producing significant posttreatment reductions in obsessive–compulsive symptoms and that these gains were maintained over a 6-month follow-up period. Enright (1991), however, found that group treatment involving cognitive (RET) and behavioral strategies resulted in only slight symptom improvement in 24 individuals with OCD. Jones and Menzies (1998) randomly assigned patients with compulsive washing to a treatment condition that included both cognitive (RET) and behavioral (ERP) components versus a wait list control. At posttreatment, patients in the 8-session group CBT condition were significantly more improved than those of the wait list control on multiple measures, and these gains held over a 3-month follow-up. Van Balkom et al. (1994) concluded in their meta-analysis of treatment effectiveness in OCD that cognitive therapy and cognitive therapy plus behavior therapy tended to be more effective than pill placebo. All three of the studies that reported on a cognitive-therapy-alone condition were based on RET. Together these studies suggest that RET can be an effective treatment for OCD.

Uncontrolled Studies of CBT

More recently, research on the effectiveness of cognitive interventions for OCD has shifted to cognitive strategies based on Beck's cognitive therapy of depression (Beck et al., 1979), as well as the theoretical formulations and treatment recommendations of Salkovskis (1985). Salkovskis and Warwick (1985) reported one of the first single-case studies in which an evidence-gathering technique was used to modify an overvalued idea ("I will give myself cancer by using contaminated cosmetics") in a woman with severe OCD who relapsed after a trial of ERP. Since this study, others have also supported the effectiveness of CBT based on the newer cognitive appraisal theories of OCD. Simos and Dimitriou (1994) used audiotaped habituation and reassessment of responsibility to reduce a harming obsession. Freeston (2001) reported on the successful treatment of a 14-year-old boy who compulsively brushed his teeth, using a cognitive-behavioral treatment rationale, modification of beliefs about perfection, and gradual introduction of response prevention. Sookman and Pinard (1999) reported substantial reductions in obsessive–compulsive symptoms, depression, and maladaptive beliefs for 6 out of 7 treatment-resistant patients with OCD who received, on average, 10 months of weekly CBT.

Ladouceur, Freeston, Gagnon, Thibodeau, and Dumont (1995) utilized a multiple baseline design to determine the effectiveness of imaginal exposure, covert response prevention, and cognitive restructuring in treating three individuals with obsessional ruminations without overt compulsions. All three clients improved, with treatment gains maintained over an 11-month follow-up period. In a subsequent study Ladouceur, Léger, Rhéaume, and Dubé (1996) employed cognitive intervention alone (no ERP) to modify inflated responsibility appraisals and beliefs in four persons with compulsive checking. Three of the four patients showed significant improvement at posttreatment, which was maintained over the 12-month follow-up period. More recently Warren and Thomas (2001) reported that CBT based on cognitive appraisal theory resulted in significant improvement in 85% of patients with OCD ($n = 26$) treated in a private practice setting. Overall, these results are encouraging for the efficacy of CBT in treating obsessions and compulsions, although it must be acknowledged that negative findings have also been reported (e.g., Black et al., 1998).

Controlled Studies of CBT

There are four controlled treatment outcome studies that are particularly important in evaluating the efficacy of CBT based on the more recent formulations of Salkovskis and others. The first study was conducted by van

Oppen et al. (1995), in which 71 individuals meeting DSM-III-R diagnostic criteria for OCD were randomly assigned to 16 sessions of cognitive therapy or 16 sessions of ERP. Cognitive therapy was based on the treatment approach described in Beck and Emery (1985) and Salkovskis (1985). Analysis revealed that the patients treated with cognitive therapy improved significantly on all outcome measures (obsessive–compulsive symptoms, anxiety, depression, and general irrational beliefs), whereas the ERP-only group improved significantly on some measures. Indices of clinically significant improvement also indicated a slight superiority of cognitive therapy over ERP alone. Moreover, only the cognitive therapy group showed a significant change on the Irrational Beliefs Questionnaire (Koopmans, Sanderman, Timmerman, & Emmelkamp, 1994).

A second major outcome study of CBT was reported by Freeston et al. (1997) for individuals with obsessional ruminations without overt compulsions. Twenty-nine participants with obsessional ruminations were randomly assigned to CBT (an average of 29 individual sessions) or wait list control (average duration was 19 weeks). Once the waiting assignment was completed, all participants were offered the active treatment condition. CBT consisted of cognitive rationale, ERP, cognitive restructuring, and relapse prevention. Outcome measures included the interview form of the YBOCS, the Current Functioning Assessment, the Padua Inventory, the Beck Anxiety Inventory (BAI), and the Beck Depression Inventory (BDI).

Posttreatment assessment revealed that the CBT group had significantly lower scores on the YBOCS, the Current Functioning Assessment, and the BAI, whereas none of the pre–post differences were significant for the wait list. When all patients were included in the analysis (including those on the wait list who crossed over into treatment), significant posttreatment reductions were evident on all measures. Furthermore, analysis of clinically significant change revealed that 67% of the total sample improved, based on the YBOCS, and this percentage dropped to 53% at the 6-month follow-up. This study is particularly important because it is the first controlled outcome treatment study to demonstrate that CBT is effective for obsessional rumination without overt compulsion, a subtype of OCD that has proven quite resistant to more behavioral treatments.

O'Connor, Todorov, Rollibard, Borgeat, and Brault (1999) examined the efficacy of CBT in 29 patients with OCD randomly assigned to CBT only, medication only, CBT plus medication, or no-treatment wait list control. CBT consisted of graded exposure, response prevention, education in faulty inferences that characterize obsessional thinking, and attempts to experientially change unrealistic inferences about reality. Participants received approximately 20 sessions of individual CBT over 5 months. Posttreatment analysis, based on the YBOCS, the National Institute of Mental Health Obsessive–Compulsive Scale, and a self-rating of efficacy to resist the compulsive urge, revealed that CBT alone, medication alone, and CBT plus medication were equally effective in significantly reducing obsessive–compulsive symptoms. All three treatment groups were significantly different from the no-treatment wait list controls. Interestingly, even though medication and CBT produced equivalent results, only CBT produced significant improvement on the primary obsession-relevant beliefs.

A final controlled study was reported by McLean et al. (2001). Seventy-six participants who met DSM-IV diagnosis for OCD were randomly assigned to 12 weeks of group CBT, ERP, or a 3-month waiting list. The latter group was offered treatment at the end of the wait list period. The CBT was based on the treatment recommendations of Salkovskis (1996a), Freeston et al. (1996), and van Oppen and Arntz (1994) and included behavioral experimentation that was similar to ERP. Outcome measures, consisting of the Thought–Action Fusion Scale, Inventory of Beliefs Related to Obsessions, Responsibility Attitude Scale, BDI, and interview-based YBOCS, were administered at posttreatment and 3-month follow-up.

Based on the YBOCS Total Score, both CBT and ERP were significantly more effective than the wait list control condition. However, direct comparison of the two treatment groups on posttreatment YBOCS, adjusting for medication usage, revealed that the ERP condition was significantly more effective than CBT, and this advantage was maintained over the 3-month follow-up. Analysis of clinically significant improvement, again based on the YBOCS, indicated that 16% of the CBT group was recovered as compared with 38% of the ERP group. At 3-month follow-up this difference proved statistically significant, with 13% of the CBT group recovered and 45% of the ERP group. The superiority of ERP was maintained even when differential dropout and refusal rates were taken into consideration.

Neither the CBT nor the ERP treatments produced significant reductions on the OCD appraisal or beliefs measures, except on the Responsibility Attitude Scale, on which both treatments led to a reduction in scores over the wait list controls. The authors concluded that although both treatments led to a significant improvement as compared with the wait list condition, ERP was consistently superior to CBT in producing treatment effects. It may be that the relatively poor results reported in this study may be due to the use of a group treatment format. Hong and Whittal (2001) found that patients with moderate to severe obsessive–compulsive symptoms may show a better response to individual, as opposed to group, therapy. Patients in the mild-to-moderate symptom range appear to respond equally well to individual and group therapy. There was also a nonsignificant trend suggesting a tendency for mild-to-moderate patients to respond better to CBT, whereas more severe patients responded better to ERP.

Summary

There is solid empirical evidence that CBT can produce significant reductions in obsessive and compulsive symptoms and that these gains are maintained over a number of months after treatment termination (see also reviews by Bouvard, 2002; Emmelkamp, van Oppen, & van Balkom, 2002; van Oppen & Emmelkamp, 2000; Steketee, Frost, Rhéaume, & Wilhem, 1998). However, as compared to psychotherapy outcome literatures for other anxiety disorders or depression, clinical trials of CBT for OCD are not sufficient in number, nor have they attained the level of design sophistication that allows one to address important questions about the effectiveness and the mechanisms of change in CBT for obsession and compulsion. For example, the longer-term efficacy of CBT has not been investigated. In addition, other important questions remain about the specificity and incremental value of CBT over existing interventions.

Does the Addition of Cognitive Strategies Significantly Improve the Effectiveness of ERP?

In Chapter 3, it was concluded that there is a strong empirical literature on the effectiveness of ERP in the treatment of OCD. If a greater emphasis is placed on the modification of dysfunctional appraisals and beliefs, will this improve our effectiveness in the treatment of this disorder? There are two ways to address this question. First, are cognitive intervention strategies more effective than behavioral strategies in reducing obsessive–compulsive symptoms? Second, is the combination of ERP plus cognitive restructuring more effective than ERP alone?

Cognitive versus Behavioral Strategies

A close examination of CBT protocols reveals that most studies include exposure and response prevention along with cognitive interventions. Only a very few studies have maintained sufficiently pure treatment integrity to afford a direct comparison of cognitive and behavioral interventions. Van Oppen et al. (1995) did not introduce behavioral experimentation into their cognitive therapy treatment condition until after the sixth session. This allowed them to compare the effects of "pure" cognitive restructuring with ERP on symptom measures administered at session 6. Analysis revealed significant reductions in obsessive–compulsive symptom scores from their pretreatment level, with no significant difference between the two treatment conditions. However, after the sixth session, behavioral experiments similar to ERP were added to the cognitive therapy condition. This resulted in a slight superiority of the CBT condition at posttreatment.

Kearney and Silverman (1990) used an alternating single-case design to compare the effectiveness of response prevention and cognitive restructuring in reducing the checking behavior of a 14-year-old boy with severe OCD. Response prevention was found to be most effective in reducing one type of checking compulsion (window checking), whereas cognitive restructuring was most effective in reducing another checking compulsion (checking his body for bat droppings).

In the first RET study, Emmelkamp et al. (1988) found that RET, in which participants were not instructed in fear exposure, was equally effective as ERP alone. In the second study, Emmelkamp and Beens (1991) randomly assigned participants to receive 6 weeks of cognitive therapy without exposure, or of ERP alone. Assessment revealed that both treatments led to similar levels of significant symptom reduction. When the RET and ERP groups received an additional six sessions of ERP, there were still no significant treatment differences between the two groups. The authors concluded that ERP with the addition of RET was no more effective than ERP alone.

In a treatment outcome study, de Haan et al. (1997) randomly assigned 99 individuals with OCD to one of four interventions: (1) cognitive therapy, (2) ERP, (3) cognitive therapy plus fluvoxamine, or (4) ERP plus fluvoxamine. All four treatment conditions produced similar reductions in symptoms at posttreatment and 6-month follow-up. Combining medication with either ERP or cognitive therapy did not significantly enhance treatment outcome (see also Franklin et al., 2002, for similar results). However, O'Connor et al. (1999) found that pharmacotherapy and CBT produced equally significant clinical improvement, but that adding CBT to the medication condition did result in significantly greater improvement on primary obsessional beliefs.

Combination versus ERP Alone

A couple of studies have compared CBT that includes exposure-based behavioral exercises with ERP alone. In one of the first clinical trials of cognitive interventions for OCD, Emmelkamp et al. (1980) found that self-instructional training plus ERP was no more effective than ERP alone. McLean et al. (2001) concluded from their study that ERP showed a consistent pattern of mild to moderate superiority over CBT. The authors noted that the less encouraging results for CBT may be due to the group treatment format, whereas the stronger effects reported by van Oppen et al. (1995) may be related to their use of individual therapy.

At this time there is no empirical evidence that adding cognitive interventions to ERP (i.e., CBT plus ERP) is clinically more effective than ERP alone for a heterogeneous sample of patients with OCD. CBT (the combined condition) appears to be no more or less effective than ERP alone. There are a number of reasons why differential treatment effects between cognitive and behavior interventions may be difficult to demonstrate. Foa, Franklin, and Kozak (1998) suggested that the question of whether cognitive interventions improve the efficacy of ERP is of little practical importance, because identification and modification of dysfunctional beliefs is part of standard exposure treatment. In addition, Foa and Kozak (1986) reasoned that one of the longer-term effects of repeated exposure to fear stimuli is the disconfirmation of erroneous threat-relevant thoughts and beliefs. Thus, cognitive change may naturally occur during ERP sessions even without direct identification of dysfunctional thinking. Moreover, cognitive interventions that are stripped of exposure to fear situations are deprived of the most potent mechanism for cognitive change. Thus, artificially splitting cognitive and behavioral interventions may be quite difficult to achieve on a practical, therapeutic level. Another possibility is that the addition of cognitive interventions may enhance treatment for only certain OCD subtypes that are less responsive to ERP.

Is CBT More Effective for Certain Subtypes of OCD?

One could argue that a more cognitive approach is unlikely to improve treatment for patients with OCD subtypes with strong phobic and avoidance symptoms such as compulsive washing and, possibly, checking. However, CBT may be particularly helpful for patients with obsessional complaints who have not shown a good response to ERP, such as those with obsessional ruminations without overt compulsions or hoarding compulsions.

Obsessional Rumination

There is considerable interest in determining whether CBT might be especially helpful in treating patients with obsessional rumination without overt compulsions. Salkovskis and Warwick (1985) first reported that the addition of cognitive restructuring was more effective in treating overvalued ideation in a woman with somatic obsessions than a previous trial of ERP alone. Other single-case studies involving patients with obsessional rumination without overt compulsion have shown that a combination of ERP and cognitive restructuring is effective in significantly alleviating obsessional complaints (Ladouceur, Freeston, Gagnon, Thibodeau, & Dumont, 1993; Ladouceur, Freeston, et al., 1995; O'Kearney, 1993). More recently, the controlled treatment outcome study of obsessional ruminators by Freeston et al. (1997) showed that 18 sessions of CBT led to significantly greater reductions in obsessive–compulsive symptoms than a no-treatment wait list control condition. Although these results are most encouraging, it is important that comparative treatment studies be conducted to determine whether CBT is more effective in treating obsessional ruminations than an alternative treatment such as pharmaco-therapy or another form of psychotherapy. Given the discussion in Chapter 3, it would be most interesting to compare CBT with thought stopping, an intervention that might be expected to intensify obsessional states according to cognitive appraisal theory.

Compulsive Checking

A couple of studies have investigated whether CBT might be differentially effective for other subtypes of OCD. Van Oppen at al. (1995) reasoned that cognitive therapy might be more effective for compulsive check-ing, given the prominent role that inflated responsibility appraisals are thought to play in this disorder (Rachman, 1993). However, analysis revealed no significant difference in effectiveness between cognitive ther-apy and ERP for patients with compulsive checking. Moreover, both treat-ments were equally effective in reducing obsessional symptoms as mea-sured by the YBOCS Obsessions subscale.

Coelho and Whittal (2001) found that individuals with compulsive cleaning rituals were less responsive to ERP or CBT than those with checking compulsions or other types of obsessions. They conclude that treatment probably needs to be tailored to specific subtypes of OCD.

Hoarding

Randy Frost and Gail Steketee developed a cognitive-behavioral treatment specifically tailored to compulsive hoarding. The intervention is based on a cognitive-behavioral model of hoarding (Frost & Hartl, 1996) and in-volves (1) presentation of the model and (2) the use of cognitive restruc-turing and behavioral experiments to modify dysfunctional beliefs and behaviors involved in the organization, acquisition, and discarding of pos-sessions (see Frost & Steketee, 1998, 1999, for description). Preliminary evaluation of the treatment package suggests that it may lead to some im-provement in hoarding compulsions (Hartl & Frost, 1999; Steketee, Frost, Wincze, Greene, & Douglas, 2000), a symptomatic behavior that has been very resistant to other forms of intervention (e.g., Black et al., 1998). For example, Hartl and Frost (1999) reported on a single-case study in which 9 months of CBT, consisting of decision-making training, ERP, and cogni-tive restructuring, resulted in a significant decline in clutter in each of the rooms targeted for treatment. Declines were also evident on self-report measures of obsessive–compulsive symptoms.

In summary, preliminary evidence suggests that CBT may be more helpful in alleviating some obsessive–compulsive subtypes such as obses-sional rumination without overt compulsion and compulsive hoarding. However, the empirical evaluation of differential effectiveness is quite ten-tative at this time. Studies involving larger samples and comparison with alternative treatments are needed before practice guidelines can be issued on CBT for specific types of OCD.

Does a Cognitive Approach Improve Treatment Compliance and Lower Dropout Rates?

Salkovskis and Warwick (1988) first suggested that cognitive techniques could be introduced early in treatment to improve acceptance of and compliance with ERP exercises that often provoke high levels of anxiety when first introduced. They suggested that the 30% refusal and dropout rate reported for ERP (i.e., Stanley & Turner, 1995) might be lowered by using cognitive restructuring strategies that modify the dysfunctional beliefs maintaining high anxiety in obsessive–compulsive-relevant situations. Salkovskis and Warwick describe the use of cognitive restructuring to address the contamination belief of a client with OCD. Because of this belief the client refused to engage in within-session exposure (touching perceived contaminants) and wished to drop out of treatment. The authors used a downward arrow probability estimate to challenge her beliefs about responsibility for spreading contamination to others. With decreases in the strength of belief in her responsibility for harm, she agreed to engage in the exposure exercises.

Unfortunately, there has been little systematic empirical research on the utility of CBT for reducing dropout and refusal rates. In the single-case study by Salkovskis and Warwick (1985), cognitive techniques were effective in maintaining a client in treatment who had refused a second trial of ERP after having a relapse in obsessive–compulsive symptoms. Van Oppen et al. (1995) reported a 20% dropout rate from their cognitive therapy condition and a 19% dropout from ERP. Freeston et al. (1997) had a CBT dropout rate of 20% ($n = 3$), whereas McLean et al. (2001) found that significantly more participants refused CBT ($n = 12$) than ERP ($n = 2$). However, more participants dropped out of ERP ($n = 8$) than out of CBT ($n = 2$), although this difference did not attain statistical significance.

From the few studies that have reported refusal and dropout rates for CBT or ERP, it does not appear that CBT is associated with a higher treatment completion rate. However, the more specific question—whether client compliance with specific treatment strategies is improved by a cognitive orientation—has not been addressed. It may be that at the individual case level, prior work on dysfunctional appraisals and beliefs will enhance a client's acceptance of the more anxiety-provoking behavioral exercises.

Are Cognitive Strategies More Effective in Directly Modifying Obsessional Appraisals and Beliefs than Behavioral Interventions?

The cognitive appraisal theories (see Chapter 5) assume that misinterpretation of an unwanted mental intrusion will lead to exaggerated efforts to control the intrusion and its associated distress through compulsive rituals, neutralization strategies, or avoidance. It is the presence of such faulty appraisal processes and neutralization responses that cause an escalation of the unwanted intrusive thought into a highly persistent and distressing obsession (see Figure 5.1). The rationale, then, for introducing cognitive intervention techniques into the treatment of OCD is to directly modify the dysfunctional thoughts, appraisals, and beliefs responsible for the persistence of the obsession. However, what evidence is there that CBT leads to symptomatic improvement in OCD by modifying obsessive–compulsive-specific faulty appraisals and beliefs? Does CBT, with its emphasis on cognition, result in more change in obsession-relevant appraisals and beliefs than standard ERP, which does not focus on the modification of cognitive content? Both of these questions address whether cognitive change is the unique and fundamental therapeutic process in CBT for OCD.

Cognitive Change in CBT versus ERP

A number of studies have investigated whether CBT produces more change on measures of obsessive–compulsive appraisals and beliefs than ERP. Emmelkamp and Beens (1991) found that RET produced significantly more reduction of scores on the Irrational Beliefs Test (a measure of general dysfunctional beliefs) than ERP. However, in their earlier study, Emmelkamp et al. (1988) reported that Irrational Belief Test scores changed more after RET than after ERP, but the difference was not statistically significant. Likewise, van Oppen et al. (1995) found that general dysfunctional beliefs improved more with cognitive therapy than with ERP, but the difference was not statistically significant.

McLean et al. (2001) administered three self-report measures of specific obsessional beliefs: the Thought–Action Fusion Scale, the Inventory of Beliefs Related to Obsessions, and the Responsibility Scale. In comparisons with the wait-list control condition, both CBT and ERP resulted in significantly more reduction on the Responsibility Scale but not on the other two obsessive–compulsive cognitive questionnaires. O'Connor et al. (1999), however, found that CBT, but not medication, produced a significant reduction in the strength of the primary and secondary obsession beliefs. In this study primary beliefs were measured by a 0–100 efficacy scale on which participants rated how confident they felt to resist the urge to perform their compulsive ritual, and a secondary belief scale assessed how strongly participants felt that something other than anxiety would occur if the ritual was or was not performed. The conclusion that can be reached from the clinical outcome studies that included cognitive change in their outcome evaluation is that CBT may result in slightly more improvement on cognitive measures than standard ERP.

Cognitive Change with CBT

A couple of treatment process studies have investigated the mechanisms of change in CBT. Ladouceur et al. (1996) examined whether the correction of inflated responsibility beliefs alone would result in symptomatic improvement in four individuals with compulsive checking rituals. A purely cognitive intervention was administered, involving the identification and modification of inflated responsibility beliefs. Ladouceur and colleagues purposely excluded behavioral interventions such as ERP. At posttreatment, one participant showed a 10% symptom reduction, one had a 65% reduction, the third a 52% decline, and the fourth a 100% decrease in obsessive–compulsive symptoms. At follow-up, two out of four participants maintained their treatment gains. All four participants had substantial reductions in their scores on the Responsibility Scale, suggesting that treatment was effective in targeting inflated responsibility beliefs.

Rhéaume and Ladouceur (2000) treated six individuals with compulsive checking rituals with 24 sessions of either cognitive therapy (excluding exposure and response prevention) or ERP (excluding cognitive interventions). Participants provided daily belief ratings on personal responsibility, perfectionism, and threat estimation. Multivariate time series analysis was performed to determine patterns of change in symptoms (a daily rating on degree of interference caused by checking behaviors) and beliefs. Analysis revealed that a decline in at least one obsessive–compulsive-relevant belief *preceded reduction* in compulsive checking in two out of three cognitive therapy clients and all three ERP clients. However, decline in checking compulsions *preceded improvement* in at least one obsessive–compulsive belief in five out of six clients.

This study indicates that both cognitive therapy and ERP can produce change in cognition that then leads to symptomatic improvement. These findings also indicate that cognitive change can be both a cause and a consequence of symptom improvement. Williams, Salkovskis, Forrester, and Allsopp (2002) reported that approximately 10 sessions of CBT focused on modification of responsibility appraisals resulted in a significant symptom improvement in six adolescents with OCD. Over the course of treatment, responsibility appraisals showed a simultaneous rate of change with change in symptom levels.

Cognitive Change with ERP

Emmelkamp et al. (2002) reported on two unpublished studies conducted in their laboratory on cognitive changes associated with ERP. In the first study, individuals with OCD completed measures of obsessive cognition and beliefs before and after treatment. Analysis revealed significant improvement on both symptom and cognition measures, and the five most improved clients obtained significantly greater reduction in obsession-related thoughts and beliefs than the five least improved individuals.

In the second study, individuals treated with ERP showed significant reductions on all subscales of the Obsessional Beliefs Questionnaire (OBQ) and the Interpretation of Intrusions Inventory (III). There was also a significant correlation between change on cognition measures and change on symptom measures. Comparison of responders and nonresponders as defined by percent change on YBOCS scores indicated that responders had significantly greater change than nonresponders on III Total Score and Importance of Thoughts and Responsibility subscales. There was no statistically significant difference between responders and nonresponders on the OBQ subscales. Ito, de Araujo, Hemsley, and Marks (1995) found that ERP produced significant change in beliefs related to participants' target compulsive rituals even though a direct cognitive intervention was not included in the treatment package. However, improvement in belief ratings was unrelated to clinical outcome. The authors concluded that ERP led to change in compulsion-related beliefs by reducing anxiety and associated emotions.

Summary

At present too few studies have investigated the therapeutic ingredients of CBT to draw firm conclusions about the mechanisms of change in this new treatment approach. However, a number of tentative observations can be made. From the preliminary studies it is evident that CBT does lead to significant change in obsessive–compulsive-specific appraisals and, to a lesser extent, beliefs. That is, more enduring beliefs that may constitute an underlying vulnerability for OCD (see Chapter 7) may be less responsive to cognitive and behavioral interventions, although this speculation is based solely on an unpublished study reported by Emmelkamp et al. (2002). Nevertheless, there is evidence that standard ERP also leads to cognitive change, with CBT showing only slight superiority over its more behavioral counterpart in effecting cognitive change. There is obviously a close relationship between cognitive change and symptom improvement. Yet Emmelkamp et al. (2002) concluded,

> [W]e do not know whether the change in specific obsessive beliefs and impulses precede, follow, or co-vary with changes in obsessive compulsive behavior. Alternatively, irrational beliefs may merely be epi-phenomena of changes in mood states rather than changes in deeper cognitive structures. Further, since we have no data from a no-treatment control group, we cannot conclude that improvements on the cognitive measures are the result of improvement in the obsessive compulsive disorder. (p. 399)

Although much remains to be learned about the mechanisms of change in CBT, there is at least some preliminary evidence that CBT does have an impact on obsessive–compulsive-relevant appraisals and beliefs, as well as provide improvement in key symptom features of the disorder.

FUTURE DIRECTIONS

The introduction of cognitive constructs into psychological models of OCD is a relatively recent application of cognitive-clinical theory to a most challenging clinical condition. The progress that cognitive-behavioral theory of OCD has attained in these few short years is noteworthy. Moreover, OCD researchers have been quick to develop theory-driven self-report measures and ingenious experimental procedures to test critical predictions of the theory. The progress achieved in understanding the cognitive basis of obsessions is substantial, providing a strong empirical foundation for cognitive-behavioral treatment.

Cognitive-Behavioral Theories

Despite the advances in our understanding of the cognitive basis of obsessions and compulsions, further research is needed on three key issues for cognitive-behavioral formulations of OCD. First, it is not clear whether the faulty appraisals and beliefs implicated in OCD are specific to the disorder or whether cognitive phenomena of this type are relevant to other clinical conditions. Are the faulty appraisals of responsibility, control of thoughts, and intolerance of uncertainty a specific feature of obsessionality, or are these appraisals a result of general distress or negative cognition? The specificity issue is important for evaluating whether the cognitive-behavioral formulations proposed by Salkovskis, Rachman, and others are distinct conceptualizations of OCD or refurbished accounts of general emotional distress.

A second important issue is whether faulty cognition is a cause, consequence, or epi-phenomenon of obsessive–compulsive symptoms (Emmelkamp et al., 2002). Although the experimental research on responsibility and TAF bias reviewed in Chapter 5 is noteworthy, we are far from establishing the causal priority of faulty appraisals, neutralization, and the escalation of obsessive–compulsive symptoms. The cognitive-behavioral theories noted in Chapters 5 and 7 assume a causal link from faulty appraisals to neutralization, and then a further escalation in the frequency and intensity of obsessional thinking. Clearly, further experimental research is needed to explore the causal status of the cognitive variables in our cognitive-behavioral formulations of OCD.

A third key issue for cognitive-behavioral models of OCD that has not been researched is whether there is a cognitive vulnerability to obsessions and compulsions. Even though cognitive vulnerability constructs have been proposed (see Chapter 7), the necessary longitudinal, prospective research has not been done. No doubt research on vulnerability to OCD is hampered by the relatively lower base rate for diagnosable OCD and the challenges in amassing a sufficiently large sample of asymptomatic highly vulnerable individuals. Nevertheless, cognitive-behavioral researchers could begin by investigating cognitive vulnerability in samples of patients with OCD who have recovered, in whom the risk for recurrence is much greater than in the general population. Until this research is undertaken, the etiological status of the cognitive constructs discussed in this book remains unknown.

Cognitive-Behavioral Therapy

The latter chapters of this book presented a detailed step-by-step description of the cognitive-behavioral assessment and treatment of OCD. The basic elements of this therapeutic approach are summarized in Table 9.3. The intervention strategies described in this treatment manual are derived from the cognitive-behavioral theories presented in Chapters 5 and 7. Moreover, each of these cognitive-behavioral tactics is scripted for the unique clinical features of OCD. This integration of theoretical tenets and clinical exigencies has led to fresh new insights into the treatment of obsessions in particular. Despite the preliminary nature of psychotherapy outcome research on CBT for OCD, a few tentative conclusions can be drawn. These are summarized in Table 13.1.

It is clear that CBT is an effective treatment for OCD, although it is still unknown whether greater emphasis on cognition increases treatment potency beyond that achieved by an exclusive emphasis on exposure and response prevention. One thing is certain: ERP must continue to be the critical therapeutic ingredient in cognitive or behavioral interventions for OCD. One of the most promising avenues for CBT is the possibility that it might improve our effectiveness in treating obsessional rumination. Moreover, future research may demonstrate that a more cognitive perspective on the treatment of OCD has a prophylactic effect, similar to that seen in cognitive therapy for depression. Emmelkamp et al. (1992) recommended that cognitive therapy techniques be added as part of a relapse prevention strategy, and Hiss et al. (1994) demonstrated that their relapse prevention package that included a prominent cognitive restructuring component was effective in maintaining recovery. Together these initial findings indicate that CBT is a viable treatment approach for obsessions and compulsions. However, many questions remain about the efficacy and therapeutic mechanisms involved in a more cognitive approach to the treatment of OCD.

TABLE 13.1. Summary of Tentative Findings on the Efficacy of CBT
for Obsessional States

- Cognitive treatment strategies can produce significant improvement in obsessive and compulsive symptoms.
- Cognitive interventions tend to produce symptom improvement equaling that of more behavioral interventions based on exposure and response prevention.
- Combining cognitive strategies with standard ERP does not improve treatment efficacy over ERP alone.
- CBT may be especially effective in certain subtypes of OCD that are more resistant to behavioral treatment, such as obsessional rumination without overt compulsions, or hoarding.
- Empirical evidence is lacking on whether CBT improves treatment compliance, lowers refusal and dropout rates, or has a prophylactic effect against future relapse and recurrence of OCD.
- CBT does lead to significant improvement in the cognitive dysfunction that characterizes obsessional states, but this cognitive effect is not treatment-specific nor does it evidence a singular linear causal relationship to symptom severity.

Over the past three decades considerable progress has been made in our understanding of OCD and its treatment. Today innovations in both pharmacological and psychological interventions offer new hope for those who suffer from this disorder. It is the intent of this book to inform the reader of the current status of cognitive-behavioral theory and research and the contribution that this perspective is making to a greater understanding of obsessional states. At the same time, this book describes new cognitive-behavioral approaches to the treatment of obsessions and compulsions. Together, cognitive theory, research, and practice clearly have much to offer in the treatment of OCD. Yet the present discussion reveals many important gaps in our theories and research of this disorder. The treatment innovations that characterize the new cognitive-behavioral therapy of OCD have yet to receive empirical verification. Moreover, the application of cognitive and behavioral interventions to obsessions and compulsions continues to present extraordinary challenges to even the most experienced practitioners. It is hoped that this book makes some contribution toward advancing our understanding of obsessional states and the effectiveness of our psychological interventions.

References

Abramowitz, J. S. (1997). Effectiveness of psychological and pharmacological treatments for obsessive–compulsive disorder: A quantitative review. *Journal of Consulting and Clinical Psychology, 65,* 44–52.

Abramowitz, J. S. (1998). Does cognitive-behavioral therapy cure obsessive–compulsive disorder?: A meta-analytic evaluation of clinical significance. *Behavior Therapy, 29,* 339–355.

Abramowitz, J. S., & Foa, E. B. (1998). Worries and obsessions in individuals with obsessive–compulsive disorder with and without comorbid generalized anxiety disorder. *Behaviour Research and Therapy, 36,* 695–700.

Abramowitz, J. S., & Foa, E. B. (2000). Does comorbid major depression influence outcome of exposure and response prevention for OCD? *Behavior Therapy, 31,* 795–800.

Abramowitz, J. S., Foa, E. B., & Franklin, M. E. (2003). Exposure and ritual prevention for obsessive–compulsive disorder: Effects of intensive versus twice-weekly sessions. *Journal of Consulting and Clinical Psychology, 71,* 394–398.

Abramowitz, J. S., Franklin, M. E., Street, G. P., Kozak, M. J., & Foa, E. B. (2000). Effects of comorbid depression on response to treatment for obsessive–compulsive disorder. *Behavior Therapy, 31,* 517–528.

Abramowitz, J. S., Huppert, J. D., Cohen, A. B., Tolin, D. F., & Cahill, S. P. (2002). Religious obsessions and compulsions in a non-clinical sample: The Penn Inventory of Scrupulosity (PIOS). *Behaviour Research and Therapy, 40,* 825–838.

Abramowitz, J. S., Schwartz, S. A., Moore, K. M., & Luenzmann, K. R. (2003). Obsessive-compulsive symptoms in pregnancy and the puerperium: A review of the literature. *Journal of Anxiety Disorders, 17,* 461–478.

Abramowitz, J. S., Tolin, D. F., & Street, G. P. (2001). Paradoxical effects of thought suppression: A meta-analysis of controlled studies. *Clinical Psychology Review, 21,* 683–703.

Abramowitz, J. S., Whiteside, S., Kalsy, S. A., & Tolin, D. F. (2003). Thought control strategies in obsessive–compulsive disorder: A replication and extension. *Behaviour Research and Therapy, 41,* 529–540.

Akhtar, S., Wig, N. N., Varma, V. K., Peershad, D., & Verma, S. K. (1975). A phenomenological analysis of symptoms in obsessive–compulsive neurosis. *British Journal of Psychiatry, 127,* 342–348.

Albert, I., & Hayward, P. (2002). Treatment of intrusive ruminations about mathematics. *Behavioural and Cognitive Psychotherapy, 30,* 223–226.

Alsobrook, J. P., & Pauls, D. L. (1998). The genetics of obsessive–compulsive disorder. In M. A. Jenike, L. Baer, & W. E. Minichiello (Eds.), *Obsessive-compulsive disorders: Practical management* (3rd ed., pp. 276–288). St. Louis: Mosby.

American Psychiatric Association (APA). (2000). *Diagnostic and statistical manual of mental disorders* (4th ed., text rev.). Washington, DC: Author.

Amir, N., Cashman, L., & Foa, E. B. (1997). Strategies of thought control in obsessive–compulsive disorder. *Behaviour Research and Therapy, 35,* 775–777.

Amir, N., Foa, E. B., & Coles, M. E. (1997). Factor structure of the Yale-Brown Obsessive–Compulsive Scale. *Psychological Assessment, 9,* 312–316.

Amir, N., Freshman, M., & Foa, E. B. (2000). Family distress and involvement in relatives of obsessive–compulsive patients. *Journal of Anxiety Disorders, 14,* 209–217.

Amir, N., Freshman, M., Ramsey, E., Neary, E., & Brigidi, B. (2001). Thought–action fusion in individuals with OCD symptoms. *Behaviour Research and Therapy, 39,* 765–776.

Amir, N., & Kozak, M. J. (2002). Information processing in obsessive compulsive disorder. In R. O. Frost & G. S. Steketee (Eds.), *Cognitive approaches to obsessions and compulsions: Theory, assessment and treatment* (pp. 165–181). Oxford, UK: Elsevier.

Andrews, G., Henderson, S., & Hall, W. (2001). Prevalence, comorbidity, disability and service utilization. Overview of the Australian National Mental Health Survey. *British Journal of Psychiatry, 178,* 145–153.

Antony, M. M. (2001). Measures for obsessive–compulsive disorder. In M. M. Antony, S. M. Orsillo, & L. Roemer (Eds.), *Practitioner's guide to empirically based measures of anxiety* (pp. 219–243). New York: Kluwer Academic/Plenum.

Antony, M. M., Downie, F., & Swinson, R. P. (1998). Diagnostic issues and epidemiology in obsessive–compulsive disorder. In R. P. Swinson, M. M. Antony, S. Rachman, & M. A. Richter (Eds.), *Obsessive–compulsive disorder: Theory, research, and treatment* (pp. 3–32). New York: Guilford Press.

Arntz, A., Rauner, M., & van den Hout, M. (1995). "If I feel anxious, there must be danger": Ex-consequential reasoning in inferring danger in anxiety disorders. *Behaviour Research and Therapy, 33,* 917–925

Baer, L. (1994). Factor analysis of symptom subtypes of obsessive compulsive disorder and their relation to personality and tic disorder. *Journal of Clinical Psychology, 55,* 18–23.

Baer, L. (2000). *Getting control: Overcoming your obsessions and compulsions* (2nd ed.). New York: Plume.

Baer, L., Brown-Beasley, W., Sorce, J., & Henriques, A. I. (1993). Computer-assisted telephone administration of a structured interview for obsessive–compulsive disorder. *American Journal of Psychiatry, 150,* 1737–1738.

Barlow, D. H. (2002). *Anxiety and its disorders: The nature and treatment of anxiety and panic* (2nd ed.). New York: Guilford Press.

Basoglu, M., Lax, T., Kasvikis, Y., & Marks, I. M. (1988). Predictors of improvement in obsessive–compulsive disorder. *Journal of Anxiety Disorders, 2,* 299–317.

Bass, B. A. (1973). An usual behavioral technique for treating obsessive ruminations. *Psychotherapy: Theory, Research and Practice, 10,* 191–192.

Beck, A. T. (1963). Thinking and depression: 1. Idiosyncratic content and cognitive distortions. *Archives of General Psychiatry, 9,* 324–333.

Beck A. T. (1967). *Depression: Causes and treatment.* Philadelphia: University of Pennsylvania Press.

Beck, A. T. (1976). *Cognitive therapy of the emotional disorders.* New York: New American Library.

Beck, A. T., & Clark, D. A. (1997). An information processing model of anxiety: Automatic and strategic processes. *Behaviour Research and Therapy, 35,* 49–58.

Beck, A.T., & Emery, G. (with Greenberg, R.L.) (1985). *Anxiety disorders and phobias: A cognitive perspective.* New York: Basic Books.

Beck, A. T., Rush, A. J., Shaw, B. F., & Emery, G. (1979). *Cognitive therapy of depression.* New York: Guilford Press.

Beck, A. T., & Steer, R. A. (1993). *Manual of the Beck Anxiety Inventory.* San Antonio, TX: Psychological Corporation.

Beck, A. T., Steer, R. A., & Brown, G. (1996). *Beck Depression Inventory manual* (2nd ed.). San Antonio, TX: Psychological Corporation.

Beck, J. S. (1995). *Cognitive therapy: Basics and beyond.* New York: Guilford Press.

Becker, E. S., Rinck, M., Roth, W. T., & Margraf, J. (1998). Don't worry and beware of white bears: Thought suppression in anxiety patients. *Journal of Anxiety Disorders, 12,* 39–55.

Beech, H. R., & Vaughan, M. (1978). *Behavioural treatment of obsessional states.* Chichester, UK: Wiley.

Beevers, C. G., Wenzlaff, R. M., Hayes, A. M., & Scott, W. D. (1999). Depression and the ironic effects of thought suppression: Therapeutic strategies for improving mental control. *Clinical Psychology: Science and Practice, 6,* 133–148.

Bellodi, L., Sciuto, G., Diaferia, G., Ronchi, P., & Smeraldi, E. (1992). Psychiatric disorders in the families of patients with obsessive–compulsive disorder. *Psychiatry Research, 42,* 111–120.

Beutler, L. E., Harwood, T. M., & Caldwell, R. (2001). Cognitive–behavioral therapy and psychotherapy integration. In K. S. Dobson (Ed.), *Handbook of cognitive–behavioral therapies* (2nd ed., pp. 138–170). New York: Guilford Press.

Bhar, S. S., & Kyrios, M. (2001). Ambivalent self-esteem as a meta-vulnerability for obsessive–compulsive disorder. In R. G. Craven & H. W. Marsh (Eds.), *Self-concept theory, research and practice: Advances for the new millennium* (pp. 143–156). Sydney, Australia: Self-concept Enhancement and Learning Facilitation (SELF) Research Centre, University of Western Sydney.

Black, A. (1974). The natural history of obsessional neurosis. In H. R. Beech (Ed.), *Obsessional states* (pp. 19–54). London: Methuen.

Black, D. W. (1998). Recognition and treatment of obsessive–compulsive spectrum disorders. In R. P. Swinson, M. M. Antony, S. Rachman, & M. A. Richter (Eds.), *Obsessive–compulsive disorder: Theory, research, and treatment* (pp. 426–457). New York: Guilford Press.

Black, D. W., Monahan, P., Gable, J., Blum, N., Clancy, G., & Baker, P. (1998). Hoarding and treatment response in 38 nondepressed subjects with obsessive–compulsive disorder. *Journal of Clinical Psychiatry, 59,* 420–425.

Bolton, D., Raven, P., Madronal-Luque, R., & Marks, I. M. (2000). Neurological and neuropsychological signs in obsessive compulsive disorder: Interaction with behavioural treatment. *Behaviour Research and Therapy, 38,* 695–708.

Borkovec, T. D. (1994). The nature, functions and origins of worry. In G. C. L. Davey & F. Tallis (Eds.), *Worrying: Perspectives on theory, assessment and treatment* (pp. 5–33). Chichester, UK: Wiley.

Bouchard, C., Rhéaume, J., & Ladouceur, R. (1999). Responsibility and perfectionism in OCD: An experimental study. *Behaviour Research and Therapy, 37,* 239–248.

Boulougouris, J. C., & Bassiakos, L. (1973). Prolonged flooding in cases with obsessive–compulsive neurosis. *Behaviour Research and Therapy, 11,* 227–231.

Boulougouris, J. C., Rabavilas, A. D., & Stefanis, C. (1977). Psychophysiological responses in obsessive–compulsive patients. *Behaviour Research and Therapy, 15,* 221–230.

Bouchard, C., Rhéaume, J., & Ladouceur, R. (1999). Responsibility and perfectionism in OCD : An experimental study. *Behaviour Research and Therapy, 37,* 239–248.

Bouvard, M. (2002). Cognitive effects of cognitive-behavior therapy for obsessive compulsive disorder. In R. O. Frost & G. S. Steketee (Eds.), *Cognitive approaches to obsessions and compulsions: Theory, assessment and treatment* (pp. 404–416). Oxford, UK: Elsevier.

Brewin, C. R., Hunter, E., Carroll, F., & Tata, P. (1996). Intrusive memories in depression: An index of schema activation? *Psychological Medicine, 26,* 1271–1276.

Bronisch, T., & Hecht, H. (1990). Major depression with and without a coexisting anxiety disorder: Social dysfunction, social integration, and personality features. *Journal of Affective Disorders, 20,* 151–157.

Brown, H. D., Kosslyn, S. M., Breiter, H. C., Baer, L., & Jenike, M. A. (1994). Can patients with obsessive–compulsive disorder discriminate between percepts and mental images?: A signal detection analysis. *Journal of Abnormal Psychology, 103*, 445–454.

Brown, T. A. (1998). The relationship between obsessive–compulsive disorder and other anxiety-based disorders. In R. P. Swinson, M. M. Antony, S. Rachman, & M. A. Richter (Eds.), *Obsessive–compulsive disorder: Theory, research, and treatment* (pp. 207–226). New York: Guilford Press.

Brown, T. A., & Barlow, D. H. (1992). Comorbidity among anxiety disorders: Implications for treatment and DSM-IV. *Journal of Consulting and Clinical Psychology, 60*, 835–844.

Brown, T. A., Campbell, L. A., Lehman, C. L., Grisham, J. R., & Mancill, R. B. (2001). Current and lifetime comorbidity of the DSM-IV anxiety and mood disorders in a large clinical sample. *Journal of Abnormal Psychology, 110*, 585–599.

Brown, T. A., Di Nardo, P. A., & Barlow, D. H. (1994). *Anxiety disorders interview schedule for DSM-IV. Client Interview Schedule.* San Antonio, TX: Graywind Publications and The Psychological Corporation.

Brown, T. A., Di Nardo, P. A., Lehman, C. L., & Campbell, L. A. (2001). Reliability of DSM-IV anxiety and mood disorders: Implications for the classification of emotional disorders. *Journal of Abnormal Psychology, 110*, 49–58.

Brown, T. A., Dowdall, D. J., Côté, G., & Barlow, D. H. (1994). Worry and obsessions: The distinction between generalized anxiety disorder and obsessive–compulsive disorder. In G. C. L. Davey & F. Tallis (Eds.), *Worrying: Perspectives on theory, assessment and treatment* (pp. 229–246). New York: Wiley.

Brown, T. A., Moras, K., Zinbarg, R. E., & Barlow, D. H. (1993). Diagnostic and symptom distinguishability of generalized anxiety disorder and obsessive–compulsive disorder. *Behavior Therapy, 24*, 227–240.

Burns, D. D., & Spangler, D. L. (2000). Does psychotherapy homework lead to improvements in depression in cognitive-behavioral therapy or does improvement lead to increased homework compliance? *Journal of Consulting and Clinical Psychology, 68*, 46–56.

Burns, G. L., Formea, G. M., Keortge, S., & Sternberger, L. G. (1995). The utilization of nonpatient samples in the study of obsessive compulsive disorder. *Behaviour Research and Therapy, 33*, 133–144.

Burns, G. L., Keortge, S. G., Formea, G. M., & Sternberger, L. G. (1996). Revision of the Padua Inventory of obsessive compulsive disorder symptoms: Distinctions between worry, obsessions and compulsions. *Behaviour Research and Therapy, 34*, 163–173.

Byers, E. S., Purdon, C., & Clark, D. A. (1998). Sexual intrusive thoughts of college students. *Journal of Sex Research, 35*, 359–369.

Calamari, J. E., Amir, N., Cassiday, K. L., Kohlbeck, P. A., Higdon, L. J., Young, P. R., et al. (1993). *Information processing in obsessive compulsive disorder.* Paper presented at the Annual Convention of the Association for the Advancement of Behavior Therapy, Atlanta.

Calamari, J. E., & Janeck, A. S. (1997). *Negative intrusive thoughts in obsessive–compulsive disorder: Appraisal and response differences.* Poster presented at the Anxiety Disorders Association of America National Convention, New Orleans, LA.

Calamari, J. E., Wiegartz, P. S., & Janeck, A. S. (1999). Obsessive–compulsive disorder subgroups: A symptom-based clustering approach. *Behaviour Research and Therapy, 37*, 113–125.

Calvocoressi, L., Lewis, B., Harris, M., Trufan, S. J., Goodman, W. K., McDougle, C. J., & Price, L. H. (1995). Family accommodation in obsessive–compulsive disorder. *American Journal of Psychiatry, 152*, 441–443.

Carr, A. T. (1974). Compulsive neurosis: A review of the literature. *Psychological Bulletin, 81*, 311–318.

Ceschi, G., Van der Linden, M., Dunker, D., Perroud, A., & Brédart, S. (2003). Further exploration of memory bias in compulsive washers. *Behaviour Research and Therapy, 41*, 737–748.

Chambless, D. L., Baker, M. J., Baucom, D. H., Beutler, L. E., Calhoun, K. S., Crits-Christoph, P., et al. (1998). Update on empirically validated therapies. II. *The Clinical Psychologist, 51,* 3–16.

Clark, D. A. (1984). *Psychophysiological, behavioural, and self-report investigations into cognitive-affective interaction within the context of potentially aversive ideation.* Unpublished doctoral dissertation, Institute of Psychiatry, University of London, UK.

Clark, D. A. (1986). Factors influencing the retrieval and control of negative cognitions. *Behaviour Research and Therapy, 24,* 151–159.

Clark, D. A. (1989). *A schema control model of negative thoughts.* Paper presented at the World Congress of Cognitive Therapy, Oxford, UK.

Clark, D. A. (1999). Cognitive behavioral treatment of obsessive–compulsive disorders: A commentary. *Cognitive and Behavioral Practice, 6,* 408–415.

Clark, D. A. (2002). A cognitive perspective on OCD and depression: Distinct and related features. In R. O. Frost & G. S. Steketee (Eds.), *Cognitive approaches to obsessions and compulsions: Theory, assessment and treatment* (pp. 233–250). Oxford, UK: Elsevier.

Clark, D. A., Antony, M. M., Beck, A. T., Swinson, R. P., & Steer, R. A. (2003). *Screening for obsessive and compulsive symptoms: Validation of the Clark–Beck Obsessive-Compulsive Inventory.* Manuscript submitted for publication.

Clark, D. A., & Beck, A. T. (with Alford, B.) (1999). *Scientific foundations of cognitive theory and therapy of depression.* New York: Wiley.

Clark, D. A., & Beck, A. T. (2002). *Manual for the Clark–Beck Obsessive Compulsive Inventory.* San Antonio, TX: Psychological Corporation.

Clark, D. A., Beck, A. T., & Stewart, B. (1990). Cognitive specificity and positive–negative affectivity: Complementary or contradictory views on anxiety and depression? *Journal of Abnormal Psychology, 99,* 148–155.

Clark, D. A., & Claybourn, M. (1997). Process characteristics of worry and obsessive intrusive thoughts. *Behaviour Research and Therapy, 35,* 1139–1141.

Clark, D. A., & de Silva, P. (1985). The nature of depressive and anxious thoughts: Distinct or uniform phenomena? *Behaviour Research and Therapy, 23,* 383–393.

Clark, D. A., & Purdon, C. L. (1993). New perspectives for a cognitive theory of obsessions. *Australian Psychologist, 28,* 161–167.

Clark, D. A., Purdon, C., & Byers, E. S. (2000). Appraisal and control of sexual and non-sexual intrusive thoughts in university students. *Behaviour Research and Therapy, 38,* 439–455.

Clark, D. A., Purdon, C., & Wang, A. (2003). The Meta-Cognitive Beliefs Questionnaire: Development of a measure of obsessional beliefs. *Behaviour Research and Therapy, 41,* 655–669.

Clark, D. M. (1986). A cognitive approach to panic. *Behaviour Research and Therapy, 24,* 461–470.

Clark, D. M. (1999). Anxiety disorders: Why they persist and how to treat them. *Behaviour Research and Therapy, 37,* S2–S27.

Clark, D. M., Ball, S., & Pape, D. (1991). An experimental investigation of thought suppression. *Behaviour Research and Therapy, 29,* 253–257.

Clark, D. M., Winton, E., & Thynn, L. (1993). A further experimental investigation of thought suppression. *Behaviour Research and Therapy, 31,* 207–210.

Clark, L. A., Watson, D., & Reynolds, S. (1995). Diagnosis and classification of psychopathology: Challenges to the current system and future directions. *Annual Review of Psychology, 46,* 121–153.

Clayton, I. C., Richards, J. C., & Edwards, C. J. (1999). Selective attention in obsessive–compulsive disorder. *Journal of Abnormal Psychology, 108,* 171–175.

Coelho, J. S., & Whittal, M. L. (2001). *Are subtypes of obsessive–compulsive disorder differentially responsive to treatment?* Paper presented at the World Congress of Behavioural and Cognitive Therapies, Vancouver, Canada.

Coles, M. E., Mennin, D. S., & Heimberg, R. G. (2001). Distinguishing obsessive features and worries: The role of thought–action fusion. *Behaviour Research and Therapy, 39,* 947–959.

Constans, J. I. (2001). Worry propensity and the perception of risk. *Behaviour Research and Therapy, 39,* 721–729.

Constans, J. I., Foa, E. B., Franklin, M. E., & Mathews, A. (1995). Memory for actual and imagined events in OC checkers. *Behaviour Research and Therapy, 33,* 665–671.

Conway, M., Howell, A., & Giannopoulos, C. (1991). Dysphoria and thought suppression. *Cognitive Therapy and Research, 15,* 153–166.

Coryell, W. (1981). Obsessive–compulsive disorder and primary unipolar depression: Comparisons of background, family history, course, and mortality. *Journal of Nervous and Mental Disease, 169,* 220–224.

Cottraux, J., Bouvard, M., Defayolle, M., & Messy, P. (1988). Validity and factorial structure of the Compulsive Activity Checklist. *Behavior Therapy, 19,* 45–53.

Cottraux, J., & Gérard, D. (1998). Neuroimaging and neuroanatomical issues in obsessive-compulsive disorder: Toward an integrative model-perceived impulsivity. In R. P. Swinson, M. M. Antony, S. Rachman, & M. A. Richter (Eds.), *Obsessive-compulsive disorder: Theory, research, and treatment* (pp. 154–180). New York: Guilford Press.

Crino, R. D., & Andrews, G. (1996). Obsessive–compulsive disorder and Axis I comorbidity. *Journal of Anxiety Disorders, 10,* 37–46.

Dalgleish, T., & Watts, F. N. (1990). Biases of attention and memory in disorders of anxiety and depression. *Clinical Psychology Review, 10,* 589–604.

Dar, R., Rish, S., Hermesh, H., Taub, M., & Fux, M. (2000). Realism of confidence in obsessive–compulsive checkers. *Journal of Abnormal Psychology, 109,* 673–678.

Davies, M. I., & Clark, D. M. (1998). Thought suppression produces a rebound effect with analogue post-traumatic intrusions. *Behaviour Research and Therapy, 36,* 571–582.

Demal, U., Lenz, G., Mayrhofer, A., Zapotoczky, H-G., & Zitterl, W. (1993). Obsessive–compulsive disorder and depression: A retrospective study on course and interaction. *Psychopathology, 26,* 145–150.

de Haan, E., van Oppen, P., van Balkom, A.J.L.M., Spinhoven, P., Hoogduin, K.A.L., & van Dyck, R. (1997). Prediction of outcome and early vs. late improvement in OCD patients treated with cognitive behaviour therapy and pharmacotherapy. *Acta Psychiatria Scandinavia, 96,* 354–361.

DeRubeis, R. J., & Crits-Christoph, P. (1998). Empirically supported individual and group psychological treatments for adult mental disorders. *Journal of Consulting and Clinical Psychology, 66,* 37–52.

de Silva, P. (1986). Obsessional–compulsive imagery. *Behaviour Research and Therapy, 24,* 333–350.

de Silva, P., & Marks, M. (1999). The role of traumatic experiences in the genesis of obsessive–compulsive disorder. *Behaviour Research and Therapy, 37,* 941–951.

de Silva, P., Menzies, R. G., & Shafran, R. (2003). Spontaneous decay of compulsive urges: The case of covert compulsions. *Behaviour Research and Therapy, 41,* 129–137.

de Silva, P., & Rachman, S. (1992). *Obsessive compulsive disorder: The facts.* Oxford, UK: Oxford University Press.

Dimidjian, S., & Dobson, K. S. (2003). Processes of change in cognitive therapy. In M. A. Reinecke & D. A. Clark (Eds.), *Cognitive therapy across the lifespan: Theory, research and practice* (pp. 477–506). Cambridge, UK: Cambridge University Press.

Ecker, W., & Engelkamp, J. (1995). Memory for actions in obsessive–compulsive disorder. *Behavioural and Cognitive Psychotherapy, 23,* 349–371.

Edwards, S., & Dickerson, M. (1987). Intrusive unwanted thoughts: A two-stage model of control. *British Journal of Medical Psychology, 60,* 317–328.

Eisen, J. L., Phillips, K. A., Baer, L., Beer, D. A., Atala, K. D., & Rasmussen, S. A. (1998). The Brown Assessment of Beliefs Scale: Reliability and validity. *American Journal of Psychiatry, 155,* 102–108.

Elliott, A. J., & Fuqua, R. W. (2000). Trichotillomania: Conceptualization, measurement, and treatment. *Behavior Therapy, 31,* 529–545.

Emmelkamp, P. M. G. (1982). *Phobic and obsessive–compulsive disorders: Theory, research and practice.* New York: Plenum Press.

Emmelkamp, P. M. G., & Aardema, A. (1999). Metacognition, specific obsessive–compulsive beliefs and obsessive–compulsive behaviour. *Clinical Psychology and Psychotherapy, 6,* 139–145.

Emmelkamp, P. M. G., & Beens, H. (1991). Cognitive therapy with obsessive–compulsive disorder: A comparative evaluation. *Behaviour Research and Therapy, 29,* 293–300.

Emmelkamp, P. M. G., & De Lange, I. (1983). Spouse involvement in the treatment of obsessive–compulsive patients. *Behaviour Research and Therapy, 21,* 341–346.

Emmelkamp, P. M. G., & Giesselbach, P. (1981). Treatment of obsessions: Relevant v. irrelevant exposure. *Behavioural Psychotherapy, 9,* 322–329.

Emmelkamp, P. M. G., & Kraanen, J. (1977). Therapist controlled exposure *in vivo* versus self-controlled exposure *in vivo*: A comparison with obsessive–compulsive patients. *Behaviour Research and Therapy, 15,* 491–495.

Emmelkamp, P. M. G., Kloek, J., & Blaauw, E. (1992). Obsessive–compulsive disorders. In P. H. Wilson (Ed.), *Principles and practice of relapse prevention* (pp. 213–234). New York: Guilford Press.

Emmelkamp, P. M. G., Kraaijkamp, H. J. M., & van den Hout, M. A. (1999). Assessment of obsessive–compulsive disorder. *Behavior Modification, 23,* 269–279.

Emmelkamp, P. M. G., & Kwee, K. G. (1977). Obsessional ruminations: A comparison between thought-stopping and prolonged exposure in imagination. *Behaviour Research and Therapy, 15,* 441–444.

Emmelkamp, P. M. G., van Linden, van den Heuvell, C. L., Ruphan, M., & Sanderman, R. (1989). Home-based treatment of obsessive–compulsive patients: Intersession interval and therapist involvement. *Behaviour Research and Therapy, 27,* 89–93.

Emmelkamp, P. M. G., van der Helm, M., van Zanten, B. L., & Plochg, I. (1980). Treatment of obsessive–compulsive patients: The contribution of self-instructional training to the effectiveness of exposure. *Behaviour Research and Therapy, 18,* 61–66.

Emmelkamp, P. M. G., van Oppen, P., & van Balkom, A. J. L. M. (2002). Cognitive changes in patients with obsessive compulsive rituals treated with exposure in vivo and response prevention. In R. O. Frost & G. S. Steketee (Eds.), *Cognitive approaches to obsessions and compulsions: Theory, assessment and treatment* (pp. 392–401). Oxford, UK: Elsevier Press.

Emmelkamp, P. M. G., Visser, S., & Hoekstra, R. J. (1988). Cognitive therapy vs exposure in vivo in the treatment of obsessive–compulsives. *Cognitive Therapy and Research, 12,* 103–114.

Enright, S. J. (1991). Group treatment of obsessive–compulsive disorder: An evaluation. *Behavioural Psychotherapy, 19,* 183–192.

Enright, S. J. (1996). Obsessive–compulsive disorder: Anxiety disorder or schizotype? In R. M. Rapee (Ed.), *Current controversies in the anxiety disorders* (pp. 161–190). New York: Guilford Press.

Enright, S. J., & Beech, A. (1990). Obsessional states: Anxiety disorders or schizotypes? An information processing and personality assessment. *Psychological Medicine, 20,* 621–627.

Enright, S. J., & Beech, A. R. (1993a) Reduced cognitive inhibition in obsessive–compulsive disorder. *British Journal of Clinical Psychology, 32,* 67–74.

Enright, S. J., & Beech, A. R. (1993b). Further evidence of reduced cognitive inhibition in obsessive–compulsive disorder. *Personality and Individual Differences, 14,* 387–395.

Eysenck, H. J., & Eysenck, M. J. (1985). *Personality and individual differences: A natural science approach.* New York: Plenum Press.

Eysenck, H. J., & Rachman, S. (1965). *The causes and cures of neurosis.* San Diego: Knapp.

Eysenck, M. W. (1992). *Anxiety: The cognitive perspective.* Hove, UK: Erlbaum.

Fallon, B. A., Rasmussen, S. A., & Liebowitz, M. R. (1993). Hypochondriasis. In E. Hollander (Ed.), *Obsessive–compulsive-related disorders* (pp. 71–92). Washington, DC: American Psychiatric Press.

Feske, U., & Chambless, D. L. (2000). A review of assessment measures for obsessive–compulsive disorder. In W. K. Goodman, M. V. Rudorfor, & J. D. Maser (Eds.), *Obsessive–compulsive disorder: Contemporary issues in treatment* (pp. 157–182). Mahwah, NJ: Erlbaum.

First, M. B., Spitzer, R. L., Gibbon, M., & Williams, J. B. W. (1996). *Structured clinical interview for DSM-IV axis I disorders–Patient edition (SCID-I/P, version 2.0)*. New York: Biometrics Research Department, New York State Psychiatric Institute.

Flavell, J. H. (1979). Metacognition and cognitive monitoring: A new area of cognitive-developmental inquiry. *American Psychologist, 34,* 906–911.

Foa, E. B. (1979). Failure in treating obsessive compulsives. *Behaviour Research and Therapy, 17,* 169–176.

Foa, E. B., Abramowitz, J. S., Franklin, M. E., & Kozak, M. J. (1999). Feared consequences, fixity of belief, and treatment outcome in patients with obsessive–compulsive disorder. *Behavior Therapy, 30,* 717–724.

Foa, E. B., Amir, N., Bogert, K. V. A., Molnar, C., & Przeworski, A. (2001). Inflated perception of responsibility for harm in obsessive–compulsive disorder. *Journal of Anxiety Disorders, 15,* 259–275.

Foa, E. B., Franklin, M. E., & Kozak, M. J. (1998). Psychosocial treatments for obsessive–compulsive disorder: Literature review. In R. P. Swinson, M. M. Antony, S. Rachman, & M. A. Richter (Eds.), *Obsessive-compulsive disorder: Theory, research, and treatment* (pp. 258–276). New York: Guilford Press.

Foa, E. B., Grayson, J. B., Steketee, G. S., Doppelt, H. G., Turner, R. M., & Latimer, P. R. (1983). Success and failure in the behavioral treatment of obsessive–compulsives. *Journal of Consulting and Clinical Psychology, 51,* 287–297.

Foa, E. B., Huppert, J. D., Leiberg, S., Langner, R., Kichic, R., Hajcak, G., & Salkovskis, P. M. (2002). The Obsessive–Compulsive Inventory: Development and validation of a short version. *Psychological Assessment, 14,* 485–496.

Foa, E. B., Ilai, D., McCarthy, P. R., Shoyer, B., & Murdock, T. (1993). Information processing in obsessive–compulsive disorder. *Cognitive Therapy and Research, 17,* 173–189.

Foa, E. B., & Kozak, M. J. (1986). Emotional processing of fear: Exposure to corrective information. *Psychological Bulletin, 99,* 20–35.

Foa, E. B., & Kozak, M. J. (1995). DSM-IV Field Trial: Obsessive–compulsive disorder. *American Journal of Psychiatry, 152,* 90–96.

Foa, E. B., & Kozak, M. J. (1996). Psychological treatment for obsessive–compulsive disorder. In M. R. Mavissakalian & R. F. Prien (Eds.), *Long-term treatments of anxiety disorders* (pp. 285–309). Washington, DC: American Psychiatric Press.

Foa, E. B., & Kozak, M. J. (1997). *Mastery of obsessive–compulsive disorder: Client workbook.* San Antonio, TX: Psychological Corporation.

Foa, E. B., Kozak, M. J., Salkovskis, P. M., Coles, M. E., & Amir, N. (1998). The validation of a new obsessive–compulsive disorder scale: The Obsessive–Compulsive Inventory. *Psychological Assessment, 10,* 206–214.

Foa, E. B., & McNally, R. J. (1986). Sensitivity to feared stimuli in obsessive–compulsives: A dichotic listening analysis. *Cognitive Therapy and Research, 10,* 477–485.

Foa, E. B., Sacks, M. B., Tolin, D. F., Przeworski, A., & Amir, N. (2002). Inflated perception of responsibility for harm in OCD patients with and without checking compulsions: A replication and extension. *Journal of Anxiety Disorders, 16,* 443–453.

Foa, E. B., & Steketee, G. (1979). Obsessive–compulsives: Conceptual issues and treatment interventions. *Progress in behavior modification* (Vol. 8, pp. 1–53). New York: Academic Press.

Foa, E. B., Steketee, G., Grayson, J. B., & Doppelt, H. G. (1983). Treatment of obsessive-compulsives: When do we fail? In E. B. Foa & P. M. G. Emmelkamp (Eds.), *Failures in behavior therapy* (pp. 10–34). New York: Wiley.

Foa, E. B., Steketee, G. S., & Ozarow, B. J. (1985). Behavior therapy with obsessive–compulsives: From theory to treatment. In M. Mavissakalian, S. M. Turner, & L. Michelson (Eds.), *Obsessive–compulsive disorder: Psychological and pharmacological treatment* (pp. 49–129). New York: Plenum Press.

Forrester, E., Wilson, C., & Salkovskis, P. M. (2002). The occurrence of intrusive thoughts transforms meaning in ambiguous situations: An experimental study. *Behavioural and Cognitive Psychotherapy, 30*, 143–152.

Franklin, M. E., Abramowitz, J. S., Bux, D. A., Zoellner, L. A., & Feeny, N. C. (2002). Cognitive-behavioral therapy with and without medication in the treatment of obsessive–compulsive disorder. *Professional Psychology: Research and Practice, 33*, 162–168.

Freeston, M. H. (2001). Cognitive-behavioral treatment of a 14-year-old teenager with obsessive–compulsive disorder. *Behavioural and Cognitive Psychotherapy, 29*, 71–84.

Freeston, M. H., & Ladouceur, R. (1993). Appraisal of cognitive intrusions and response style: Replication and extension. *Behaviour Research and Therapy, 31*, 185–191.

Freeston, M. H., & Ladouceur, R. (1997a). *The cognitive behavioral treatment of obsessions: A treatment manual.* Unpublished manuscript, École de Psychologie, Université Laval, Québec, Canada.

Freeston, M. H., & Ladouceur, R. (1997b). What do patients do with their obsessive thoughts? *Behaviour Research and Therapy, 35*, 335–348.

Freeston, M. H., & Ladouceur, R. (1999). Exposure and response prevention for obsessional thoughts. *Cognitive and Behavioral Practice, 6*, 362–383.

Freeston, M. H., Ladouceur, R., Gagnon, F., & Thibodeau, N. (1993). Beliefs about obsessional thoughts. *Journal of Psychopathology and Behavioral Assessment, 15*, 1–21.

Freeston, M. H., Ladouceur, R., Gagnon, F., Thibodeau, N., Rhéaume, J., Letarte, H., & Bujold, A. (1997). Cognitive-behavioral treatment of obsessive thoughts: A controlled study. *Journal of Consulting and Clinical Psychology, 65*, 405–413.

Freeston, M. H., Ladouceur, R., Letarte, H., Rhéaume, J., Thibodeau, N., & Gagnon, F. (1992). *Information processing of responsibility, anxiety and depression related words in OCD patients and low and high anxiety controls.* Paper presented at the annual meeting of the Association for Advancement of Behavior Therapy, Boston.

Freeston, M. H., Ladouceur, R., Provencher, M., & Blais, F. (1995). Strategies used with intrusive thoughts: Context, appraisal, mood, and efficacy. *Journal of Anxiety Disorders, 9*, 201–215.

Freeston, M. H., Ladouceur, R., Rhéaume, J., Letarte, H., Gagnon, F., & Thibodeau, N. (1994). Self-report of obsessions and worry. *Behaviour Research and Therapy, 32*, 29–36.

Freeston, M. H., Ladouceur, R., Thibodeau, N., & Gagnon, F. (1991). Cognitive intrusions in a non-clinical population. I. Response style, subjective experience, and appraisal. *Behaviour Research and Therapy, 29*, 585–597.

Freeston, M. H., Ladouceur, R., Thibodeau, N., & Gagnon, F. (1992). Cognitive intrusions in a non-clinical population. II. Associations with depressive, anxious, and compulsive symptoms. *Behaviour Research and Therapy, 30*, 263–271.

Freeston, M. H., Rhéaume, J., & Ladouceur, R. (1996). Correcting faulty appraisals of obsessional thoughts. *Behaviour Research and Therapy, 34*, 433–446.

Freud, S. (1959). Character and eroticism. In J. Strachey (Ed. and Trans.), *The standard edition of the complete psychological works of Sigmund Freud* (Vol. 9, pp. 167–175). London: Hogarth Press. (Original work published 1908)

Freund, B., & Steketee, G. (1989). Sexual history, attitudes and functioning of obsessive–compulsive patients. *Journal of Sex and Marital Therapy, 15*, 31–41.

Freund, B., Steketee, G. S., & Foa, E. B. (1987). Compulsive Activity Checklist (CAC): Psychometric analysis with obsessive–compulsive disorder. *Behavioral Assessment, 9*, 67–79.

Frost, R. O., & Gross, R. C. (1993). The hoarding of possessions. *Behaviour Research and Therapy, 31,* 367–381.

Frost, R. O., & Hartl, T. L. (1996). A cognitive-behavioral model of compulsive hoarding. *Behaviour Research and Therapy, 34,* 341–350.

Frost, R. O., Kim, H-J., Morris, C., Bloss, C., Murray-Close, M., & Steketee, G. (1998). Hoarding, compulsive buying and reasons for saving. *Behaviour Research and Therapy, 36,* 657–664.

Frost, R. O., Krause, M., & Steketee, G. (1996). Hoarding and obsessive compulsive symptoms. *Behavior Modification, 20,* 116–132.

Frost, R. O., Meagher, B. M., & Riskind, J. H. (2001). Obsessive–compulsive features in pathological lottery and scratch-ticket gamblers. *Journal of Gambling Studies, 17,* 5–19.

Frost, R. O., Novara, C., & Rhéaume, J. (2002). Perfectionism in obsessive compulsive disorder. In R. O. Frost & G. Steketee (Eds.), *Cognitive approaches to obsessions and compulsions: Theory, assessment and treatment* (pp. 92–105). Oxford, UK: Elsevier.

Frost, R. O., & Steketee, G. (1997). Perfectionism in obsessive–compulsive disorder patients. *Behaviour Research and Therapy, 35,* 291–296.

Frost, R. O., & Steketee, G. (1998). Hoarding: Clinical aspects and treatment strategies. In M. A. Jenike, L. Baer, & W. E. Minichiello (Eds.), *Obsessive–compulsive disorder: Practical management* (3rd ed., pp. 533–554). St. Louis: Mosby.

Frost, R. O., & Steketee, G. (1999). Issues in the treatment of compulsive hoarding. *Cognitive and Behavioral Practice, 6,* 397–407.

Frost, R. O., & Steketee, G. (Eds.). (2002). *Cognitive approaches to obsessions and compulsions: Theory, assessment, and treatment.* Amsterdam: Elsevier Science.

Frost, R. O., Steketee, G., & Greene, K. A. I. (1999). Cognitive and behavioral treatment of compulsive hoarding. Unpublished manuscript, Department of Psychology, Smith College, Northampton, MA.

Frost, R. O., Steketee, G., Krause, M. S., & Trepanier, K. L. (1995). The relationship of the Yale-Brown Obsessive–Compulsive Scale (YBOCS) to other measures of obsessive compulsive symptoms in a nonclinical population. *Journal of Personality Assessment, 65,* 158–168.

Gaskell, S. L., Wells, A., & Calam, R. (2001). An experimental investigation of thought suppression and anxiety in children. *British Journal of Clinical Psychology, 40,* 45–56.

Gibbs, N. A. (1996). Nonclinical populations in research on obsessive–compulsive disorder: A critical review. *Clinical Psychology Review, 16,* 729–773.

Gibbs, N. A., & Oltmanns, T. F. (1995). The relation between obsessive–compulsive personality traits and subtypes of compulsive behavior. *Journal of Anxiety Disorders, 9,* 397–410.

Gittleson, N. L. (1966). The phenomenology of obsessions in depressive psychosis. *British Journal of Psychiatry, 112,* 261–264.

Goldsmith, T., Shapira, N. A., Phillips, K. A., & McElroy, S. L. (1998). Conceptual foundations of obsessive–compulsive spectrum disorders. In R. P. Swinson, M. M. Antony, S. Rachman, & M. A. Richter (Eds.), *Obsessive–compulsive disorder: Theory, research, and treatment* (pp. 397–425). New York: Guilford Press.

Goodman, W. K., Price, L. H., Rasmussen, S. A., Mazure, C., Fleischmann, R. L., Hill, C. L., Heninger, G. R., & Charney, D. S. (1989a). The Yale-Brown Obsessive–Compulsive Scale I. Development, use, and reliability. *Archives of General Psychiatry, 46,* 1006–1011.

Goodman, W. K., Price, L. H., Rasmussen, S. A., Mazure, C., Delgado, P., Heninger, G. R., & Charney, D. S. (1989b). The Yale-Brown Obsessive–Compulsive Scale II. Validity. *Archives of General Psychiatry, 46,* 1012–1016.

Gotlib, I. H., & Neubauer, D. L. (2000). Information-processing approaches to the study of cognitive biases in depression. In S. L. Johnson, A. M. Hayes, T. M. Field, N. Sclneiderman, & P. M. McCabe (Eds.), *Stress, coping and depression* (pp. 117–143). Mahwah, NJ: Erlbaum.

Greenberger, D., & Padesky, C. A. (1995). *Mind over mood: A cognitive therapy treatment manual for clients.* New York: Guilford Press.

Greisberg, S., & McKay, D. (2003). Neuropsychology of obsessive–compulsive disorder: A review and treatment implications. *Clinical Psychology Review, 23,* 95–117.

Guidano, V. F., & Liotti, G. (1983). *Cognitive processes and emotional disorders: A structural approach to psychotherapy.* New York: Guilford Press.

Gurnani, P. D., & Vaughan, M. (1981). Changes in frequency and distress during prolonged repetition of obsessional thoughts. *British Journal of Clinical Psychology, 20,* 79–81.

Haaga, D. A. F., Dyck, M. J., & Ernst, D. (1991). Empirical status of cognitive theory of depression. *Psychological Bulletin, 110,* 215–236.

Hackman, A., & McLean, C. (1975). A comparison of flooding and thought stopping in the treatment of obsessional neurosis. *Behaviour Research and Therapy, 13,* 263–269.

Hanna, G. L. (2000). Clinical and family-genetic studies of childhood obsessive–compulsive disorder. In W. K. Goodman, M. V. Rudorfor, & J. D. Maser (Eds.), *Obsessive–compulsive disorder: Contemporary issues in treatment* (pp. 87–103). Mahwah, NJ: Erlbaum.

Hartl, T. L., & Frost, R. O. (1999). Cognitive-behavioral treatment of compulsive hoarding: A multiple baseline experimental case study. *Behaviour Research and Therapy, 37,* 451–461.

Harvey, A. G., & Bryant, R. A. (1998). The effect of attempted thought suppression in acute stress disorder. *Behaviour Research and Therapy, 36,* 583–590.

Harvey, A. G., & Bryant, R. A. (1999). The role of anxiety in attempted thought suppression following exposure to distressing or neutral stimuli. *Cognitive Therapy and Research, 23,* 39–52.

Hazlett-Stevens, H., Zucker, B. G., & Craske, M. G. (2002). The relationship of thought-action fusion to pathological worry and generalized anxiety disorder. *Behaviour Research and Therapy, 40,* 1199–1204.

Headland, K., & McDonald, B. (1987). Rapid audio-tape treatment of obsessional ruminations: A case report. *Behavioural Psychotherapy, 15,* 188–192.

Hermans, D., Martens, K., De Cort, K., Pieters, G., & Eelen, P. (2003). Reality monitoring and metacognitive beliefs related to cognitive confidence in obsessive–compulsive disorder. *Behaviour Research and Therapy, 41,* 383–401.

Hiss, H., Foa, E. B., & Kozak, M. J. (1994). Relapse prevention program for treatment of obsessive–compulsive disorder. *Journal of Consulting and Clinical Psychology, 62,* 801–808.

Hodgson, R.J., & Rachman, S. J. (1972). The effects of contamination and washing in obsessional patients. *Behaviour Research and Therapy, 10,* 111–117.

Hodgson, R. J., & Rachman, S. J. (1977). Obsessional compulsive complaints. *Behaviour Research and Therapy, 15,* 389–395.

Hodgson, R. J., Rachman, S., & Marks, I. M. (1972). The treatment of chronic obsessive-compulsive neurosis: Follow-up and further findings. *Behaviour Research and Therapy, 10,* 181–189.

Hollander, E. (1993). Introduction. In E. Hollander (Ed.), *Obsessive–compulsive-related disorders* (pp. 1–16). Washington, DC: American Psychiatric Press.

Hollander, E., & Wong, C. M. (2000). Spectrum, boundary, and subtyping issues: Implications for treatment-refractory obsessive–compulsive disorder. In W. K. Goodman, M. V. Rudorfor, & J. D. Maser (Eds.) *Obsessive–compulsive disorder: Contemporary issues in treatment* (pp. 3–22). Mahwah, NJ: Erlbaum.

Hollon, S. D., & Beck, A. T. (1986). Cognitive and cognitive-behavioral therapies. In S. L. Garfield & A. E. Bergin (Eds.), *Handbook of psychotherapy and behavior change* (3rd ed., pp. 443–482). New York: Wiley.

Hollon, S. D., & Beck, A. T. (1986). Cognitive and cognitive-behavioral therapies. In S. L. Garfield & A. E. Bergin (Eds.), *Handbook of psychotherapy and behavior change* (3rd ed., pp. 443–481). New York: Wiley.

Hong, J. L., & Whittal, M. L. (2001). *Varying levels of symptom severity in obsessive–compulsive disorder patients: Differential response to treatment type and format?* Paper presented at the World Congress of Behavioral and Cognitive Therapies, Vancouver, Canada.

Höping, W., & de Jong-Meyer, R. (2003). Differentiating unwanted intrusive thoughts from thought suppression: What does the White Bear Suppression Inventory measure? *Personality and Individual Differences, 34,* 1049–1055.

Horowitz, M. J. (1975). Intrusive and repetitive thoughts after experimental stress: A summary. *Archives of General Psychiatry, 32,* 1457–1463.

Ingram, I. M. (1961a). The obsessional personality and obsessional illness. *American Journal of Psychiatry, 117,* 1016–1019.

Ingram, I. M. (1961b). Obsessional illness in mental health patients. *Journal of Mental Science, 197,* 382–402.

Ingram, R. E., & Kendall, P. C. (1986). Cognitive clinical psychology: Implications of an information processing perspective. In R. E. Ingram (Ed.), *Information processing approaches to clinical psychology* (pp. 3–21). Orlando, FL: Academic Press.

Ingram, R. E., & Price, J. M. (2001). The role of vulnerability in understanding psychopathology. In R. E. Ingram & J. M. Price (Eds.), *Vulnerability to psychopathology: Risk across the lifespan* (pp. 3–19). New York: Guilford Press.

Insel, T. R., & Akiskal, H. S. (1986). Obsessive–compulsive disorder with psychotic features: A phenomenologic analysis. *American Journal of Psychiatry, 143,* 1527–1533.

Ito, L. M., de Araujo, L, A. Hemsley, D., & Marks, I. M. (1995). Beliefs and resistance in obsessive–compulsive disorder: Observations from a controlled study. *Journal of Anxiety Disorders, 9,* 269–281.

Jakes, I. (1989a). Salkovskis on obsessional–compulsive neurosis: A critique. *Behaviour Research and Therapy, 27,* 673–675.

Jakes, I. (1989b). Salkovskis on obsessional–compulsive neurosis: A rejoinder. *Behaviour Research and Therapy, 27,* 683–684.

Janeck, A. S., & Calamari, J. E. (1999). Thought suppression in obsessive–compulsive disorder. *Cognitive Therapy and Research, 23,* 497–509.

Janeck, A. S., Calamari, J. E., Riemann, B. C., & Heffelfinger, S. K. (2003). Too much thinking about thinking?: Metacognitive differences in obsessive–compulsive disorder. *Journal of Anxiety Disorders, 17,* 181–195.

Jaspers, K. (1963). *General psychopathology* (J. Hoenig & M. W. Hamilton, Trans.). Chicago: University of Chicago Press.

Johnson, M. K., & Raye, C. L. (1981). Reality monitoring. *Psychological Review, 88,* 67–85.

Jones, M. K., & Menzies, R. G. (1997). The cognitive mediation of obsessive–compulsive handwashing. *Behaviour Research and Therapy, 35,* 843–850.

Jones, M. K., & Menzies, R. G. (1998). Danger ideation reduction therapy (DIRT) for obsessive–compulsive washers: A controlled trial. *Behaviour Research and Therapy, 36,* 959–970.

Kampman, M., Keijsers, G. P. J., Verbraak, M. J. P. M., Naring, G., & Hoogduin, C. A. L. (2002). The emotional Stroop: A comparison of panic disorder patients, obsessive-compulsive patients, and normal controls, in two experiments. *Journal of Anxiety Disorders, 16,* 425–441.

Karno, M., & Golding, J. M. (1991). Obsessive compulsive disorder. In L. N. Robins & D. A. Regier (Eds.), *Psychiatric disorders in America: The Epidemiologic Catchment Area Study* (pp. 204–219). New York: Free Press.

Karno, M., Golding, J. M., Sorenson, S. B., & Burnam, A. (1988). The epidemiology of obsessive–compulsive disorder in five US communities. *Archives of General Psychiatry, 45,* 1094–1099.

Kearney, C. A., & Silverman, W. K. (1990). Treatment of an adolescent with obsessive–compulsive disorder by alternating response prevention and cognitive therapy: An empirical analysis. *Journal of Behavior Therapy and Experimental Psychiatry, 21,* 39–47.

Kelly, A. E., & Kahn, J. H. (1994). Effects of suppression of personal intrusive thoughts. *Journal of Personality and Social Psychology, 66,* 998–1006.

Kendell, R. E., & Discipio, W. J. (1970). Obsessional symptoms and obsessional personality traits in patients with depressive illness. *Psychological Medicine, 1,* 65–72.

Kline, P. (1968). Obsessional traits, obsessional symptoms and anal eroticism. *British Journal of Medical Psychology, 41,* 299–304.

Koopmans, P. C., Sanderman, R., Timmerman, I., & Emmelkamp, P. M. G. (1994). The Irrational Beliefs Inventory: Development and psychometric evaluation. *European Journal of Psychological Assessment, 10,* 15–27.

Kozak, M. J. (1999). Evaluating treatment efficacy for obsessive–compulsive disorder: Caveat practitioner. *Cognitive and Behavioral Practice, 6,* 422–426.

Kozak, M. J., & Foa, E. B. (1994). Obsessions, overvalued ideas, and delusions in obsessive–compulsive disorder. *Behaviour Research and Therapy, 32,* 343–353.

Kozak, M. J., & Foa, E. B. (1997). *Mastery of obsessive–compulsive disorder: A cognitive-behavioral approach. Therapist Guide.* San Antonio, TX: Graywind.

Kozak, M. J., Foa, E. B., & McCathy, P. (1988). Obsessive–compulsive disorder. In C. G. Last & M. Hersen (Eds.), *Handbook of anxiety disorders* (pp. 87–108). New York: Pergamon Press.

Kozak, M. J., Liebowitz, M. R., & Foa, E. B. (2000). Cognitive behavior therapy and pharmacotherapy for obsessive–compulsive disorder: The NIMH-Sponsored Collaborative Study. In W. K. Goodman, M. V. Rudorfor, & J. D. Maser (Eds.), *Obsessive-compulsive disorder: Contemporary issues in treatment* (pp. 501–530). Mahwah, NJ: Erlbaum.

Kringlen, E., Torgersen, S., & Cramer, V. (2001). A Norwegian psychiatric epidemiological study. *American Journal of Psychiatry, 158,* 1091–1098.

Kyrios, M., & Bhar, S. (1997). *An experimental manipulation of inflated responsibility: Behavioural effects in clinical and non-clinical groups.* Unpublished manuscript, Department of Psychology, University of Melbourne.

Kyrios, M., Bhar, S., & Wade, D. (1996). The assessment of obsessive–compulsive phenomena: Psychometric and normative data on the Padua Inventory from an Australian non-clinical student sample. *Behaviour Research and Therapy, 34,* 85–95.

Kyrios, M., & Iob, M. (1998). Automatic and strategic processing in obsessive–compulsive disorder: Attentional bias, cognitive avoidance or more complex phenomena? *Journal of Anxiety Disorders, 12,* 271–292.

Ladouceur, R., Freeston, M. H., Gagnon, F., Thibodeau, N., & Dumont, J. (1993). Idiographic considerations in the behavioral treatment of obsessional thoughts. *Journal of Behavior Therapy and Experimental Psychiatry, 24,* 301–310.

Ladouceur, R., Freeston, M. H., Gagnon, F., Thibodeau, N., & Dumont, J. (1995). Cognitive-behavioral treatment of obsessions. *Behavior Modification, 19,* 247–257.

Ladouceur, R., Freeston, M. H., Rheaume, J., Dugas, M. J., Gagnon, F., Thibodeau, N., & Fournier, S. (2000). Strategies used with intrusive thoughts: A comparison of OCD patients with anxious and community controls. *Journal of Abnormal Psychology, 109,* 179–187.

Ladouceur, R., Léger, E., Rhéaume, J., & Dubé, D. (1996). Correction of inflated responsibility in the treatment of obsessive–compulsiuve disorder. *Behaviour Research and Therapy, 34,* 767–774.

Ladouceur, R., Rhéaume, J., Freeston, M. H., Aublet, F., Jean, K., Lachance, S., et al. (1995). Experimental manipulations of responsibility: An analogue test for models of obsessive–compulsive disorder. *Behaviour Research and Therapy, 33,* 937–946.

Lang, P. J., & Lazovik, A. D. (1963). Experimental desensitization of a phobia. *Journal of Abnormal and Social Psychology, 66,* 519–525.

Langlois, F., Freeston, M. H., & Ladouceur, R. (2000a). Differences and similarities between obsessive intrusive thoughts and worry in a non-clinical population: Study 1. *Behaviour Research and Therapy, 38,* 157–173.

Langlois, F., Freeston, M. H., & Ladouceur, R. (2000b). Differences and similarities between obsessive intrusive thoughts and worry in a non-clinical population: Study 2. *Behaviour Research and Therapy, 38,* 175–189.

Lavey, E. H., & van den Hout, M. A. (1990). Thought suppression induces intrusions. *Behavioural Psychotherapy, 18,* 251–258.

Lavy, E. H., van Oppen, P., & van den Hout, M. (1994). Selective processing of emotional information in obsessive compulsive disorder. *Behaviour Research and Therapy, 32,* 243–246.

Leahy, R. (2001). *Overcoming resistance in cognitive therapy.* New York: Guilford Press.

Leckman, J. F. (1993). Tourette's syndrome. In E. Hollander (Ed.), *Obsessive–compulsive-related disorders* (pp. 113–137). Washington, DC: American Psychiatric Press.

Leckman, J. F., Grice, D. E., Boardman, J., Zhang, H., Vitale, A., Bondi, C., et al. (1997). Symptoms of obsessive–compulsive disorder. *American Journal of Psychiatry, 154,* 911–917.

Leckman, J. F., McDougle, C. J., Pauls, D. L., Peterson, B. S., Grice, D. E., King, R. A., et al. (2000). Tic-related versus non-tic-related obsessive–compulsive disorder. In W. K. Goodman, M. V. Rudorfer, & J. D. Maser (Eds.), *Obsessive–compulsive disorder: Contemporary issues in treatment* (pp. 43–68). Mahwah, NJ: Erlbaum.

Lee, H.-J., & Kwon, S.-M. (2003). Two different types of obsession: Autogenous obsessions and reactive obsessions. *Behaviour Research and Therapy, 41,* 11–29.

Leger, L. A. (1978). Spurious and actual improvement in the treatment of preoccupying thoughts by thought-stopping. *British Journal of Clinical Psychology, 17,* 373–377.

Lelliott, P. T., Noshirvani, H. F., Basoglu, M., Marks, I. M., & Monteiro, W. O. (1988). Obsessive–compulsive beliefs and treatment oucome. *Psychological Medicine, 18,* 697–702.

Lensi, P., Cassano, G. B., Correddu, G., Ravagli, S., Kunovac, J. L., & Akiskal, H. S. (1996). Obsessive–compulsive disorder: Familial-developmental history, symptomatology, comorbidity and course with special reference to gender-related differences. *British Journal of Psychiatry, 169,* 101–107.

Lewis, A. (1936). Problems of obsessional illness. *Proceedings of the Royal Society of Medicine, 24,* 13–24.

Likierman, H., & Rachman, S. (1982). Obsessions: An experimental investigation of thought-stopping and habituation training. *Behavioural Psychotherapy, 10,* 324–338.

Lo, W. H. (1967). A follow-up of obsessional neurotics in Hong Kong Chinese. *British Journal of Psychaitry, 113,* 823–832.

Lopatka, C., & Rachman, S. (1995). Perceived responsibility and compulsive checking: An experimental analysis. *Behaviour Research and Therapy, 33,* 673–684.

MacDonald, P. A., Antony, M. M., MacLeod, C. M., & Richter, M. A. (1997). Memory and confidence in memory judgments among individuals with obsessive compulsive disorder and non-clinical controls. *Behaviour Research and Therapy, 35,* 497–505.

MacDonald, P. A., Antony, M. M., MacLeod, C. M., & Swinson, R. P. (1999). Negative priming for obsessive–compulsive checkers and non-checkers. *Journal of Abnormal Psychology, 108,* 679–686.

MacLeod, C. (1993). Cognition in clinical psychology: Measures, methods or models? *Behaviour Change, 10,* 169–195.

Maki, W. S., O'Neill, H. K., & O'Neill, G. W. (1994). Do nonclinical checkers exhibit deficits in cognitive control? Tests of an inhibitory control hypothesis. *Behaviour Research and Therapy, 32,* 183–192.

Mancini, F., D'Olimpio, F., del Genio, M., Didonna, F., & Prunetti, E. (2002). Obsessions and compulsions and intolerance for uncertainty in a non-clinical sample. *Journal of Anxiety Disorders, 16,* 401–411.

March, J. S., Frances, A., Carpenter, D., & Kahn, D. A. (1997). Expert Consensus Guideline for Treatment of Obsessive-Compulsive Disorder. *The Journal of Clinical Psychiatry, 58*(Suppl. 4), 5–72.

March, J. S., & Mulle, K. (1998). *OCD in children and adolescents: A cognitive-behavioral treatment manual.* New York: Guilford Press.

Markowitz, L. J., & Borton, J. L. S. (2002). Suppression of negative self-referent and neutral thoughts: A preliminary investigation. *Behavioural and Cognitive Psychotherapy, 30,* 271–277.

Marks, I. M., Hallam, R. S., Connolly, J., & Philpott, R. (1977). *Nursing in behavioural psychotherapy.* London: Royal College of Nursing of the United Kingdom.

Marks, I. M., O'Dwyer, A. M., Meehan, O., Greist, J., Baer, L., & McGuire, P. (2000). Subjective imagery in obsessive–compulsive disorder before and after exposure therapy. *British Journal of Psychiatry, 176,* 387–391.

Marks, I. M., Stern, R. S., Mawson, D., Cobb, J., & McDonald, R. (1980). Clomipramine and exposure for obsessive–compulsive rituals: I. *British Journal of Psychiatry, 136,* 1–25.

Martin, C., & Tarrier, N. (1992). The importance of cultural factors in the exposure to obsessional ruminations: A case example. *Behavioural Psychotherapy, 20,* 181–184.

Maser, J. D., & Cloninger, C. R. (1990). Comorbidity of anxiety and mood disorders: Implications and overview. *Comorbidity of mood and anxiety disorders* (pp. 3–12). Washington, DC: American Psychiatric Press.

Mathews, A. (1990). Why worry? The cognitive function of worry. *Behaviour Research and Therapy, 28,* 455–468.

Mathews, A. (1997). Information-processing biases in emotional disorders. In D. M. Clark & C. G. Fairburn (Eds.), *Science and practice of cognitive behavior therapy* (pp. 47–66). Oxford, UK: Oxford University Press.

Mathews, A., & MacLeod, C. (1994). Cognitive approaches to emotion and emotional disorders. *Annual Review of Psychology, 45,* 25–50.

McFall, M. E., & Wollersheim, J. P. (1979). Obsessive–compulsive neurosis: A cognitive-behavioral formulation and approach to treatment. *Cognitive Therapy and Research, 3,* 333–348.

McKay, D. (1997). A maintenance program for obsessive–compulsive disorder using exposure with response prevention: 2-year follow-up. *Behaviour Research and Therapy, 35,* 367–369.

McKay, D., Danyko, S., Neziroglu, F., & Yaryura-Tobias, J. A. (1995). Factor structure of the Yale–Brown Obsessive–Compulsive Scale: A two dimensional measure. *Behaviour Research and Therapy, 33,* 865–869.

McKeon, J., Roa, B., & Mann, A. (1984). Life events and personality traits in obsessive–compulsive neurosis. *British Journal of Psychiatry, 144,* 185–189.

McLean, P. D., Whittal, M. L., Sochting, I., Koch, W. J., Paterson, R., Thordarson, D. S., et al. (2001). Cognitive versus behavior therapy in the group treatment of obsessive–compulsive disorder. *Journal of Consulting and Clinical Psychology, 69,* 205–214.

McLean, P. D., & Woody, S. R. (2001). *Anxiety disorders in adults: An evidence-based approach to psychological treatment.* Oxford, UK: Oxford University Press.

McNally, R. J. (2000). Information-processing abnormalities in obsessive–compulsive disorder. In W. K. Goodman, M. V. Rudorfor, & J. D. Maser (Eds.), *Obsessive–compulsive disorder: Contemporary issues in treatment* (pp. 105–116). Mahwah, NJ: Erlbaum.

McNally, R. J. (2001a). On the scientific status of cognitive appraisal models of anxiety disorder. *Behaviour Research and Therapy, 39,* 513–521.

McNally, R. J. (2001b). Vulnerability to anxiety disorders in adulthood. In R. E. Ingram & J. M. Price (Eds.), *Vulnerability to psychopathology: Risk across the lifespan* (pp. 304–321). New York: Guilford Press.

McNally, R. J., Amir, N., Louro, C. E., Lukach, B. M., Riemann, B., & Calamari, J. E. (1994). Cognitive processing of idiographic emotional information in panic disorder. *Behaviour Research and Therapy, 32,* 119–122.

McNally, R. J., & Kohlbeck, P. A. (1993). Reality monitoring in obsessive–compulsive disorder. *Behaviour Research and Therapy, 31,* 249–253.

McNally, R. J., & Ricciardi, J. N. (1996). Suppression of negative and neutral thoughts. *Behavioural and Cognitive Psychotherapy, 24,* 17–25.

McNally, R. J., Wilhem, S., Buhlmann, U., & Shin, L. M. (2001). Cognitive inhibition in obsessive–compulsive disorder: Application of a valenced-based negative priming paradigm. *Behavioural and Cognitive Psychotherapy, 29,* 103–106.

Meichenbaum, D. (1977). *Cognitive-behavior modification: An integrative approach.* New York: Plenum.

Menzies, R. G., Harris, L. M., Cumming, S. R., & Einstein, D. A. (2000). The relationship between inflated personal responsibility and exaggerated danger expectancies in obsessive–compulsive concerns. *Behaviour Research and Therapy, 38,* 1029–1037.

Merckelbach, H., Muris, P., van den Hout, M., & de Jong, P. (1991). Rebound effects of thought suppression: Instruction-dependent? *Behavioural Psychotherapy, 19,* 225–238.

Meyer, V. (1966). Modifications of expectations in cases with obsessional rituals. *Behaviour Research and Therapy, 4,* 273–280.

Meyer, V., Levy, R., & Schnurer, A. (1974). The behavioural treatment of obsessive–compulsive disorders. In H. R. Beech (Ed.), *Obsessional states* (pp. 233–258). London: Methuen.

Mineka, S., & Sutton, S. K. (1992). Cognitive biases and the emotional disorders. *Psychological Science, 3,* 65–69.

Moritz, S., Birkner, C., Kloss, M., Jacobsen, D., Fricke, S., Bothern, A., & Iver, H. (2001). Impact of comorbid depressive symptoms on neuropsychological performance in obsessive–compulsive disorder. *Journal of Abnormal Psychology, 110,* 653–657.

Mowrer, O. H. (1939). A stimulus–response analysis of anxiety and its role as a reinforcing agent. *Psychological Review, 46,* 553–565.

Mowrer, O. H. (1953). Neurosis, psychotherapy, and two-factor learning theory. In O. H. Mowrer (Ed.), *Psychotherapy theory and research* (pp. 140–149). New York: Ronald Press.

Mowrer, O. H. (1960). *Learning theory and behavior.* New York: Wiley.

Muris, P., Meesters, C., Rasssin, E., Merckelbach, H., & Campbell, J. (2001). Thought–action fusion and anxiety disorders symptoms in normal adolescents. *Behaviour Research and Therapy, 39,* 843–852.

Muris, P., Merckelbach, H., & Clavan, M. (1997). Abnormal and normal compulsions. *Behaviour Research and Therapy, 35,* 249–252.

Muris, P., Merckelbach, H., & de Jong, P. (1993). Verbalization and environmental cuing in thought suppression. *Behaviour Research and Therapy, 31,* 609–612.

Muris, P., Merckelbach, H., van den Hout, M., & de Jong, P. (1992). Suppression of emotional and neutral material. *Behaviour Research and Therapy, 30,* 639–642.

Nakagawa, A., Marks, I. M., Takei, N., De Araujo, L. A., & Ito, L. M. (1996). Comparisons among the Yale–Brown Obsessive–Compulsive Scale, Compulsion Checklist, and other measures of obsessive–compulsive disorder. *British Journal of Psychiatry, 169,* 108–112.

Nestadt, G., Samuels, J. F., Romanoski, A. J., Folstein, M. F., & McHugh, P. R. (1994). Obsessions and compulsions in the community. *Acta Psychiatrica Scandinavica, 89,* 219–224.

Newth, S., & Rachman, S. (2001). The concealment of obsessions. *Behaviour Research and Therapy, 39,* 457–464.

Neziroglu, F., Anemone, R., & Yaryura-Tobias, J. A. (1992). Onset of obsessive–compulsive disorder in pregnancy. *American Journal of Psychiatry, 149,* 947–950.

Neziroglu, F., McKay, D., Yaryura-Tobias, J. A., Stevens, K. P., & Todaro, J. (1999). The overvalued ideas scale: Development, reliability and validity in obsessive–compulsive disorder. *Behaviour Research and Therapy, 37,* 881–902.

Neziroglu, F., & Stevens, K. P. (2002). Insight: Its conceptualization and assessment. In R. O. Frost & G. Steketee (Eds.), *Cognitive approaches to obsessions and compulsions: Theory, assessment and treatment* (pp. 183–193). Oxford, UK: Elsevier.

Neziroglu, F., Stevens, K. P., McKay, D., & Yaryura-Tobia, J. A. (2001). Predictive validity of the overvalued ideas scale: outcome in obsessive–compulsive and body dysmorphic disorders. *Behaviour Research and Therapy, 39,* 745–756.

Neziroglu, F., Stevens, K. P., Yaryura-Tobias, J. A., & Hoffman, J. H. (1999). Assessment, treatment prevalence, and prognostic indicators for patients with obsessive-compulsive spectrum disorders. *Cognitive and Behavioral Practice, 6,* 345–350.

Niler, E. R., & Beck, S. J. (1989). The relationship among guilt, anxiety and obsessions in a normal population. *Behaviour Research and Therapy, 27,* 213–220.

Obsessive Compulsive Cognitions Working Group (OCCWG). (1997). Cognitive assessment of obsessive–compulsive disorder. *Behaviour Research and Therapy, 35,* 667–681.

Obsessive Compulsive Cognitions Working Group (OCCWG). (2001). Development and initial validation of the Obsessive Beliefs Questionnaire and the Interpretation of Intrusions Inventory. *Behaviour Research and Therapy, 39,* 987–1006.

Obsessive Compulsive Cognitions Working Group (OCCWG). (2003a). Psychometric validation of the Obsessive Beliefs Questionnaire and the Interpretation of Intrusions Inventory: Part I. *Behaviour Research and Therapy, 41,* 863–878.

Obsessive Compulsive Cognitions Working Group (OCCWG). (2003b). Psychometric validation of the Obsessive Beliefs Questionnaire and the Interpretation of Intrusions Inventory: Part II. Factor analyses and testing a brief version. Manuscript submitted for publication.

O'Connor, K. P. (2001). Clinical and psychological features distinguishing obsessive–compulsive and chronic tic disorders. *Clinical Psychology Review, 21,* 631–660.

O'Connor, K. P. (2002). Intrusions and inferences in obsessive compulsive disorder. *Clinical Psychology and Psychotherapy, 9,* 38–46.

O'Connor, K. P., & Robillard, S. (1995). Inference processes in obsessive–compulsive disorder: Some clinical observations. *Behaviour Research and Therapy, 33,* 887–896.

O'Connor, K. P., & Robillard, S. (1999). A cognitive approach to the treatment of primary inferences in obsessive–compulsive disorder. *Journal of Cognitive Psychotherapy: An International Quarterly, 13,* 359–375.

O' Connor, K., Todorov, C., Robillard, S., Borgeat, F., & Brault, M. (1999). Cognitive-behaviour therapy and medication in the treatment of obsessive–compulsive disorder: A controlled study. *Canadian Journal of Psychiatry, 44,* 64–71.

O'Dwyer, A.-M., & Marks, I. (2000). Obsessive–compulsive disorder and delusions revisited. *British Journal of Psychiatry, 176,* 281–284.

O'Kearney, R. (1993). Additional considerations in the cognitive-behavioral treatment of obsessive–compulsive ruminations: A case study. *Journal of Behavior Therapy and Experimental Psychiatry, 24,* 357–365.

O'Rourke, D. A., Wurtman, J. J., Wurtman, R. J., Tsay, R., Gleason, R., Baer, L., & Jenike, M. A. (1994). Aberrant snacking patterns and eating disorders in patients with obsessive compulsive disorder. *Journal of Clinical Psychiatry, 5,* 445–447.

Padesky, C. A. (with Greenberger, D.) (1995). *Clinician's guide to "mind over mood."* New York: Guilford Press.

Parkinson, L., & Rachman, S. J. (1980). Are intrusive thoughts subject to habituation? *Behaviour Research and Therapy, 18,* 409–418.

Parkinson, L., & Rachman, S. J. (1981a). Part II. The nature of intrusive thoughts. *Advances in Behaviour Research and Therapy, 3,* 101–110.

Parkinson, L., & Rachman, S. J. (1981b). Part III. Intrusive thoughts: The effects of an uncontrived stress. *Advances in Behaviour Research and Therapy, 3,* 111–118.

Persons, J. B. (1989). *Cognitive therapy in practice: A case formulation approach.* New York: Norton.

Persons, J. B., & Davidson, J. (2001). Cognitive-behavioral case formulation. In K. S. Dobson (Ed.), *Handbook of cognitive-behavioral therapies* (2nd ed., pp. 86–110). New York: Guilford Press.

Philpott, R. (1975). Recent advances in the behavioural measurement of obsessional illness: Difficulties common to these and other measures. *Scottish Medical Journal, 20,* 33–40.

Pollak, J. M. (1979). Obsessive–compulsive personality: A review. *Psychological Bulletin, 86,* 225–241.

Pollard, C. A., Henderson, J. G., Frank, M., & Margolis, R. B. (1989). Help-seeking patterns of anxiety-disordered individuals in the general population. *Journal of Anxiety Disorders, 3,* 131–138.

Pollitt, J. (1957). Natural history of obsessional states: A study of 150 cases. *British Medical Journal, 1,* 194–198.

Purcell, R., Maruff, P., Kyrios, M., & Pantcils, C. (1998). Neuropsychological deficits in obsessive–compulsive disorder: A comparison with unipolar depression, panic disorder, and normal controls. *Archives of General Psychiatry, 55,* 415–423.

Purdon, C. (1997). *The role of thought suppression and meta-cognitive beliefs in the persistence of obsession-like intrusive thoughts.* Unpublished doctoral dissertation, University of New Brunswick, Canada.

Purdon, C. (1999). Thought suppression and psychopathology. *Behaviour Research and Therapy, 37,* 1029–1054.

Purdon, C. (2001). Appraisal of obsessional thought recurrences: Impact on anxiety and mood state. *Behavior Therapy, 32,* 47–64.

Purdon, C. (2002). Cognitive behavioral models of obsessive compulsive disorder. Unpublished manuscript, University of Waterloo, Canada.

Purdon, C., & Clark, D. A. (1993). Obsessive intrusive thoughts in nonclinical subjects. Part I. Content and relation with depressive, anxious and obsessional symptoms. *Behaviour Research and Therapy, 31,* 713–720.

Purdon, C. L., & Clark, D.A. (1994a). Obsessive intrusive thoughts in nonclinical subjects. Part II. Cognitive appraisal, emotional response and thought control strategies. *Behaviour Research and Therapy, 32,* 403–410.

Purdon, C. L., & Clark, D. A. (1994b). Perceived control and appraisal of obsessional intrusive thoughts: A replication and extension. *Behavioural and Cognitive Psychotherapy, 22,* 269–285.

Purdon, C. L., & Clark, D. A. (1999). Metacognition and obsessions. *Clinical Psychology and Psychotherapy, 6,* 102–110.

Purdon, C. L., & Clark, D. A. (2000). White bears and other elusive phenomena: Assessing the relevance of thought suppression for obsessional phenomena. *Behavior Modification, 24,* 425–453.

Purdon, C. L., & Clark, D. A. (2001). Suppression of obsession-like thoughts in nonclinical individuals. Part I. Impact on thought frequency, appraisal and mood state. *Behaviour Research and Therapy, 39,* 1163–1181.

Purdon, C. L., & Clark, D. A. (2002). The need to control thoughts. In R. O. Frost & G. Steketee (Eds.), *Cognitive approaches to obsessions and compulsions: Theory, assessment and treatment* (pp. 29–43). Oxford, UK: Elsevier.

Purdon, C. L., Rowa, K., & Antony, M. (2002). *Daily records of thought suppression attempts by individuals with obsessive–compulsive disorder.* Manuscript submitted for publication.

Rabavilas, A. D., & Boulougouris, J. C. (1974). Physiological accompaniments of ruminations, flooding and thought-stopping in obsessive patients. *Behaviour Research and Therapy, 12,* 239–243.

Rachman, S. J. (1971). Obsessional ruminations. *Behaviour Research and Therapy, 9,* 229–235.

Rachman, S. J. (1974). Primary obsessional slowness. *Behaviour Research and Therapy, 12,* 9–18.

Rachman, S. J. (1976a). The modification of obsessions: A new formulation. *Behaviour Research and Therapy, 14,* 437–443.

Rachman, S. J. (1976b). The passing of the two-stage theory of fear and avoidance: Fresh possibilities. *Behaviour Research and Therapy, 14,* 125–131.

Rachman, S. (1977). The conditioning theory of fear-acquisition: A critical examination. *Behaviour Research and Therapy, 15,* 375–387.

Rachman, S. J. (1978). An anatomy of obsessions. *Behavioural Analysis and Modification, 2,* 253–278.

Rachman, S. J. (1981). Part I. Unwanted intrusive cognitions. *Advances in Behaviour Research and Therapy, 3,* 89–99.

Rachman, S. J. (1983). Obstacles to the successful treatment of obsessions. In E. B. Foa & P. M. G. Emmelkamp (Eds.), *Failures in behavior therapy* (pp. 35–57). New York: Wiley.

Rachman, S. J. (1985). An overview of clinical and research issues in obsessional–compulsive disorders. In M. Mavissakalian, S. M. Turner, & L. Michelson (Eds.), *Obsessive–compulsive disorder: Psychological and pharmacological treatment* (pp. 1–47). New York: Plenum Press.

Rachman, S. J. (1993). Obsessions, responsibility and guilt. *Behaviour Research and Therapy, 31,* 149–154.

Rachman, S. J. (1997). A cognitive theory of obsessions. *Behaviour Research and Therapy, 35,* 793–802.

Rachman, S. J. (1998). A cognitive theory of obsessions: Elaborations. *Behaviour Research and Therapy, 36,* 385–401.

Rachman, S. J. (2002). A cognitive theory of compulsive checking. *Behaviour Research and Therapy, 40,* 625–639.

Rachman, S. J. (2003). *The treatment of obsessions.* Oxford, UK: Oxford University Press.

Rachman, S. J., Cobb, J., Grey, S., McDonald, B., Mawson, D., Sartory, G., & Stern, R. (1979). The behavioural treatment of obsessional–compulsive disorders, with and without clomipramine. *Behaviour Research and Therapy, 17,* 467–478.

Rachman, S. J., & de Silva, P. (1978). Abnormal and normal obsessions. *Behaviour Research and Therapy, 16,* 233–248.

Rachman, S. J., de Silva, P., & Roper, G. (1976). The spontaneous decay of compulsive urges. *Behaviour Research and Therapy, 14,* 445–453.

Rachman, S. J., & Hodgson, R. J. (1980). *Obsessions and compulsions.* Englewood Cliffs, NJ: Prentice-Hall.

Rachman, S. J., Hodgson, R., & Marks, I. M. (1971). The treatment of chronic obsessive-compulsive neurosis. *Behaviour Research and Therapy, 9,* 237–247.

Rachman, S. J., Marks, I. M., & Hodgson, R. (1973). The treatment of obsessive–compulsive neurotics by modelling and flooding *in vivo. Behaviour Research and Therapy, 11,* 463–471.

Rachman, S. J., & Shafran, R. (1998). Cognitive and behavioral features of obsessive–compulsive disorder. In R. P. Swinson, M. M. Antony, S. Rachman, & M. A. Richter (Eds.), *Obsessive–compulsive disorder: Theory, research, and treatment* (pp. 51–78). New York: Guilford Press.

Rachman, S. J., & Shafran, R. (1999). Cognitive distortions: Thought–action fusion. *Clinical Psychology and Psychotherapy, 6,* 80–85.

Rachman, S. J., Shafran, R., Mitchell, D., Trant, J., & Teachman, B. (1996). How to remain neutral: An experimental analysis of neutralization. *Behaviour Research and Therapy, 34,* 889–898.

Rachman, S. J., Thordarson, D. S., & Radomsky, A. S. (1995). *A revision of the Maudsley Obsessional Compulsive Inventory (MOCI-R).* Poster presented at the World Congress of Behavioural and Cognitive Therapies, Copenhagen, Denmark.

Rachman, S. J., Thordarson, D. S., Shafran, R., & Woody, S. R. (1995). Perceived responsibility: Structure and significance. *Behaviour Research and Therapy, 33,* 779–784.

Radomsky, A. S., & Rachman, S. (1999). Memory bias in obsessive–compulsive disorder (OCD). *Behaviour Research and Therapy, 37,* 605–618.

Radomsky, A. S., Rachman, S., & Hammond, D. (2001). Memory bias, confidence and responsibility in compulsive checking. *Behaviour Research and Therapy, 39,* 813–822.

Rasmussen, S. A., & Eisen, J. L. (1992). The epidemiology and clinical features of obsessive compulsive disorder. *Psychiatric Clinics of North America, 15,* 743–758.

Rasmussen, S. A., & Eisen, J. L. (1998). The epidemiology and clinical features of obsessive–

compulsive disorder. In M. A. Jenike & W. E. Minichiello (Eds.), *Obsessive–compulsive disorders: Practical management* (pp. 12–43). St. Louis: Mosby.

Rasmussen, S. A., & Tsuang, M. T. (1986). Clinical characteristics and family history in DSM-III obsessive–compulsive disorder. *American Journal of Psychiatry, 143,* 317–322.

Rassin, E. (2001). The contribution of thought–action fusion and thought suppression in the development of obsession-like intrusions in normal participants. *Behaviour Research and Therapy, 39,* 1023–1032.

Rassin, E., Diepstraten, P., Merckelbach, H., & Muris, P. (2001). Thought–action fusion and thought suppression in obsessive–compulsive disorder. *Behaviour Research and Therapy, 39,* 757–764.

Rassin, E., & Koster, E. (2003). The correlation between thought–action fusion and religiosity in a normal sample. *Behaviour Research and Therapy, 41,* 361–368.

Rassin, E., Mercekelbach, H., & Muris, P. (2000). Paradoxical and less paradoxical effects of thought suppression: A critical review. *Clinical Psychology Review, 20,* 973–995.

Rassin, E., Merckelbach, H., Muris, P., & Schmidt, H. (2001). The Thought-Action Fusion Scale: Further evidence for its reliability and validity. *Behaviour Research and Therapy, 39,* 537–544.

Rassin, E., Merckelbach, H., Muris, P., & Spaan, V. (1999). Thought–action fusion as a causal factor in the development of intrusions. *Behaviour Research and Therapy, 37,* 231–237.

Rassin, E., Merckelbach, H., Muris, P., & Stapert, S. (1999). Suppression and ritualistic behaviour in normal participants. *British Journal of Clinical Psychology, 38,* 195–201.

Rassin, E., Muris, P., Schmidt, H., & Merckelbach, H. (2000). Relationships between thought–action fusion, thought suppression and obsessive–compulsive symptoms: A structural equation modeling approach. *Behaviour Research and Therapy, 38,* 889–897.

Reed, G. F. (1968). Some formal qualities of obsessional thinking. *Psychiatric Clinics, 1,* 382–392.

Reed, G. F. (1985). *Obsessional experience and compulsive behavior: A cognitive-structural approach.* Orlando, FL: Academic Press.

Regier, D. A., Narrow, W. E., Rae, D. S., Manderscheid, R. W., Locke, B. Z., & Goodwin, F. K. (1993). The de facto US mental and addictive disorders service system: Epidemiologic Catchment Area prospective 1 year prevalence rates of disorders and services. *Archives of General Psychiatry, 50,* 85–94.

Rettew, D. C., Swedo, S. E., Leonard, H. L., Lenane, M. C., & Rapoport, J. L. (1992). Obsessions and compulsions across time in 79 children and adolescents with obsessive–compulsive disorder. *Journal of the American Academy of Child and Adolescent Psychiatry, 31,* 1050–1056.

Reynolds, M., & Salkovskis, P. M. (1991). The relationship among guilt, dysphoria, anxiety and obsessions in a normal population: An attempted replication. *Behaviour Research and Therapy, 29,* 259–265.

Reynolds, M., & Salkovskis, P. M. (1992). Comparison of positive and negative intrusive thoughts and experimental investigation of the differential effects of mood. *Behaviour Research and Therapy, 30,* 273–281.

Rhéaume, J., Freeston, M. H., Dugas, M. J., Letarte, H., & Ladouceur, R. (1995). Perfectionism, responsibility and obsessive–compulsive symptoms. *Behaviour Research and Therapy, 33,* 785–794.

Rhéaume, J., Freeston, M. H., Léger, E., & Ladouceur, R. (1998). Bad luck: An underestimated factor in the development of obsessive–compulsive disorder. *Clinical Psychology and Psychotherapy, 5,* 1–12.

Rhéaume, J., & Ladouceur, R. (2000). Cognitive and behavioural treatments of checking behaviours: An examination of individual cognitive change. *Clinical Psychology and Psychotherapy, 7,* 118–127.

Rhéaume, J., Ladouceur, R., Freeston, M. H., & Letarte, H. (1994). Inflated responsibility in obsessive–compulsive disorder: Psychometric studies of a semiidiographic measure. *Journal of Psychopathology and Behavioral Assessment, 16,* 265–276.

Ricciardi, J. N., & McNally, R. J. (1995). Depressed mood is related to obsessions, but not to compulsions in obsessive–compulsive disorder. *Journal of Anxiety Disorders, 9,* 249–256.

Richards, H. C. (1995). *The cognitive phenomenology of OCD repeated rituals.* Poster presented at the World Congress of Behavioural and Cognitive Therapies, Copenhagen, Denmark.

Richter, M. A., Cox, B. J., & Direnfeld, D. M. (1994). A comparison of three assessment instruments for obsessive–compulsive symptoms. *Journal of Behavior Therapy and Experimental Psychiatry, 25,* 143–147.

Robertson, J., Wendiggensen, P., & Kaplan, I. (1983). Towards a comprehensive treatment for obsessional thoughts. *Behaviour Research and Therapy, 21,* 347–356.

Roemer, L., & Borkovec, T. D. (1994). Effects of suppressing thoughts about emotional material. *Journal of Abnormal Psychology, 103,* 467–474.

Roper, G., & Rachman, S. J. (1976). Obsessional–compulsive checking: Experimental replication and development. *Behaviour Research and Therapy, 14,* 25–32.

Roper, G., Rachman, S. J., & Hodgson, R. (1973). An experiment on obsessional checking. *Behaviour Research and Therapy, 11,* 271–277.

Roper, G., Rachman, S., & Marks, I. M. (1975). Passive and participant modelling in exposure treatment of obsessive–compulsive neurotics. *Behaviour Research and Therapy, 13,* 271–279.

Rosenberg, C. M. (1968). Obsessional neurosis. *Australian and New Zealand Journal of Psychiatry, 2,* 33–38.

Rosenfeld, R., Dar, R., Anderson, D., Kobak, K. A., & Greist, J. H. (1992). A computer-administered version of the Yale–Brown Obsessive–Compulsive Scale. *Psychological Assessment, 4,* 329–332.

Rowa, K., & Purdon, C. (2003). Why are certain intrusive thoughts more upsetting than others? *Behavioural and Cognitive Psychotherapy, 31,* 1–11.

Rubenstein, C. S., Peynircioglu, Z. F., Chambless, D. L., & Pigott, T. A. (1993). Memory in sub-clinical obsessive–compulsive checkers. *Behaviour Research and Therapy, 31,* 759–765.

Rutledge, P. C. (1998). Obsessionality and the attempted suppression of unpleasant personal intrusive thoughts. *Behaviour Research and Therapy, 36,* 403–416.

Rutledge, P. C., Hancock, R. A., & Rutledge, J. H. (1996). Predictors of thought rebound. *Behaviour Research and Therapy, 34,* 555–562.

Rutledge, P. C., Hollenberg, D., & Hancock, R. A. (1993). Individual differences in the Wegner rebound effect: Evidence for a moderator variable in thought rebound following thought suppression. *Psychological Reports, 72,* 867–880.

Salkovskis, P. M. (1983). Treatment of an obsessional patient using habituation to audiotaped ruminations. *British Journal of Clinical Psychology, 22,* 311–313.

Salkovskis, P. M. (1985). Obsessional–compulsive problems: A cognitive-behavioural analysis. *Behaviour Research and Therapy, 23,* 571–583.

Salkovskis, P. M. (1989a). Cognitive-behavioural factors and the persistence of intrusive thoughts in obsessional problems. *Behaviour Research and Therapy, 27,* 677–682.

Salkovskis, P. M. (1989b). Obsessions and compulsions. In J. Scott, J. Mark, G. Williams, & A. T. Beck (Eds.), *Cognitive therapy in clinical practice: An illustrative casebook* (pp. 50–77). New York: Routledge.

Salkovskis, P. M. (1996a). Cognitive-behavioral approaches to the understanding of obsessional problems. In R. M. Rapee (Ed.), *Current controversies in the anxiety disorders* (pp. 103–133). New York: Guilford Press.

Salkovskis, P. M. (1996b). The cognitive approach to anxiety: Threat beliefs, safety-seeking behavior, and the special case of health anxiety and obsession. In P. M. Salkovskis (Ed.), *Frontiers of cognitive therapy* (pp. 48–74). New York: Guilford Press.

Salkovskis, P. M. (1996c). Understanding of obsessive–compulsive disorder is not improved by redefining it as something else: Reply to Pigott et al. and to Enright. In R. M. Rapee (Ed.), *Current controversies in the anxiety disorders* (pp. 191–200). New York: Guilford Press.

Salkovskis, P. M. (1998). Psychological approaches to the understanding of obsessional problems. In R. P. Swinson, M. M. Antony, S. Rachman, & M. A. Richter (Eds.), *Obsessive–compulsive disorder: Theory, research, and treatment* (pp. 33–50). New York: Guilford Press.

Salkovskis, P. M. (1999). Understanding and treating obsessive–compulsive disorder. *Behaviour Research and Therapy, 37,* S29–S52.

Salkovskis, P. M., & Campbell, P. (1994). Thought suppression induces intrusion in naturally occurring negative intrusive thoughts. *Behaviour Research and Therapy, 32,* 1–8.

Salkovskis, P. M., & Forrester, E. (2002). Responsibility. In R. O. Frost & G. Steketee (Eds.), *Cognitive approaches to obsessions and compulsions: Theory, assessment and treatment* (pp. 45–61). Oxford, UK: Elsevier Science.

Salkovskis, P. M., & Freeston, M. H. (2001). Obsessions, compulsions, motivation, and responsibility for harm. *Australian Journal of Psychology, 53,* 1–6.

Salkovskis, P. M., & Harrison, J. (1984). Abnormal and normal obsessions: A replication. *Behaviour Research and Therapy, 22,* 1–4.

Salkovskis, P. M., & Kirk, J. (1989). Obsessional disorder. In K. Hawton, P. M. Salkovskis, J. Kirk, & D. M. Clark (Eds.), *Cognitive behaviour therapy for psychiatric problems: A practical guide* (pp. 129–168). Oxford, UK: Oxford University Press.

Salkovskis, P. M., & Reynolds, M. (1994). Thought suppression and smoking cessation. *Behaviour Research and Therapy, 32,* 193–201.

Salkovskis, P. M., Richards, H. C., & Forrester, E. (1995). The relationship between obsessional problems and intrusive thoughts. *Behavioural and Cognitive Psychotherapy, 23,* 281–299.

Salkovskis, P. M., Shafran, R., Rachman, S., & Freeston, M. H. (1999). Multiple pathways to inflated responsibility beliefs in obsessional problems: Possible origins and implications for therapy and research. *Behaviour Research and Therapy, 37,* 1055–1072.

Salkovskis, P. M., & Wahl, K. (2003). Treating obsessional problems using cognitive-behavioural therapy. In M. Reinecke & D. A. Clark (Eds.), *Cognitive therapy across the lifespan: Theory, research and practice* (138–171). Cambridge, UK: Cambridge University Press.

Salkovskis, P. M., & Warwick, H. M. C. (1985). Cognitive therapy of obsessive–compulsive disorder: Treating treatment failures. *Behavioural Psychotherapy, 13,* 243–255.

Salkovskis, P. M., & Warwick, H. M. C. (1988). Cognitive therapy of obsessive–compulsive disorder. In C. Perris, I. M. Blackburn, & H. Perris (Eds.), *Cognitive psychotherapy: Theory and Practice* (pp. 376–395). Berlin: Springer-Verlag.

Salkovskis, P. M., & Westbrook, D. (1989). Behaviour therapy and obsessional ruminations: Can failure be turned into success? *Behaviour Research and Therapy, 27,* 149–160.

Salkovskis, P. M., Westbrook, D., Davis, J., Jeavons, A., & Gledhill, A. (1997). Effects of neutralizing on intrusive thoughts: An experiment investigating the etiology of obsessive–compulsive disorder. *Behaviour Research and Therapy, 35,* 211–219.

Salkovskis, P. M., Wroe, A. L., Gledhill, A., Morrison, N., Forrester, E., Richards, C., et al. (2000). Responsibility attitudes and interpretations are characteristic of obsessive compulsive disorder. *Behaviour Research and Therapy, 38,* 347–372.

Samuels, J., Nestadt, G., Bienvenu, O. J., Costa, P. T., Riddle, M. A., Liang, K-Y., et al. (2000). Personality disorders and normal personality dimensions in obsessive–compulsive disorder. *British Journal of Psychiatry, 177,* 457–462.

Sanavio, E. (1988). Obsessions and compulsions: The Padua Inventory. *Behaviour Research and Therapy, 26,* 169–177.

Sandler, J., & Hazari, A. (1960). The "obsessional": On the psychological classification of obsessional character traits and symptoms. *British Journal of Medical Psychology, 33,* 113–122.

Savage, C. R. (1998). Neuropsychology of obsessive–compulsive disorder: Reserwach findings and treatment implications. In M. A. Jenike & W. E. Minichiello (Eds.), *Obsessive–compulsive disorders: Practical management* (pp. 254–275). St. Louis: Mosby.

Savage, C. R., Baer, L., Keuthen, N. J., Brown, H. D., Rauch, S. L., & Jenike, M. A. (1999). Organizational strategies mediate nonverbal memory impairment in obsessive–compulsive disorder. *Biological Psychiatry, 45,* 905–916.

Scherer, K. R. (1999). Appraisal theory. In T. Dalgleish & M. Power (Eds.), *Handbook of cognition and emotion* (pp. 637–663). Chichester, UK: Wiley.

Schut, A. J., Castonguay, L. G., & Borkovec, T. D. (2001). Compulsive checking behaviors in generalized anxiety disorders. *Journal of Clinical Psychology, 57,* 705–715.

Shafran, R. (1997). The manipulation of responsibility in obsessive–compulsive disorder. *British Journal of Clinical Psychology, 36,* 397–407.

Shafran, R., & Tallis, F. (1996). Obsessive–compulsive hoarding: A cognitive-behavioral approach. *Behavioural and Cognitive Psychotherapy, 24,* 209–221.

Shafran, R., Thordarson, D. S., & Rachman, S. J. (1996). Thought–action fusion in obsessive compulsive disorder. *Journal of Anxiety Disorders, 10,* 379–391.

Shafran, R., Watkins, E., & Charman, T. (1996). Guilt in obsessive–compulsive disorder. *Journal of Anxiety Disorders, 10,* 509–516.

Sher, K., Frost, R., Kushner, M., Crews, T., & Alexander, J. (1989). Memory deficits in compulsive checkers: Replication and extension in a clinical sample. *Behaviour Research and Therapy, 27,* 65–69.

Sher, K., Frost, R. O., & Otto, R. (1983). Cognitive deficits in compulsive checkers: An exploratory study. *Behaviour Research and Therapy, 21,* 357–363.

Sica, C., Coradeschi, D., Sanavio, E., Dorz, S., Manchisi, D., & Novara, C. (in press). A study of the psychometric properties of the Obsessive Beliefs Inventory and Interpretations of Intrusions Inventory on clinical Italian individuals. *Journal of Anxiety Disorders.*

Sica, C., Novara, C., & Sanavio, E. (2002). Religiousness and obsessive–compulsive cognitions and symptoms in an Italian population. *Behaviour Research and Therapy, 40,* 813–823.

Simonds, L. M., Thorpe, S. J., & Elliott, S. A. (2000). The Obsessive Compulsive Inventory: Psychometric properties in a nonclinical student sample. *Behavioural and Cognitive Psychotherapy, 28,* 153–159.

Simos, G., & Dimitriou, E. (1994). Cognitive-behavioural treatment of culturally bound obsessional ruminations: A case report. *Behavioural and Cognitive Psychotherapy, 22,* 325–330.

Skoog, G., & Skoog, I. (1999). A 40-year follow-up of patients with obsessive–compulsive disorder. *Archives of General Psychiatry, 56,* 121–127.

Smári, J., Birgisdóttir, A. B., & Brynjólfsdóttir, B. (1995). Obsessive–compulsive symptoms and suppression of personally relevant unwanted thoughts. *Personality and Individual Differences, 18,* 621–625.

Smári, J., Glyfadóttir, T., & Halldórsdóttir, G. L. (2003). Responsibility attitudes and different types of obsessive–compulsive symptoms in a student population. *Behavioural and Cognitive Psychotherapy, 31,* 45–51.

Smári, J., & Hólmsteinsson, H. E. (2001). Intrusive thoughts, responsibility attitudes, thought–action fusion, and chronic thought suppression in relation to obsessive–compulsive symptoms. *Behavioural and Cognitive Psychotherapy, 29,* 13–20.

Smári, J., Sigurjónsdóttir, H., & Saémundsdóttir, I. (1994). Thought suppression and obsession–compulsion. *Psychological Reports, 75,* 227–235.

Solyom, L., Garza-Perez, J., Ledwidge, B. L., & Solyom, C. (1972). Paradoxical intention in the treatment of obsessive thoughts: A pilot study. *Comprehensive Psychiatry, 13,* 291–297.

Sookman, D., & Pinard, G. (1999). Integrative cognitive therapy for obsessive compulsive disorder: A focus on multiple schemas. *Cognitive and Behavioral Practice, 6,* 351–361.

Sookman, D., & Pinard, G. (2002). Overestimation of threat and intolerance of uncertainty in obsessive compulsive disorder. In R. O. Frost & G. Steketee (Eds). *Cognitive approaches to obsessions and compulsions: Theory, assessment and treatment.* (pp. 63–89). Oxford, UK: Elsevier.

Sookman, D., Pinard, G., & Beck, A. T. (2001). Vulnerability schemas in obsessive–compulsive disorder. *Journal of Cognitive Psychotherapy: An International Quarterly, 15,* 109–130.

Stanley, M. A., & Turner, S. M. (1995). Current status of pharmacological and behavioral treatment of obsessive–compulsive disorder. *Behavior Therapy, 26,* 163–186.

Stein, D. J., & Hollander, E. (1993). The spectrum of obsessive–compulsive-related disorders. In E. Hollander (Ed.), *Obsessive-compulsive-related disorders* (pp. 241–271). Washington, DC: American Psychiatric Press.

Stein, M. B., Forde, D. R., Anderson, G., & Walker, J. R. (1997). Obsessive–compulsive disorder in the community: An epidemiologic survey with clinical reappraisal. *American Journal of Psychiatry, 154,* 1120–1126.

Steiner, J. (1972). A questionnaire study of risk-taking in psychiatric patients. *British Journal of Medical Psychology, 45,* 365–374.

Steketee, G. S. (1993). *Treatment of obsessive compulsive disorder.* New York: Guilford Press.

Steketee, G. S. (1994). Behavioral assessment and treatment planning with obsessive compulsive disorder: A review emphasizing clinical application. *Behavior Therapy, 25,* 613–633.

Steketee, G. (1999). *Overcoming obsessive–compulsive disorder: A behavioral and cognitive protocol for the treatment of OCD.* Oakland, CA: New Harbinger.

Steketee, G., & Barlow, D. H. (2002). Obsessive–compulsive disorder. In D. H. Barlow, *Anxiety and its disorders: The nature and treatment of anxiety and panic* (2nd ed., pp. 516–550). New York: Guilford Press.

Steketee, G., Chambless, D. L., Tran, G. Q., Worden, H., & Gillis, M. A. (1996). Behavioral avoidance test for obsessive compulsive disorder. *Behaviour Research and Therapy, 34,* 73–83.

Steketee, G. S., & Freund, B. (1993). Compulsive Activity Checklist (CAC): Further psychometric analyses and revision. *Behavioural Psychotherapy, 21,* 13–25.

Steketee, G. S., & Frost, R. O. (1994). Measurement of risk-taking in obsessive–compulsive disorder. *Behavioural and Cognitive Psychotherapy, 22,* 287–298.

Steketee, G. S., Frost, R. O., & Bogart, K. (1996). The Yale–Brown Obsessive–Compulsive Scale: Interview versus self-report. *Behaviour Research and Therapy, 34,* 675–684.

Steketee, G. S., Frost, R. O., & Cohen, I. (1998). Beliefs in obsessive–compulsive disorder. *Journal of Anxiety Disorders, 12,* 525–537.

Steketee, G., Frost, R. O., Rhéaume, J., & Wilhelm, S. (1998). Cognitive theory and treatment of obsessive–compulsive disorder. In M. A. Jenike, L. Baer, & W. E. Minichiello (Eds.), *Obsessive-compulsive disorders: Practical management* (3rd ed., pp. 368–399). St. Louis: Mosby.

Steketee, G., Frost, R., & Wilson, K. (2002). Studying cognition in obsessive compulsive disorder: Where to from here? In R. O. Frost & G. Steketee (Eds.), *Cognitive approaches to obsessions and compulsions: Theory, assessment, and treatment* (pp. 466–473). Amsterdam: Elsevier Science.

Steketee, G., Frost, R. O., Wincze, J., Greene, K. A. I., & Douglas, H. (2000). Group and individual treatment of compulsive hoarding: A pilot study. *Behavioural and Cognitive Psychotherapy, 28,* 259–268.

Steketee, G. S., Grayson, J. B., & Foa, E. B. (1985). Obsessive–compulsive disorder: Differences between washers and checkers. *Behaviour Research and Therapy, 23,* 197–201.

Steketee, G. S., Grayson, J. B., & Foa, E. B. (1987). A comparison of characteristics of obsessive–compulsive disorder and other anxiety disorders. *Journal of Anxiety Disorders, 1,* 325–335.

Steketee, G., Quay, S., & White, K. (1991). Religion and guilt in OCD patients. *Journal of Anxiety Disorders, 5,* 359–367.

Steketee, G., & Shapiro, L. J. (1995). Predicting behavioral treatment outcome for agoraphobia and obsessive compulsive disorder. *Clinical Psychology Review, 15,* 317–346.

Stengel, E. (1945). A study on some clinical aspects of the relationship between obsessional neurosis and psychotic reaction types. *Journal of Mental Science, 91,* 166–187.

Stern, R. (1970). Treatment of a case of obsessional neurosis using thought-stopping technique. *British Journal of Psychiatry, 117,* 441–442.

Stern, R. S., & Cobb, J. P. (1978). Phenomenology of obsessive–compulsive neurosis. *British Journal of Psychiatry, 132,* 233–239.

Stern, R. S., Lipsedge, M. S., & Marks, I. M. (1973). Obsessive ruminations: A controlled trial of thought stopping. *Behaviour Research and Therapy, 11,* 659–662.

Sternberger, L. G., & Burns, G. L. (1990a). Compulsive Activity Checklist and the Maudsley Obsessional–Compulsive Inventory: Psychometric properties of two measures of obsessive–compulsive disorder. *Behavior Therapy, 21,* 117–127.

Sternberger, L. G., & Burns, G. L. (1990b). Obsessions and compulsions: Psychometric properties of the Padua Inventory with an American population. *Behaviour Research and Therapy, 28,* 341–345.

Suarez, L., & Bell-Dolan, D. (2001). The relationship of child worry to cognitive biases: Threat interpretation and likelihood of event occurrence. *Behavior Therapy, 32,* 425–442.

Summerfeldt, L. J. (2001). Obsessive–compulsive disorder: A brief overview and guide to assessment. In M. M. Antony, S. M. Orsillo, & L. Roemer (Eds.), *Practitioner's guide to empirically based measures of anxiety* (pp. 211–217). New York: Kluwer Academic/Plenum.

Summerfeldt, L. J., & Antony, M. M. (2002). Structured and semistructured diagnostic interviews. In M. M. Antony & D. H. Barlow (Eds.), *Handbook of assessment and treatment planning for psychological disorders* (pp. 3–37). New York: Guilford Press.

Summerfeldt, L. J., & Endler, N. S. (1998). Examining the evidence for anxiety-related cognitive biases in obsessive–compulsive disorder. *Journal of Anxiety Disorders, 12,* 579–598.

Summerfeldt, L. J., Huta, V., & Swinson, R. P. (1998). Personality and obsessive–compulsive disorder. In R. P. Swinson, M. M. Antony, S. Rachman, & M. A. Richter (Eds.), *Obsessive–compulsive disorder: Theory, research, and treatment* (pp. 79–119). New York: Guilford Press.

Summerfeldt, L. J., Richter, M. A., Antony, M. M., & Swinson, R. P. (1999). Symptom structure in obsessive–compulsive disorder: A confirmatory factor-analytic study. *Behaviour Research and Therapy, 37,* 297–311.

Sutherland, G., Newman, B., & Rachman, S. (1982). Experimental investigations of the relations between mood and intrusive unwanted cognitions. *British Journal of Medical Psychology, 55,* 127–138.

Swedo, S. E. (1993). Trichotillomania. In E. Hollander (Ed.), *Obsessive–compulsive-related disorders* (pp. 93–111). Washington, DC: American Psychiatric Press.

Tallis, F. (1995). *Obsessive compulsive disorder: A cognitive and neuropsychological perspective.* Chichester, UK: Wiley.

Tallis, F. (1997). The neuropsychology of obsessive–compulsive disorder: A review and consideration of clinical implications. *British Journal of Clinical Psychology, 36,* 3–20.

Tallis, F., & de Silva, P. (1992). Worry and obsessional symptoms: A correlational analysis. *Behaviour Research and Therapy, 30,* 103–105.

Tallis, F., Pratt, P., & Jamani, N. (1999). Obsessive compulsive disorder, checking, and nonverbal memory: A neuropsychological investigation. *Behaviour Research and Therapy, 37,* 161–166.

Tallis, F., Rosen, K., & Shafran, R. (1996). Investigation into the relationship between personality traits and OCD: A replication employing a clinical population. *Behaviour Research and Therapy, 34,* 649–653.

Tata, P. R., Leibowitz, J. A., Prunty, M., Cameron, M., & Pickering, A. D. (1996). Attentional bias in obsessional compulsive disorder. *Behaviour Research and Therapy, 34,* 53–60.

Taylor, S. (1995). Assessment of obsessions and compulsions: Reliability, validity, and sensitivity to treatment effects. *Clinical Psychology Review, 15,* 261–296.

Taylor, S. (1998). Assessment of obsessive–compulsive disorder. In R. P. Swinson, M. M. Antony, S. Rachman, & M. A. Richter (Eds.), *Obsessive–compulsive disorder: Theory, research, and treatment* (pp. 229–257). New York: Guilford Press.

Taylor, S. (2002) Cognition in obsessive–compulsive disorder: An overview. In R. O. Frost & G. Steketee (Eds.), *Cognitive approaches to obsessions and compulsions: Theory, assessment and treatment* (pp. 1–12). Oxford, UK: Elsevier.

Taylor, S., Thordarson, D. S., & Söchting, I. (2002). Obsessive–compulsive disorder. In M. M. Antony & D. H. Barlow (Eds.), *Handbook of assessment and treatment planning for psychological disorders* (pp. 182–214). New York: Guilford Press.

Teasdale, J. D. (1974). Learning models of obsessional–compulsive disorder. In H. R. Beech (Ed.), *Obsessional states* (pp. 197–229). London: Methuen.

Tellegen, A. (1985). Structures of mood and personality and their relevance to assessing anxiety with an emphasis on self-report. In A. H. Tuma & J.D. Maser (Eds.), *Anxiety and the anxiety disorders* (pp. 681–706). Hillsdale, NJ: Erlbaum.

Thomsen, P. H. (1995). Obsessive–compulsive disorder in children and adolescents: Predictors in childhood for long-term phenomenological course. *Acta Psychiatrica Scandinavica, 92,* 255–259.

Thordarson, D. S., & Shafran, R. (2002). Importance of thoughts. In R. O. Frost & G. Steketee (Eds.), *Cognitive approaches to obsessions and compulsions: Theory, assessment and treatment* (pp. 15–28). Oxford, UK: Elsevier.

Tolin, D. F., Abramowitz, J. S., Brigidi, B. D., Amir, N., Street, G. P., & Foa, E. B. (2001). Memory and memory confidence in obsessive–compulsive disorder. *Behaviour Research and Therapy, 39,* 913–927.

Tolin, D. F., Abramowitz, J. S., Brigidi, B. D., & Foa, E. B. (2003). Intolerance of uncertainty in obsessive–compulsive disorder. *Journal of Anxiety Disorders, 17,* 233–242.

Tolin, D. F., Abramowitz, J. S., Hamlin, C., & Synodi, D. S. (2002). Attributions for thought suppression failure in obsessive–compulsive disorder, *Cognitive Therapy and Research, 26,* 505–517.

Tolin, D. F., Abramowitz, J. S., Kozak, M. J., & Foa, E. B. (2001). Fixity of belief, perceptual aberration, and magical ideation in obsessive–compulsive disorder. *Journal of Anxiety Disorders, 15,* 501–510.

Tolin, D. F., Abramowitz, J. S., Przeworski, A., & Foa, E. B. (2002). Thought suppression in obsessive–compulsive disorder. *Behaviour Research and Therapy, 40,* 1255–1274.

Trinder, H., & Salkovskis, P. M. (1994). Personally relevant intrusions outside the laboratory: Long-term suppression increases intrusion. *Behaviour Research and Therapy, 32,* 833–842.

Tryon, G. S., & Palladino, J. J. (1979). Thought stopping: A case study and observations. *Journal of Behavior Therapy and Experimental Psychiatry, 10,* 151–154.

Türksoy, N., Tükel, R., Özdemir, Ö., & Karali, A. (2002). Comparison of clinical characteristics in good and poor insight obsessive–compulsive disorder. *Journal of Anxiety Disorders, 16,* 413–423.

Turner, S. M., Beidel, D. C., & Stanley, M. A. (1992). Are obsessional thoughts and worry different cognitive phenomena? *Clinical Psychology Review, 12,* 257–270.

van Balkom, A. J. L. M., van Oppen, P., Vermeulen, A. W. A., van Dyck, R., Nauta, M. C. E., & Vorst, H. C. M. (1994). A meta-analysis on the treatment of obsessive compulsive disorder: A comparison of antidepressants, behavior, and cognitive therapy. *Clinical Psychology Review, 14,* 359–381.

van den Hout, M., & Kindt, M. (2003a). Repeated checking causes memory distrust. *Behaviour Research and Therapy, 41,* 301–316.

van den Hout, M., & Kindt, M. (2003b). Phenomenological validity of an OCD-memory model and the remember/know distinction. *Behaviour Research and Therapy, 41,* 369–378.

van Oppen, P. (1992). Obsessions and compulsions: Dimensional structure, reliability, convergent and divergent validity of the Padua Inventory. *Behaviour Research and Therapy*, *30*, 631–637.

van Oppen, P., & Arntz, A. (1994). Cognitive therapy for obsessive–compulsive disorder. *Behaviour Research and Therapy*, *32*, 79–87.

van Oppen, P., de Haan, E., van Balkom, A. J. L. M., Spinhoven, P., Hoogduin, K., & van Dyck, R. (1995). Cognitive therapy and exposure *in vivo* in the treatment of obsessive compulsive disorder. *Behaviour Research and Therapy*, *33*, 379–390.

van Oppen, P., & Emmelkamp, P. M. G. (2000). Issues in cognitive treatment of obsessive-compulsive disorder. In W. K. Goodman, M. V. Rudorfor, & J. D. Maser (Eds.), *Obsessive-compulsive disorder: Contemporary issues in treatment* (pp. 117–132). Mahwah, NJ: Erlbaum.

van Oppen, P., Hoekstra, R. J., & Emmelkamp, P. M. G. (1995). The structure of obsessive-compulsive symptoms. *Behaviour Research and Therapy*, *33*, 15–23.

Veale, D. (2002). Over-valued ideas: A conceptual analysis. *Behaviour Research and Therapy*, *40*, 383–400.

Vogel, W., Peterson, L. E., & Broverman, I. K. (1982). A modification of Rachman's habituation technique for treatment of the obsessive–compulsive disorder. *Behaviour Research and Therapy*, *20*, 101–104.

Volans, P. J. (1976). Styles of decision-making and probability appraisal in selected obsessional and phobic patients. *British Journal of Social and Clinical Psychology*, *15*, 305–317.

Warren, R., & Thomas, J. C. (2001). Cognitive-behavior therapy of obsessive–compulsive disorder in private practice: An effectiveness study. *Journal of Anxiety Disorders*, *15*, 277–285.

Watson, D., & Clark, L. A. (1984). Negative affectivity: The disposition to experience aversive emotional states. *Psychological Bulletin*, *96*, 465–490.

Watson, D., Clark, L. A., & Carey, G. (1988). Positive and negative affectivity and their relation to anxiety and depressive disorders. *Journal of Abnormal Psychology*, *97*, 346–353.

Watson, D., Clark, L. A., & Harkness, A. R. (1994). Structures of personality and their relevance to psychopathology. *Journal of Abnormal Psychology*, *103*, 18–31.

Wegner, D. M. (1994a). *White bears and other unwanted thoughts: Suppression, obsession, and the psychology of mental control.* New York: Guilford Press.

Wegner, D. M. (1994b). Ironic processes of mental control. *Psychological Review*, *101*, 34–52.

Wegner, D. M., & Erber, R. (1992). The hyperaccessibility of suppressed thoughts. *Journal of Personality and Social Psychology*, *63*, 903–912.

Wegner, D. M., Schneider, D. J., Carter, S. R., & White, T. L. (1987). Paradoxical effects of thought suppression. *Journal of Personality and Social Psychology*, *53*, 5–13.

Wegner, D. M., Schneider, D. J., Knutson, B., & McMahon, S. R. (1991). Polluting the stream of consciousness: The effect of thought suppression on the mind's environment. *Cognitive Therapy and Research*, *15*, 141–152.

Wegner, D. M., Shortt, J. W., Blake, A. W., & Page, M. S. (1990). The suppression of exciting thoughts. *Journal of Personality and Social Psychology*, *58*, 409–418.

Wegner, D. M., & Zanakos, S. (1994). Chronic thought suppression. *Journal of Personality*, *62*, 615–640.

Weissman, M. M., Bland, R. C., Canino, G. J., Greenwald, S., Hwu, H.- G., Lee, C. K., et al. (1994). The cross national epidemiology of obsessive compulsive disorder. *Journal of Clinical Psychiatry*, *3*(Suppl.), 5–10.

Welkowitz, L. A., Struening, E. L., Pittman, J., Guardino, M., & Welkowitz, J. (2000). Obsessive–compulsive disorder and comorbid anxiety problems in a National Anxiety Screening sample. *Journal of Anxiety Disorders*, *14*, 471–482.

Wells, A. (1997). *Cognitive therapy of anxiety disorders: A practice manual and conceptual guide.* Chichester, UK: Wiley.

Wells, A., & Davies, M. I. (1994). The Thought Control Questionnaire: A measure of individual differences in the control of unwanted thoughts. *Behaviour Research and Therapy, 32,* 871–878.

Wells, A., & Matthews, G. (1994). *Attention and emotion: A clinical perspective.* Hove, UK: Erlbaum.

Wells, A., & Morrison, A. P. (1994). Qualitative dimensions of normal worry and normal obsessions: A comparative study. *Behaviour Research and Therapy, 32,* 867–870.

Wells, A., & Papageorgiou, C. (1998). Relationships between worry, obsessive–compulsive symptoms and meta-cognitive beliefs. *Behaviour Research and Therapy, 36,* 899–913.

Welner, A., Reich, T., Robins, E., Fishman, R., & van Doren, T. (1976). Obsessive–compulsive neurosis: Record, follow-up, and family studies. I. Inpatient record study. *Comprehensive Psychiatry, 17,* 527–539.

Wenzlaff, R. M., & Wegner, D. M. (2000). Thought suppression. *Annual Review of Psychology, 51,* 59–91.

Wenzlaff, R. M., Wegner, D. M., & Roper, D. W. (1988). Depression and mental control: The resurgence of unwanted negative thoughts. *Journal of Personality and Social Psychology, 55,* 882–892.

Whisman, M. A. (1993). Mediators and moderators of change in cognitive therapy of depression. *Psychological Bulletin, 114,* 248–265.

Whittal, M. L., & McLean, P. D. (1999). CBT for OCD: The rationale, protocol, and challenges. *Cognitive and Behavioral Practice, 6,* 383–396.

Whittal, M. L., & McLean, P. D. (2002). Group cognitive behavioral therapy for obsessive compulsive disorder. In R. O. Frost & G. Steketee (Eds.), *Cognitive approaches to obsessions and compulsions: Theory, assessment, and treatment* (pp. 417–433). Amsterdam: Elsevier Science.

Wilhem, S., McNally, R. J., Baer, L., & Florin, I. (1996). Directed forgetting in obsessive–compulsive disorder. *Behaviour Research and Therapy, 34,* 633–641.

Williams, J. B. W., Gibbon, M., First, M. B., Spitzer, R. L., Davies, M., Borus, J., et al. (1992). The Structured Clinical Interview for DSM-III-R (SCID) II. Multisite test–retest reliability. *Archives of General Psychiatry, 49,* 630–636.

Williams, J. M. G., Watts, F. N., MacLeod, C., & Mathews, A. (1997). *Cognitive psychology and emotional disorders* (2nd ed.). Chichester, UK: Wiley.

Williams, T. I., Salkovskis, P. M., Forrester, E. A., & Allsopp, M. A. (2002). Changes in symptoms of OCD and appraisal of responsibility during cognitive behavioural treatment: A pilot study. *Behavioural and Cognitive Psychotherapy, 30,* 69–78.

Wilson, K. A., & Chambless, D. L. (1999). Inflated perceptions of responsibility and obsessive–compulsive symptoms. *Behaviour Research and Therapy, 37,* 325–335.

Wolpe, J. (1958). *Psychotherapy by reciprocal inhibition.* Stanford, CA: Stanford University Press.

Woods, C. M., Frost, R. O., & Steketee, G. (2002). Obsessive compulsive (OC) symptoms and subjective severity, probability, and coping ability estimations of future negative events. *Clinical Psychology and Psychotherapy, 9,* 104–111.

Woody, S. R., Steketee, G., & Chambless, D. L. (1995). Reliability and validity of the Yale–Brown Obsessive–Compulsive Scale. *Behaviour Research and Therapy, 33,* 597–605.

Wroe, A. L., Salkovskis, P. M., & Richards, H. C. (2000). "Now I know it could happen, I have to prevent it": A clinical study of the specificity of intrusive thoughts and the decision to prevent harm. *Behavioural and Cognitive Psychotherapy, 28,* 63–70.

Yamagami, T. (1971). The treatment of an obsession by thought stopping. *Journal of Behavior Therapy and Experimental Psychiatry, 2,* 133–135.

Yaryura-Tobias, J. A., Grunes, M. S., Todaro, J., McKay, D., Neziroglu, F. A., & Stockman, R. (2000). Nosological insertion of Axis I disorders in the etiology of obsessive–compulsive disorder. *Journal of Anxiety Disorders, 14,* 19–30.

Index

313